ATLAS OF
LAPAROSCOPIC
SURGERY

ATLAS OF
LAPAROSCOPIC
SURGERY

Garth H. Ballantyne, M.D., F.A.C.S., F.A.S.C.R.S.

Professor of Surgery

Director of Minimally Invasive Surgery

Hackensack University Medical Center

Hackensack, New Jersey

W.B. SAUNDERS COMPANY

A Harcourt Health Sciences Company

Philadelphia   London   New York   St. Louis   Sydney   Toronto

W.B. SAUNDERS COMPANY
A Harcourt Health Sciences Company

The Curtis Center
Independence Square West
Philadelphia, Pennsylvania 19106

Library of Congress Cataloging-in-Publication Data

Atlas of laparoscopic surgery / [edited by] Garth H. Ballantyne.—1st ed.

p.   cm.

ISBN 0–7216–6326–5

1. Endoscopic surgery Atlases.   2. Laparoscopic surgery Atlases.
   I. Ballantyne, Garth H.   [DNLM: 1. Surgical Procedures, Laparoscopic—
   methods Atlases.   WO517 A8799 2000]

RD33.53.A862 2000   617′.05—DC21

DNLM/DLC   99–31883

Editor: Lisette Bralow
Designer: Gene Harris
Production Manager: Natalie Ware
Project Supervisor: Tina K. Rebane
Illustration Coordinator: Peg Shaw

ATLAS OF LAPAROSCOPIC SURGERY   ISBN 0–7216–6326–5

Printed in the United States of America.

Last digit is the print number: 9   8   7   6   5   4   3   2   1

I dedicate this tome to my wife,
Helen Francis Ballantyne.
She faced and overcame the
challenges of the real world so that
I could spend the time to shepherd
the growth of this Atlas.

NOTICE

Surgery is an ever-changing field. Standard safety precautions must be followed, but as new research and clinical experience broaden our knowledge, changes in treatment and drug therapy become necessary or appropriate. Readers are advised to check the product information currently provided by the manufacturer of each drug to be administered to verify the recommended dose, the method and duration of administration, and contraindications. It is the responsibility of the treating physician, relying on experience and knowledge of the patient, to determine dosages and the best treatment for the patient. Neither the publisher nor the editor assumes any responsibility for any injury and/or damage to persons or property.

THE PUBLISHER

Contributors

Kranthi Achanta, M.D.
Clinical Instructor of Surgery, University of Southern California School of Medicine; Laparoscopic Fellow, University of Southern California Medical Center, Los Angeles, California
Laparoscopic Management of Complications of Peptic Ulcer Disease

Joseph F. Amaral, M.D., F.A.C.S
Associate Professor of Surgery, Brown University School of Medicine; Director of Laparoscopic Surgery, The Rhode Island Hospital, Providence, Rhode Island
Laparoscopic Nissen Fundoplication with Laparoscopic Coagulating Shears; Laparoscopic Vertical Banded Gastroplasty

Wayne L. Ambrose, M.D., F.A.C.S., F.A.S.C.R.S.
Georgia Colon and Rectal Surgical Clinic, Atlanta, Georgia
Laparoscopic Total Proctocolectomy with Ileoanal Anastomosis

David N. Armstrong, M.D., F.R.C.S., F.A.C.S., F.A.S.C.R.S.
Program Director, Georgia Colon and Rectal Surgical Clinic, Atlanta, Georgia
Laparoscopic Total Proctocolectomy with Ileoanal Anastomosis

Garth H. Ballantyne, M.D., F.A.C.S., F.A.S.C.R.S.
Professor of Surgery, and Director of Minimally Invasive Surgery, Hackensack University Medical Center, Hackensack, New Jersey
Laparoscopic Highly Selective Vagotomy; Laparoscopic-Assisted Sigmoid Colectomy for Benign Disease; Laparoscopic Closure of a Hartmann's Pouch

David Bartolo, M.D., F.R.C.S.
Consultant Colorectal Surgeon, Royal Infirmary of Edinburgh, Edinburgh, United Kingdom
Laparoscopic-Assisted Anterior Resection for Rectal Prolapse

Ross Bremner, M.D.
Department of Surgery, University of Southern California, School of Medicine, Los Angeles, California
Laparoscopic Management of Complications of Peptic Ulcer Disease

David C. Brooks, M.D.
Associate Professor of Surgery, Harvard Medical School; Senior Surgeon and Associate Chief of Surgery, Brigham and Women's Hospital, Boston, Massachusetts
Laparoscopic Repair of Paraesophageal Hernias

Philip F. Caushaj, M.D., F.A.C.S., F.A.S.C.R.S.
Professor of Surgery, Temple University School of Medicine, Philadelphia; Chairman, Department of Surgery, Western Pennsylvania Hospital, Pittsburgh, Pennsylvania
Laparoscopic Appendectomy

Anthony V. Coletta, M.D.
Formerly Associate Director, Surgical Residency Program, Thomas Jefferson University Hospital, Philadelphia; Attending Surgeon, Bryn Mawr Hospital, Bryn Mawr, Pennsylvania
Laparoscopic Drainage of a Diverticular Abscess

Kevin C. Conlon, M.D., M.B.A.
Associate Professor of Surgery, Director of Endosurgery Program, Memorial Sloan-Kettering Cancer Center, New York, New York
Pancreatic and Gastric Cancer Staging

Avram M. Cooperman, M.D.
Professor of Surgery, New York Medical
College, Valhalla; Director, The Center for
Hepatobiliary and Pancreatic Surgery, Dobbs
Ferry Community Hospital, Dobbs Ferry, New
York
Laparoscopic Cholecystectomy; Laparoscopic-Assisted
Ileocolectomy for Inflammatory Bowel Disease

John D. Corbitt, Jr., M.D.
Clinical Assistant Professor, Nova University;
Chief of Surgery, John F. Kennedy Medical
Center, Atlantis, Florida
Laparoscopic Transabdominal Transperitoneal Patch Hernia
Repair

John M. Cosgrove, M.D.
Associate Professor of Clinical Surgery, Albert
Einstein College of Medicine, Bronx; Chief of
Surgery, Long Island Jewish-North Shore
University Hospital at Forest Hills, Forest
Hills, New York
Laparoscopic Plication of a Perforated Duodenal Ulcer

Bernard Dallemagne, M.D.
Department of Surgery, Les Cliniques Saint
Joseph, 4000 Liege, Belgium
Laparoscopic Nissen Fundoplication

Jose Antonio Diaz-E, M.D.
Attending, Instituto Tecnológico y De
Estudios Superiores de Monterrey, Hospital
San José de Monterrey, and Texas Endosurgery
Institute, San Antonio, Texas
Laparoscopic Left Hemicolectomy with Transanal Extraction
of the Specimen

**Michael Edye, M.B., B.S., F.R.A.C.S.,
F.A.C.S.**
Associate Professor of Surgery, New York
University School of Medicine; Chief, Division
of Minimally Invasive Surgery, New York
University Medical Center, New York, New
York
Laparoscopic Choledochoduodenostomy

Steve Eubanks, M.D.
Assistant Professor of Surgery, Director of
Surgical Endoscopy and Endoscopy Center,
and Endosurgery Fellowship Program;
Director, Duke University Medical Center,
Durham, North Carolina
Laparoscopic Heller Myotomy

John L. Flowers, M.D.
Associate Professor of Surgery, University of
Maryland School of Medicine; Chief, Division
of General Surgery, and Director, Maryland
Center for Videoscopic Surgery, Baltimore,
Maryland
Anterior Approach to Laparoscopic Splenectomy

Dennis L. Fowler, M.D.
Associate Professor of Surgery, MCP
Hahnemann University School of Medicine;
Director, Allegheny Center for Laparoscopic
and Minimally Invasive Surgery, Allegheny
General Hospital, Pittsburgh, Pennsylvania
Laparoscopic Gastrectomy

Morris E. Franklin, Jr., M.D.
Professor of Surgery, University of Texas
Health Science Center, and Director, Texas
Endosurgery Institute, San Antonio, Texas
Laparoscopic Left Hemicolectomy with Transanal Extraction
of the Specimen

Melanie M. Friedlander, M.D.
Clinical Instructor of Surgery, University of
Southern California School of Medicine;
Laparoscopic Fellow, University of Southern
California Medical Center, Los Angeles,
California
Laparoscopic Management of Complications of Peptic Ulcer
Disease

Michel Gagner, M.D., F.R.C.S.C., F.A.C.S.
Professor of Surgery, Mount Sinai School of
Medicine; Chief, Laparoscopic Surgery, Mount
Sinai Medical Center, New York, New York
Laparoscopic Adrenalectomy

W. Peter Geis, M.D.
Minimally Invasive Surgery Training Institute,
St. Joseph Medical Center, Baltimore,
Maryland
Laparoscopic Resection of Benign Gastric Tumors

Steve W. Grant, M.D.
Clinical Instructor of Surgery, University of
Southern California School of Medicine;
Laparoscopic Fellow, University of Southern
California Medical Center, Los Angeles,
California
Laparoscopic Management of Complications of Peptic Ulcer
Disease

Frederick L. Greene, M.D.
Chairman, Department of General Surgery,
Carolinas Medical Center, Charlotte; Clinical
Professor of Surgery, University of North
Carolina School of Medicine, Chapel Hill,
North Carolina
Laparoscopic Staging of Lymphomas

John E. Hartley, M.B., B.Sc.
Lecturer in Surgery, University of Hull, Hull,
United Kingdom
Laparoscopic Abdominoperineal Resection

Lucius D. Hill, M.D., F.A.C.S.
Swedish Hospital Medical Center, Seattle,
Washington
Laparoscopic Hill Repair

Namir Katkhouda, M.D., F.A.C.S.
Associate Professor of Surgery, University of
Southern California School of Medicine;
Chief, Division of Emergency Nontrauma and
Minimally Invasive Surgery, USC Los Angeles
County Medical Center, Los Angeles,
California
Laparoscopic Management of Complications of Peptic Ulcer
Disease

William E. Kelley, Jr., M.D., F.A.C.S.
Director, Laparoendoscopic Surgery
Fellowship, Richmond Surgical Group,
Richmond, Virginia
Laparoscopic Left Hemicolectomy

**Samuel P. Y. Kwok, F.R.C.S.(Ed.), F.R.A.C.S.,
F.H.K.Am. (Surgery)**
Adjunct Associate Professor, Department of
Surgery, The Chinese University of Hong
Kong, Shatin; Chief of Service and Consultant
Surgeon, Department of Surgery, United
Christian Hospital, Kowloon, Hong Kong
Laparoscopic-Assisted Sigmoid Colectomy for Colon Cancer

Michael J. Mastrangelo, Jr., M.D.
Assistant Professor of Surgery, University of
Kentucky School of Medicine, Lexington,
Kentucky
Anterior Approach to Laparoscopic Splenectomy

David E. Mazza, M.D.
Ryan Hill Research Foundation Fellow,
Swedish Hospital Medical Center, Seattle,
Washington
Laparoscopic Hill Repair

**John R. T. Monson, M.D., F.R.C.S.I.,
F.A.C.S.**
Professor of Surgery, University of Hull,
Academic Surgical Unit; Head, Department of
Colorectal Surgery, Castle Hill Hospital, Hull,
United Kingdom
Laparoscopic Abdominoperineal Resection

Jean Mouiel, M.D., F.A.C.S.
Professor of Surgery, University of Nice
School of Medicine; Chairman, Department of
Surgery, University Hospital of Nice, Hospital
L'Archet, Nice, France
Laparoscopic Management of Complications of Peptic Ulcer
Disease

Adrian Ortega, M.D.
Department of Surgery, University of
Southern California School of Medicine, Los
Angeles, California
Laparoscopic Management of Complications of Peptic Ulcer
Disease

David M. Ota, M.D.
Professor of Surgery, University of
Missouri–Columbia School of Medicine, and
Medical Director and Chief of Surgery, Ellis
Fischel Cancer Center, Columbia, Missouri
Laparoscopic-Assisted Right Hemicolectomy for Malignancy

Richard Perry, M.D.
Honorary Clinical Lecturer, Christchurch
Clinical School of Medicine, University of
Otago; Clinical Director, Bowel and Digestion
Centre, Oxford Clinic, Christchurch, New
Zealand
Laparoscopic Proctopexy

Jeffrey H. Peters, M.D., F.A.C.S.
Associate Professor of Surgery, University of
Southern California School of Medicine, and
Chief, Section of General Surgery, USC
University Hospital, Los Angeles, California
Techniques of Laparoscopic Enteral Access

Johann Pfeifer, M.D.
Department of Colorectal Surgery, Cleveland
Clinic, Florida, Fort Lauderdale, Florida
Laparoscopic-Assisted Total Abdominal Colectomy

Jean W. Saleh, M.D.
Associate Clinical Professor of Medicine,
Columbia University College of Physicians and
Surgeons; Attending Physician, St.
Luke's–Roosevelt Medical Center, New York,
New York
Diagnostic Laparoscopy

Barry A. Salky, M.D., F.A.C.S.
Clinical Professor of Surgery, Mt. Sinai School
of Medicine, New York, New York
Laparoscopic Distal Pancreatectomy

J. Stephen Scott, M.D.
Clinical Assistant Professor of Surgery,
University of Missouri–Columbia, Columbia;
Adjunct Clinical Faculty, St. Louis University,
St. Louis, Missouri
Endoscopic Total Extraperitoneal Hernia Repair with Balloon
Dissection

Stephen J. Shapiro, M.D., F.A.C.S.
Assistant Clinical Professor of Surgery,
University of California at Los Angeles,
School of Medicine; Attending Surgeon,
Cedars-Sinai Medical Center, Los Angeles,
California
Laparoscopic Transcystic Common Duct Exploration

Constantino Stratoulias, M.D.
Minimally Invasive Surgical Training Institute,
St. Joseph Medical Center, Baltimore,
Maryland
Laparoscopic Resection of Benign Gastric Tumors

Lee L. Swanström, M.D.
Clinical Professor of Surgery, Oregon Health
Sciences University; Director, Department of
Minimally Invasive Surgery, Legacy Health
System, Portland, Oregon
Laparoscopic Toupet Partial Fundoplication

Scott C. Thornton, M.D.
Assistant Clinical Professor of Surgery, Yale
University School of Medicine, New Haven;
Director of Colorectal Teaching, Bridgeport
Hospital, Bridgeport, Connecticut
Laparoscopic-Assisted Perineoabdominal Resection

Roger A. de la Torre, M.D.
Clinical Assistant Professor of Surgery,
University of Missouri–Columbia, Columbia;
Adjunct Clinical Faculty, St. Louis University,
St. Louis; Chief of Surgery, Doctors Hospital,
Wertzville, Missouri
Endoscopic Total Extraperitoneal Hernia Repair with Balloon
Dissection

Joseph F. Uddo, Jr., M.D., F.A.C.S.
Clinical Assistant Professor of Surgery,
Louisiana State University Medical School,
Metaire, Louisiana
Laparoscopic Partial Gastrectomy and Billroth II
Gastrojejunostomy; Laparoscopic Right Hemicolectomy with
Intracorporeal Anastomosis

Ron Verham, M.D.
Department of Surgery, University of
Southern California School of Medicine, Los
Angeles, California
Laparoscopic Management of Complications of Peptic Ulcer
Disease

Thomas J. Watson, M.D.
Department of Surgery, University of
Southern California School of Medicine, Los
Angeles, California
Techniques of Laparoscopic Enteral Access

Steven D. Wexner, M.D.
Professor of Surgery, Cleveland Clinic
Foundation Health Sciences of the Ohio State
University, Cleveland, Ohio; Clinical
Professor, Department of Surgery, University
of South Florida College of Medicine;
Chairman and Residency Program Director,
Department of Colorectal Surgery, and
Chairman, Division of Research and
Education, Cleveland Clinic Florida, Fort
Lauderdale, Florida
Laparoscopic-Assisted Total Abdominal Colectomy

Karl A. Zucker, M.D.
Professor of Clinical Surgery, University of
Arizona, Phoenix, Arizona
Laparoscopic Cholecystectomy for Acute Cholecystitis

Preface

Surgeons have rapidly embraced advances within their profession throughout the modern era. When Vesalius (1514–1564) accurately unlocked the secrets of human anatomy and depicted them in his *De Humani Corporis Fabrica*, published in 1543, his students rapidly transmitted his teachings to other surgeons throughout Europe. John Caius (1510–1573), an English surgeon, for example, lived in Vesalius's house for eight months during the time period of the preparation of *de Fabrica*. Caius soon returned to London, where he demonstrated the teachings of Vesalius to his fellow members of the Barber Surgeons of London. The first Latin edition of *De Humani Corporis Fabrica* appeared in England by 1545, and the first edition translated into English appeared by 1553. In France, Ambroise Paré (1510–1590) similarly recognized the importance of Vesalius's anatomy and made his anatomical discoveries available to French surgeons in his textbook of anatomy, *Anatomie Universelle du Corps Humain*, published in 1561. Paré wrote the text of this atlas in vernacular French rather than in academic Latin, which made the work much more accessible to working surgeons, many of whom were not fluent in Latin. The same phenomenon was seen when gastrointestinal surgery blossomed in the late 19th century. American surgeons such as William Stewart Halstead visited the great surgical clinics of Europe and immediately introduced the new surgical techniques that they observed into practice. The rapid spread and evolution of laparoscopic surgery has been stoked by this same spirit.

Laparoscopic surgery burst into the practice of general surgery in 1989 when Jacques Perissat showed a videotape of a laparoscopic cholecystectomy at the Society of American Gastrointestinal Endoscopic Surgeons (SAGES). Later in the same year, Eddie J. Reddick displayed another videotape of a laparoscopic cholecystectomy at the Fall meeting of the American College of Surgeons. The dramatic visualization of surgical anatomy in these videotapes convinced many surgeons of the utility of video laparoscopy in the performance of abdominal surgery.

The technology used in video laparoscopic surgery facilitated the revolutionary introduction of laparoscopic cholecystectomy into surgical practice. The ease with which operations could be viewed, videotaped, projected, and telecast rejuvenated the historical tendency of surgeons to exchange and share techniques. Surgeons once again commonly traveled to the operating rooms of other surgeons to view and learn these new techniques. Live operations were commonly telecast at regional, national, and international meetings. As a result, in the span of only a couple of years, laparoscopic cholecystectomy became the standard of practice in many hospitals in the world.

Over the past decade, laparoscopic surgery has been applied to virtually every general surgery abdominal procedure. Although the use of laparoscopic techniques has not supplanted traditional incisions in all procedures as rapidly as it did in laparoscopic cholecystectomy, the percentage of general surgery operations accomplished laparoscopically is steadily increasing. Indeed, one can envision the day when the term laparoscopic general surgery will be redundant since all general surgery will be accomplished using the video laparoscope or related technology.

The purpose of *Atlas of Laparoscopic Surgery* is to present to surgeons the techniques of laparoscopic general surgery operations. Each chapter has been presented in the same format. Important preoperative, intraoperative, and postoperative issues have been reviewed by our faculty of internationally known experts in a succinct and uniform manner. Each chapter lists in outline form the indications, contraindications, factors important in patient selection, and preoperative preparations. Similarly, issues regarding choice of anesthesia, accessory devices required for the operation, and the instruments and telescopes used in the procedure are listed. The heart of this work is the illustrations. Each step of the operation is clearly depicted with pen and ink drawings and described with the surgeon's narrative. Finally, each surgeon describes his or her preferences of postoperative medications, the rate of advancement of diet, the determinants of discharge, and the instructions on return to normal activities or work.

Atlas of Laparoscopic Surgery is divided into seven parts. The first part, Diagnostic Laparoscopy, shows the use of laparoscopy in the diagnosis of liver diseases, in the staging of gastric and pancreatic carcinomas, and in the staging of lymphomas. The second part, Laparoscopic Hepatobiliary Surgery, portrays laparoscopic cholecystectomy for chronic cholecystitis and acute cholecystitis. In addition, the techniques of laparoscopic common bile duct exploration and laparoscopic construction of a choledochoduodenostomy are shown. In the third part, Laparoscopic Surgery of the Esophagus, laparoscopic esophageal surgery is addressed. Four laparoscopic techniques for the treatment of gastroesophageal reflux disease are illustrated. These in-

clude two methods of constructing a Nissen fundoplication, the Toupet fundoplication, and the Hill fundoplication. Techniques for the repair of a paraesophageal hernia and performance of a Heller myotomy for achalasia are illustrated. Laparoscopic surgery of the stomach is covered in the fourth part. Techniques for highly selective vagotomy, posterior vagotomy, and anterior fundic seromyotomy, various types of gastrectomy and vertical banded gastropexy are presented. The fifth part describes other laparoscopic operations of the upper gastrointestinal tract. These operations include plication of a perforated duodenal ulcer, placement of a feeding gastrostomy or jejunostomy, distal pancreatectomy, splenectomy, and adrenalectomy. Laparoscopic surgery of the lower gastrointestinal tract is illustrated in the sixth and most extensive part of the book. Laparoscopic appendectomy and 15 different techniques of laparoscopic bowel resection are illustrated. These include operations for treatment of Crohn's disease, chronic ulcerative colitis, rectal prolapse, diverticulitis, colon cancer, and rectal cancer. The final section, Laparoscopic Repairs of Inguinal Hernias, shows transabdominal and preperitoneal techniques.

Most of the illustrations published in this tome have been drawn by the artists of Visible Productions, headed by Thomas McCracken, in Fort Collins, Colorado. A few of the drawings were published previously in *Laparoscopic Surgery* (W.B. Saunders Company, Philadelphia, 1994). These, too, were drawn by Thomas McCracken and associates. We owe thanks to the United States Surgical Corporation for permission to reprint these previously published drawings.

Garth H. Ballantyne, M.D., F.A.C.S., F.A.S.C.R.S.

Contents

Part I

DIAGNOSTIC LAPAROSCOPY

Chapter 1

Diagnostic Laparoscopy

JEAN W. SALEH, M.D.

I. Indications

A. General indications for diagnostic laparoscopy
 1. When other diagnostic techniques have
  failed
   a. Laboratory tests are undecisive
   b. Sonography or computed tomogra-
    phy (CT) is inconclusive
   c. Sonography and CT are discordant
   d. Cholangiography is too hazardous
    and ERCP is unsuccessful
 2. When intra-abdominal disease remains
  obscure, as shown by
   a. Persistent pain
   b. Ill-defined mass or organomegaly
   c. Intrahepatic versus extrahepatic jaun-
    dice
   d. Fever
   e. Cachexia
 3. When deciding for or against laparotomy
   a. Staging for lymphomas
   b. Pelvic inflammatory disease versus
    appendicitis
   c. Venous or lymphatic obstruction
   d. Acute gallbladder disease
   e. Severe blunt abdominal trauma
 4. When performing helpful ancillary techniques
   a. Transcholecystocholangiography
   b. Transhepatocholangiography
   c. Splenoportography
   d. Laparotomography
B. Present indications for diagnostic laparoscopy

 1. Liver diseases
   a. Cirrhosis
   b. Portal hypertension
   c. Primary biliary cirrhosis
   d. Congestive liver disease
   e. Primary or secondary tumors
   f. Parasitic diseases
 2. Suspected carcinoma
   a. Diffuse or localized filling defects of
    the liver
   b. Peritoneal carcinomatosis
   c. Hepatic metastases
   d. Pelvic carcinoma
 3. Ill-defined infections
   a. Tuberculous peritonitis
   b. Periodic polyseritis
   c. *Chlamydia trachomatis* perihepatitis
   d. Fever of unknown origin
   e. Acquired immunodeficiency syn-
    drome (AIDS)
   f. Parasitosis
 4. Jaundice
   a. Prehepatic, hepatic, posthepatic
   b. Infectious, mitotic
 5. Ascites
   a. Infectious or mitotic
   b. Decompensated cirrhosis
   c. Peritoneal reaction
 6. Special indications
   a. Staging of lymphomas
   b. Abdominal emergencies
   c. Unresolved intra-abdominal pain or
    mass
   d. Gallbladder disease
   e. Pancreatic disease

7. Miscellaneous conditions
   a. Removal of intra-abdominal foreign bodies
   b. Monitoring of dialysis or chemotherapy in patients with intra-abdominal tumors
   c. Evaluation of omentum for breast prosthesis

II. Contraindications

A. Absolute contraindications
   1. Blood dyscrasias
      a. Prothrombin time (PT) 5 seconds above control
      b. Platelet count below 70,000
   2. Acute abdomen
   3. Acute and recent myocardial infarction
   4. Severe chronic obstructive lung disease
   5. Advanced pregnancy
   6. Massive abdominal or diaphragmatic hernias
   7. Uncooperative patient
B. Relative contraindications
   1. Massive ascites
   2. Multiple abdominal scars
   3. Extensive organomegaly
   4. Large abdominal hernias
   5. Congestive heart failure

III. Factors Important in Patient Selection

A. Obese patients
   1. Cannot always distend the abdominal wall.
   2. Require special custom-made longer needles for the induction of pneumoperitoneum.
   3. Need a double or triple layer closure of the abdominal wall.
B. Organomegaly should be avoided after very careful delineation and assessment.
C. Ascites should be evacuated almost entirely before the procedure if it is an exudate; it should be evacuated very slowly before the procedure if it is a transudate.
D. Hernias, whether parietal or inguinal, are not absolute contraindications of the procedure. They can be taped tightly without any untoward effects. In the event of a large eventration a hernia may constitute a clear contraindication. On occasion a hernia that communicates with the abdominal cavity may show some secondary distention owing to the insufflated abdominal air, all without major consequence.
E. Scars should be avoided because very often they harbor underlying severe adhesions.
F. Adhesions may be vascular or avascular, limited or extensive, loculating or diffuse. They are often the source of abdominal pain and can be lysed easily if they are avascular.
G. In children, laparoscopy is better performed under general anesthesia because the operator can very seldom ensure a meaningful level of cooperation with local anesthesia.
H. Situs inversus can be very frustrating and occasionally can be a complicating situation if it is unknown before the procedure. Since laparoscopy is a second-line technique after CT scan or ultrasound, the anatomy is usually known beforehand.

V. Choice of Anesthesia

Premedications

Following informed consent signed by a responsible patient and the rehearsal at bedside of the abdominal distention maneuver, the patient is quickly oriented in the endoscopy suite and introduced to the staff. Since one of the main advantages of laparoscopy is that it is performed under local anesthesia, the premedications used are aimed at alleviating anxiety, subduing perceptions, relieving pain, and, most of all, ensuring the patient's comfort and cooperation.

- *Atropine sulfate*, 0.4 mg intramuscularly (IM), is used essentially to counteract any possibility of vasovagal reflex and to promote the needed stillness of the intestinal loops. In the presence of tachycardia, atropine should not be used, and many laparoscopists do not consider this option at all.
- *Meperidine*, 50 to 75 mg IM, is usually given after the procedure in the event of pain due to entrapped air or gas or for occasional severe discomfort at the site of a liver or peritoneal biopsy. In most instances, however, local anesthesia and a sound technique should render the procedure totally painless and pain medication unwarranted. In very apprehensive and nocioceptive patients, some laparoscopists may use meperidine intravenously (IV) before the procedure.

- *Diazepam*, 5 to 10 mg IM, may be used for the relief of anxiety, muscle spasm, and acute awareness. Drowsiness and superficial narcosis are also desirable effects. In some instances, it may be dispensed and titrated IV.

Personally, I have always used a combination of atropine and diazepam half an hour before the procedure and meperidine after the procedure but only pro re nata. Other laparoscopists may use a different regimen or combination including atropine and meperidine IM with a slow titration of diazepam IV.

Phenobarbital and meperidine are used without atropine, and diazepam and meperidine can be administered IV. These are only a few examples of the many possible drug combinations that one can use to achieve sedation and relaxation. Deep sedation is to be avoided, however, before the initiation of pneumoperitoneum because the patient in this condition will not be able to tense his or her abdominal wall, and this is essential for the safe introduction and induction of the pneumoperitoneum needle.

VI. Accessory Devices

None required

VII. Instruments and Telescopes

(Fig. 1–1)

A. There are two orders of optical instruments
   1. Light- and image-transmitted fiberoptic or quartz instruments
   2. Video laparoscope (most widely used)
B. Scalpel with different size blades for skin incision
C. One 10-ml and one 20-ml syringe
D. Two or four small curved hemostatic forceps
E. Four straight-tip large forceps
F. Two stainless steel cupulas for lidocaine (Xylocaine) and alcohol with Betadine
G. Two 22-gauge, 10-cm long needles (spinal) for local anesthesia
H. One 21-gauge, 3.5-cm long needle for skin anesthesia
I. One pair of scissors
J. Curved needle with mounted 3–0 silk thread for skin closure
K. Sharp trocar and trocar sleeve with trumpet valve for air contention
L. Laparoscope (Fig. 1–2)
M. Insulating needles
   1. Veress needle with spring release for peritoneal "pop"

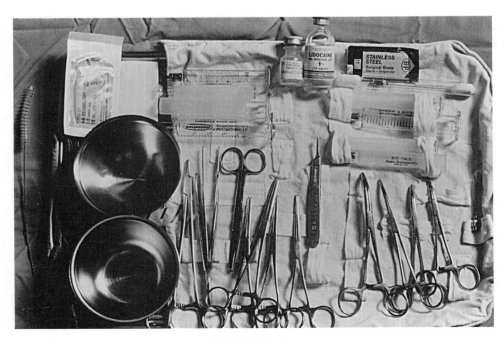

FIGURE 1–1

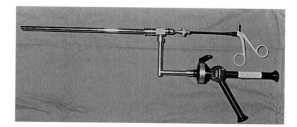

FIGURE 1-2

2. Foures needle in different lengths, with smaller diameter and fore and lateral holes for safety

VIII. Position of Monitors and Placement of Trocars

FIGURE 1-3. Laparoscopy is the transgression of the abdominal wall under local anesthesia for the purpose of examining and sampling the intra-abdominal organs following distention of the abdominal cavity with gas or air. Pneumoperitoneum without doubt is the most essential if not the most critical step in performing perforating laparoscopy. The entire feasibility and safety of the examination depend on successful insertion of the pneumoperitoneum needle and symmetrical distention of the abdomen. This process ensures the proper introduction of the trocar and the telescope, thus allowing an adequate and complete examination. The needle may be inserted in the left or right midclavicular line at its intersection with a line joining the umbilicus to the anterosuperior iliac spine. It is also commonly introduced periumbilically to the left and above or in the midline below. These sites of introduction should remain flexible but should always avoid any vascular pathway, namely the epigastric artery, any organomegaly, or a scar.

Following local anesthesia of the skin and the parietal peritoneum with 1 per cent lidocaine,

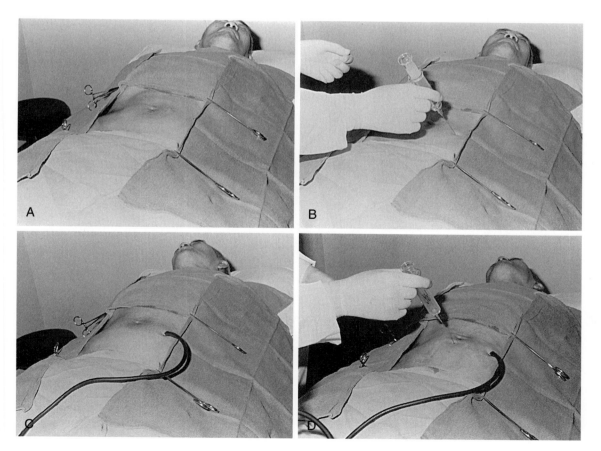

FIGURE 1-3

the patient is asked to protrude the anterior abdominal wall while keeping the back flat on the table. This Valsalva maneuver distances the intra-abdominal organs from the parietal wall and ensures the safe introduction of the pneumoperitoneum needle in this enhanced virtual space. Once the needle has transgressed the peritoneum (as felt by the classic "pop") and the 360-degree rotation of the tip of the needle is free from any encroachment, insufflation of the abdomen may proceed with room air, carbon dioxide, or nitrous oxide until the abdomen is symmetrically distended and the prehepatic dullness has disappeared. The thickness of the "air cushion" can be appreciated by drawing back the plunger of the lidocaine syringe while pulling it out of the abdominal cavity. The influx of air bubbles into the syringe during this maneuver gives a clear idea of the measure of the air cushion.

Once pneumoperitoneum has been adequately induced, the telescope can be introduced through the trocar sleeve using one of the following methods.

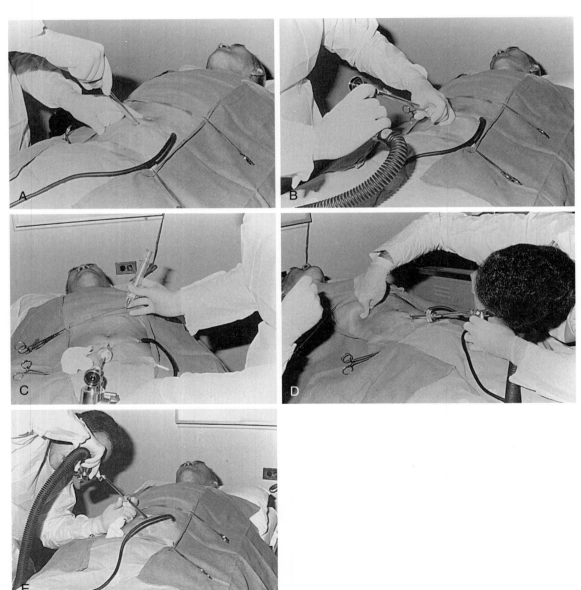

FIGURE 1-4

"One-Site Technique." Using the conical or pyramidal trocar with its sleeve, the parietal wall is transgressed at the site of the induction of pneumoperitoneum.

FIGURE 1–4. "Two-Site Technique" Following the induction of pneumoperitoneum in any safe part of the abdomen, the laparoscope is introduced in the trocar sleeve at another location than the one used for local anesthesia. The same procedure is used for the second puncture for probe measurement, biopsy, or the introduction of a second telescope.

IX. Narrative of Surgical Technique
The Clinical Situations

1. IN THE EVALUATION OF LIVER DISEASE

FIGURE 1–5. Laparoscopy remains of paramount importance in the diagnosis of cirrhosis because the liver surface is readily accessible for directed biopsy of the fibrotic tracts rather than of the regenerating nodules. The presence and severity of ancillary portal hypertension are also easily assessed. Furthermore, the nature and origin of the surface lesion can be determined with great accuracy whether it is due to micro- or macronodular cirrhosis, changes secondary to congestive liver or heart disease, or biliary cirrhosis. Sclerosing cholangitis, congenital disease, aging, infectious or parasitic disease, or mitotic implant or transformations will not escape the scrutiny of the experienced eye. All these changes, which may be manifest by a lesion as small as 0.5 mm, are immediately accessible for evaluation, directed biopsy, and/or brushing.

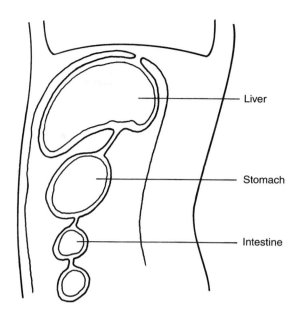

FIGURE 1–6

2. IN SUSPECTED INTRA-ABDOMINAL CARCINOMA

FIGURE 1–6. Laparoscopy can determine with proven detail whether the heterogeneous uptake by the liver seen on scintiscans, whether localized or diffuse, is benign or is already infiltrated with malignant transformation. It also remains the only valid technique used for the diagnosis of peritoneal involvement in patients with carcinomatosis and should be undertaken whenever this condition is suggested by clinical symptoms or suspicious ascites. In patients with pelvic carcinoma, laparoscopy is the ultimate procedure not only for local diagnosis and therapy but also for the evaluation of local and distant dissemination. In any of these situations, the laparoscopic surgeon can immediately recognize the true nature of the lesions involving these structures and can confirm the diagnosis through directed biopsies. Finally, this simple technique eliminates the need for laparotomy and general anesthesia.

In general, if the patient has a suspicious lesion on the surface of the liver by computed tomography (CT) or ultrasound and if the initial directed biopsy is not conclusive, laparoscopy may represent the technique of choice for visualization and sampling. However, if through

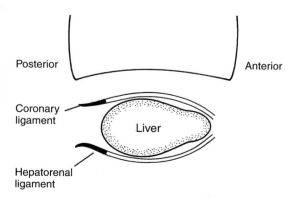

FIGURE 1–5

these imaging techniques the lesion is shown to be more in the core of the liver, a CT or ultrasound-directed biopsy is more appropriate. In any of these situations, all techniques remain complementary and should be used whenever the more indicated one has failed to achieve a decisive diagnosis.

3. IN ILL-DEFINED INFECTION

Laparoscopy remains an important recourse for visual evaluation of organ transformation and for the collection of adequate samples. Tuberculous peritonitis is now undergoing a clinical reactivation and may mimic several pathologic conditions before it is decisively diagnosed through peritoneal, visceral, and parietal sampling under direct vision. Periodic serositis may display similar findings albeit without the equally sized "millet seed" implants so typical of tuberculosis. In this serious condition, laparoscopy can determine, through the diffuse aspect of peritoneal hyperemia, intestinal spasm, distention, and padding, the origin of the illness and set the stage for successful medical treatment while avoiding the need for an exploratory laparotomy with occasional intestinal resection.

In patients with fever of unknown origin, laparoscopy may disclose the cause of the hyperthermia. In a patient with a striking Fitz-Hugh-Curtis syndrome with its ancillary right upper quadrant pain, "violin-string-like" adhesions may be seen on the surface of the liver and within the neighboring organs. Biopsies and cultures will reveal the responsible agent, gonococcus or *Chlamydia*, or a complicated condition in a patient known to be positive for human immunodeficiency virus (HIV). Alternatively, the fever may represent the early manifestation of hepatitis or the only clinical symptom of diffuse intra-abdominal carcinomatosis. Lymphomas of Hodgkin's or non-Hodgkin's origin, either limited to the liver or already disseminated, may be manifested early by organomegaly and fever. In these difficult situations laparoscopy can redirect the diagnosis and set the treatment in its proper perspective.

4. IN THE EVALUATION OF JAUNDICE

Laparoscopy is no longer considered a first-choice procedure for the refined determination of prehepatic, hepatic, or posthepatic jaundice. However, in patients with prehepatic jaundice with hemolysis, the liver is normal in color and consistency, and transparent biliary stones may be seen in the gallbladder. In hepatic jaundice the liver may be normal in color and anatomy in the early phase of biliary retention, but in the later phase it may show lakes of bile retention with some surface modification and fibrosis. In posthepatic jaundice, which most of the time is due to extrahepatic obstruction, the liver is yellow or typically green with some degree of nodularity if the obstruction is chronic. Laparoscopy remains a stand-by technique in patients with complicated jaundice and should be performed only when the choice is between an infectious process and a mitotic one. This consideration becomes important if surgery is contemplated.

5. IN THE EVALUATION OF ASCITES

Laparoscopy may be the best procedure for determining the origin of a peritoneal reaction, especially when the reaction is exudative, borderline, or undetermined. It may also unveil an unsuspected cirrhosis or a complicated congestive liver disease. If ascites is large and is determined to be exudative, it can be evacuated almost in toto the night before the procedure. If ascites is large and is a transudate, careful monitoring and a small amount of evacuation over a 48-hour period is the rule to avoid brusque intravascular depletion and shock. However, some studies have shown that a large transudate can be totally evacuated in a short period of time with no complication. In some cases, ascites is minimal and is seen on the scan only in dependent areas of the abdomen. Laparoscopy in this situation is an important procedure because often a blind attempt at paracentesis will fail. During the procedure and under direct vision, the remote accumulation is tapped, the intra-abdominal structures are examined, and a diagnosis is reached as to whether the collection is from the upper or lower abdominal cavity.

Termination of Procedure

After a final evaluation of the abdominal cavity and documentation and sampling of the lesions, the laparoscope is retrieved, leaving the trocar sleeve in situ. The trumpet valve is then depressed to allow the intra-abdominal insufflated air or gas to escape freely. This egress is further facilitated by external abdominal compression, having the patient sit up halfway, and repeated coughing efforts. The trocar sleeve is then re-moved, the area is cleansed again, and the small incision is closed in one or two layers with 3–0 silk thread.

Specimen Collection

Organ sampling is achieved using a needle or special forceps. The needle, Menghini or oth-ers, may be introduced transcutaneously under direct vision or through the ancillary channel of the operating telescope. This channel is also used mainly for forceps biopsy, or one may resort to a more convenient second puncture. Tissue collection in the core of solid organs or masses is usually painless but could be accompa-nied by severe pain if the parietal peritoneum is involved. This structure should always be anes-thetized before sampling is performed.

Documentation of Lesions

When abnormal pathology is discovered, docu-mentation is necessary for three major reasons:

- Permanent visual record of the lesions or pa-thology
- Teaching and reference file
- Legal necessity

Documentation can be achieved either by still photographs using 400 ASA Ektachrome or any similar high-speed slide film in a 35-mm camera or by video endoscopy for a more "live" re-cording. Photographic and video equipment should be thoroughly checked before the proce-dure begins to avoid unpleasant surprises such as absence of film, a blown-up bulb, or a nonre-cording VCR.

Limitations of Laparoscopy

FIGURE 1–7. Most of the limitations encoun-tered in peritoneoscopy are subject to the visual boundaries of the intra-abdominal anatomy and to the skill, dexterity, and experience of the operator. The possible structural modifications of the intra-abdominal organs following a dif-fuse inflammatory process, metastases, or prior surgery may sometimes limit the field of visual-ization. We are indeed far, however, from being able to examine adequately the posterior surface of the liver, retroperitoneum, and renal and ad-renal areas, as well as, to some extent, the pan-

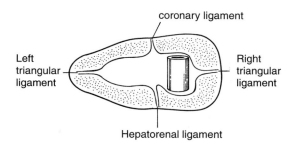

FIGURE 1–7

creas, porta hepatis, and periaortic nodes. Moreover, 75 per cent of the liver surface, the anterior and lateral parietal peritoneum, the fal-ciform ligament, the anterior aspect of the stomach and omentum, portions of the large and small intestines, a tumoral pancreas, and the pelvic organs are readily accessible. With added expertise and modification of the patient's position together with external manipulation of the organs with a probe, more extensive areas can be explored, including the inferior aspect of the liver, the head of the pancreas, the appendix, and the spleen.

X. Postoperative Medications

Meperidine is usually given after the procedure if pain due to trapped air or gas is present or for occasional severe discomfort at the site of a liver or peritoneal biopsy.

XI. Advancement of Diet

A. Patients are allowed to eat clear liquids when they are alert.
B. They are allowed to eat a regular diet once they are discharged to home.

XII. Determinants of Discharge

Patients are discharged to home when:

1. Their vital signs are stable.
2. They have voided.
3. They are tolerating liquids.

XIII. Return to Normal Activity

Patients can resume their normal activities within 1 to 2 days.

Chapter 2

Pancreatic and Gastric Cancer Staging

KEVIN C. CONLON, M.D., M.B.A.

I. Indications

A. Staging of abdominal malignancies
   1. Pancreatic carcinoma
   2. Gastric carcinoma
B. Assessment of primary tumor
C. Identification of hepatic metastases
D. Diagnosis of regional nodal metastases
E. Detection of small-volume peritoneal disease unappreciated by other noninvasive staging modalities such as computed tomography (CT), magnetic resonance imaging (MRI), or ultrasonography

II. Contraindications

A. Patients with known disseminated disease
B. Patients who cannot tolerate general anesthesia

III. Factors Important in Patient Selection

Adenocarcinoma of the pancreas remains a lethal disease. Despite advances in detection, the majority of patients continue to present with advanced disease. Unfortunately, because of the inability of sophisticated diagnostic modalities such as CT, MRI, and ultrasound to accurately assess the extent of disease, many of these patients still undergo surgical exploration for accurate staging or palliation. In many cases, an open palliative procedure is not warranted, the exploratory procedure confers no benefit, and it may be associated with significant morbidity and mortality affecting both the quality and duration of survival.

Pancreatic Cancer

Patients with a suspected peripancreatic malignancy should undergo a contrast-enhanced, dynamic CT scan of the abdomen with 5-mm cuts of the pancreas. This examination has been shown to be highly sensitive in determining local regional extension and vascular encasement of the tumor. Those patients who are considered to have "radiologically" resectable disease should then undergo laparoscopic staging prior to open exploration.

Gastric Cancer

For patients with gastric cancer, accurate pretherapeutic staging has become increasingly important with the advent of a multidisciplinary approach to therapy. Patients are now offered choices between surgical extirpation, radiation therapy, investigational neoadjuvant chemotherapy, palliative chemotherapy and/or radiotherapy, or supportive palliative care alone. Laparoscopic staging is indicated for the majority of patients with gastric cancer who have no obstruction and no bleeding. Patients with "early" tumors (T1, T2) have a low risk of disseminated disease and should proceed directly to open operation. The remainder undergo an operative approach similar to that described for patients with pancreatic cancer. Preliminary experience from centers in the United States and Europe suggests that laparoscopic examination can accurately identify intraperitoneal dissemination and avoid unnecessary exploration.

IV. Preoperative Preparation

A. Preoperative staging
   1. Computed tomography
   2. Magnetic resonance imaging
   3. Ultrasonography
B. Patients are admitted on the day of surgery.
C. Routine premedication is administered according to the type of anesthesia given.

D. Bowel preparation
   1. Clear liquid diet on the day before surgery
   2. Magnesium citrate for bowel preparation the day before surgery

V. Choice of Anesthesia

All patients require general anesthesia.

VI. Accessory Devices

A. Warming blanket
B. Laparoscopic articulated ultrasound probe

VII. Instruments and Telescopes

A. 10-mm 30-degree telescope
B. 5-mm laparoscopic scissors
C. 5-mm laparoscopic atraumatic grasping forceps
D. Laparoscopic retractor
E. Endosurgical biopsy forceps

Laparoscopic surgical techniques should adhere to standard surgical oncologic principles and should replicate as far as possible the equivalent open operation. The following section describes the operative technique for laparoscopic staging as practiced at Memorial Sloan-Kettering Cancer Center.

Pancreatic Cancer

VIII. Position of Monitors and Placement of Trocars

FIGURE 2-1. All procedures are performed with the patient under general anesthesia. The patient is placed supine on the operating table. Two monitors are used, placed at the level of the patient's shoulders. The surgeon stands on the right side. The first assistant stands on the left side (with a camera operator, if one is present, also on this side). A warming blanket is used to maintain normal body temperature. An "open" surgical technique for carbon dioxide insufflation is used in all cases. A 21-cm subumbilical incision is made, exposing the abdominal wall fascia. The peritoneum is opened under direct vision, and a 10/11-mm Hasson-type trocar is inserted. This is attached to a high-flow carbon dioxide insufflator. Carbon dioxide insufflation is commenced through this trocar to an intra-abdominal pressure of 14 mm Hg. If there is a prior history of a midline laparotomy, the initial port may be placed in either the right or left upper quadrant of the abdomen. A 30-degree angled telescope is used for laparoscopic examination. A 10/12-mm port is placed laterally in the right upper quadrant. This is used for the laparoscopic ultrasound probe. Additional ports are placed as shown in the figure. If on initial exploration, carcinomatosis or liver metastases are seen, a single 5-mm port is placed to allow biopsy specimens to be taken.

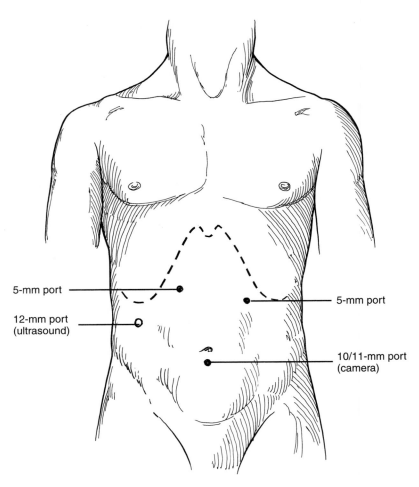

5-mm port

12-mm port (ultrasound)

5-mm port

10/11-mm port (camera)

FIGURE 2-1

FIGURE 2–2

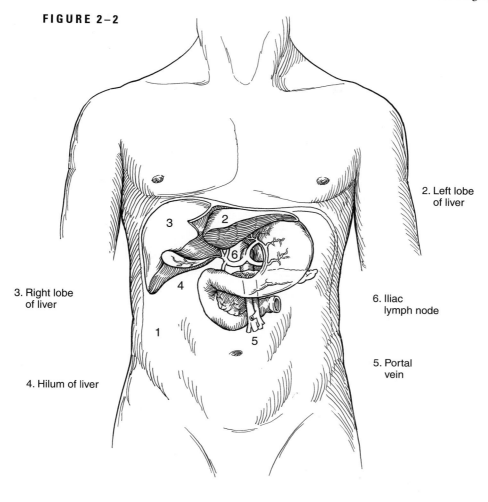

2. Left lobe
of liver

3. Right lobe
of liver

6. Iliac
lymph node

4. Hilum of liver

5. Portal
vein

1. Peritoneal cavity

IX. Narrative of Surgical Technique

FIGURE 2–2. A systematic examination is performed that mimics the routine exploration at open operation. Intraperitoneal adhesions, if present, are divided. The primary tumor is assessed, and its local extent, size, and fixation are noted. Extension to contiguous organs such as the colon, duodenum, liver, spleen, or stomach is identified if present. The sequence of examination is shown.

FIGURE 2–3. The patient is then placed in 20 degrees of reverse Trendelenburg position with 10 degrees of left lateral tilt. Examination begins with visualization of the anterior and posterior surfaces of the left lateral segment of the liver and the anterior and inferior surfaces of its right lobe. "Palpation" of the liver is achieved by using a 10-mm instrument along with a 5-mm grasping forceps.

FIGURE 2–4. The hilum of the liver is visualized by using the PEER retractor to elevate the liver. By correctly positioning the 30-degree telescope, the foramen of Winslow can be examined, and biopsies of the periportal lymph nodes can be taken if required. This positioning is also used to facilitate ultrasound examination of the hepatoduodenal ligament as demonstrated in this figure. This portion of the examination can be helped by gentle retraction of the duodenum with a nontraumatic grasper.

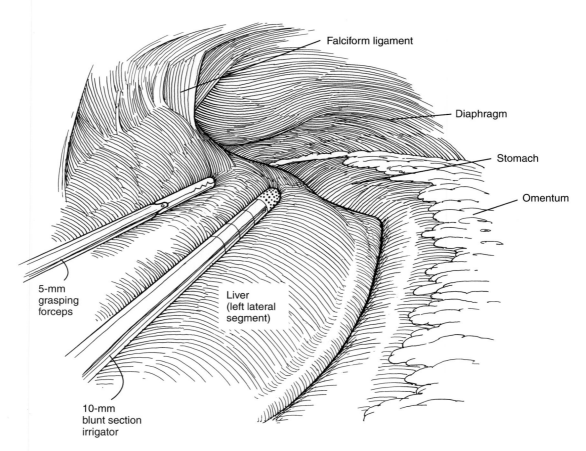

FIGURE 2–3

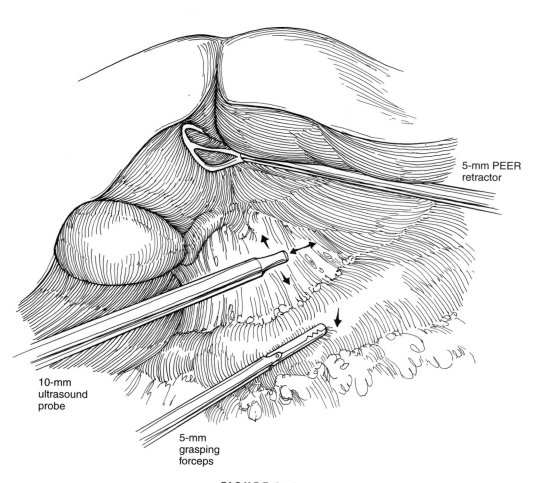

5-mm PEER
retractor

10-mm
ultrasound
probe

5-mm
grasping
forceps

FIGURE 2–4

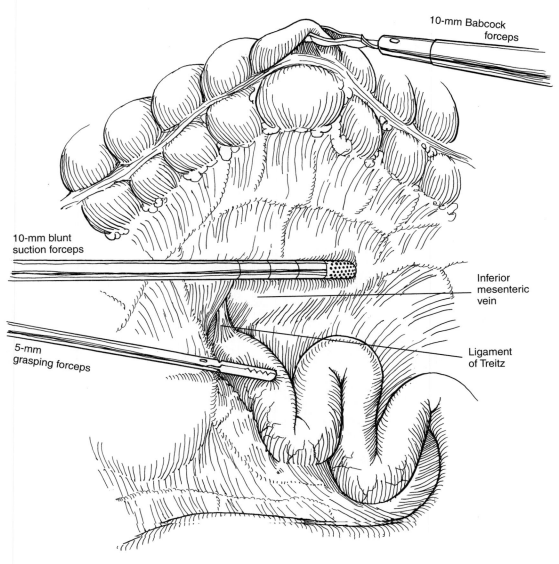

10-mm Babcock
forceps

10-mm blunt
suction forceps

5-mm
grasping forceps

Inferior
mesenteric
vein

Ligament
of Treitz

FIGURE 2–5

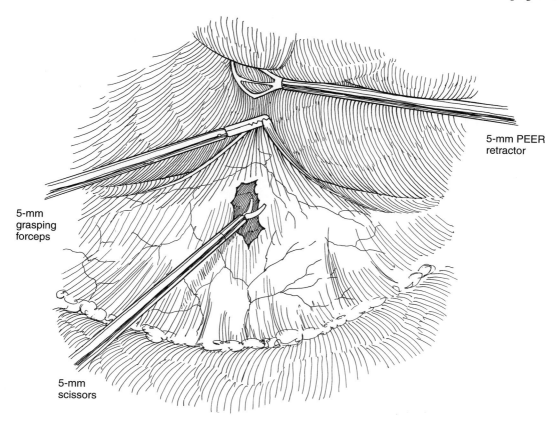

5-mm PEER
retractor

5-mm
grasping
forceps

5-mm
scissors

FIGURE 2–6

FIGURE 2–5. The patient is then placed in 10 degrees of Trendelenburg position without lateral tilt. The omentum is identified and retracted toward the left upper quadrant, allowing the ligament of Treitz to be identified. The mesocolon can now be easily inspected, paying particular attention to the mesocolic vein, which is normally quite visible.

FIGURE 2–6. On completion of the mesocolic examination, the patient is replaced in the supine position. By elevating the left lateral segment of the liver with a PEER retractor, the gastrohepatic omentum is put under stretch and is clearly visible. This is then incised, exposing

the caudate lobe of the liver, the vena cava, and the celiac axis. Hemostasis is achieved using cautery. Care is taken to preserve any anomalous left hepatic arteries.

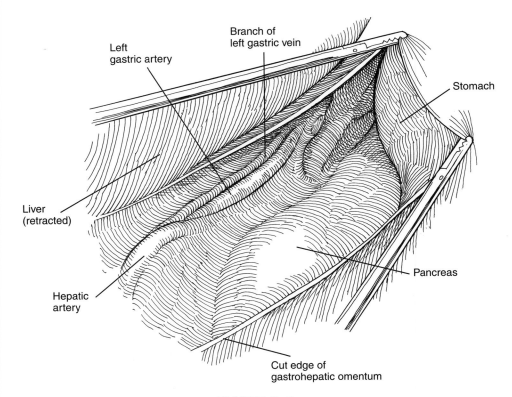

FIGURE 2-7

FIGURE 2-7. The lesser sac can be inspected in most cases through this approach. Celiac, portal, or perigastric lymph nodes are sampled if required. The hepatic artery is identified and its course to the porta hepatis visualized. The celiac axis is also visualized with this maneuver. During the examination samples of any suspicious lesions are taken for biopsy using endosurgical biopsy forceps; the samples are then sent for frozen section analysis.

FIGURE 2-8. Ultrasonography is then performed. The articulated laparoscopic ultrasound probe is inserted through the 10-mm or 12-mm laparoscopic port placed in either the right or left upper quadrant. In the majority of patients the right side is used because this position facilitates scanning of the hepatoduodenal ligament.

The examination commences with the probe placed transversely over the left lateral segment. Using Couinaud's description of the segmental anatomy of the liver as a guide, segments I, II, and III are examined in turn. The ultrasound probe is then placed over the dome of the right liver as demonstrated in the figure. The liver is examined sequentially by moving and rotating the probe slowly over the surface of each of the hepatic segments. The portal vein (PV) and hepatic veins are identified. The gallbladder and right kidney are examined using the liver as an acoustic window with the ultrasound probe placed on segment V. The hepatoduodenal ligament is examined with the transducer probe placed transversely across the ligament. The common hepatic duct, common bile duct, portal vein, and hepatic arteries are identified during this part of the examination. Identification of these structures is aided by the use of both pulse and color-flow Doppler.

When this portion of the examination has been completed, the superior mesenteric artery (SMA) and the confluence of the PV and SMA are examined. This is accomplished by placing the transducer transversely on the gastrocolic omentum. In most patients the confluence of the PV and SMA is readily identified, and the relationship, if any, of a tumor to this structure and the SMA is assessed. Next, the pancreas itself, the celiac axis, and the proximal hepatic artery are scanned by placing the probe directly on the surface of the pancreas. At any point

during the examination samples of any suspicious lesion can be taken with a Tru-Cut needle or biopsy forceps under sonographic guidance.

A tumor is determined to be unresectable if one of the following is present and is proved histologically:

1. Metastases: hepatic, serosal, or peritoneal
2. Extrapancreatic extension of tumor (i.e., mesocolic involvement)
3. Celiac or portal nodal involvement
4. Invasion or encasement of the celiac axis or hepatic artery
5. Encasement by tumor of the portal or superior mesenteric vein and/or the superior mesenteric artery

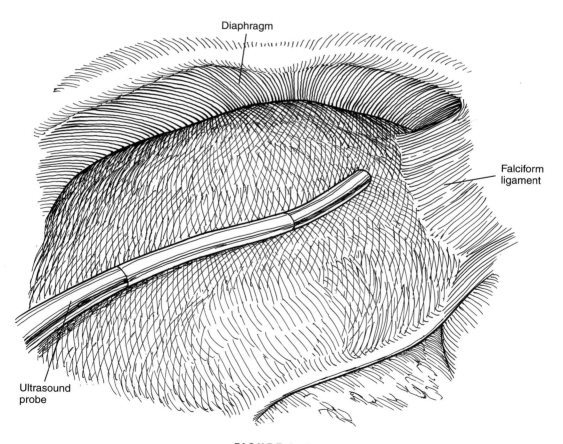

Diaphragm

Falciform ligament

Ultrasound probe

FIGURE 2–8

FIGURE 2–9A

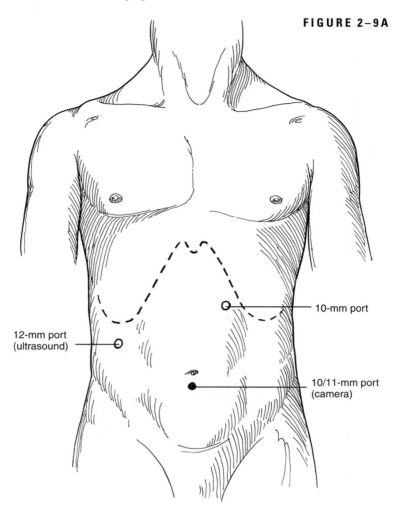

12-mm port
(ultrasound)

10-mm port

10/11-mm port
(camera)

Gastric Cancer

VIII. Position of Monitors and Size of Trocars

FIGURE 2–9A. Access to the abdomen is achieved as described earlier in Figure 2–1. Ports are placed in the right and left upper quadrants. Currently, three 10-mm ports are used. However, if laparoscopic ultrasonography is not being performed, smaller (i.e., 3- or 5-mm) ports can be inserted.

IX. Narrative of Surgical Technique

FIGURE 2–9B. The sequence of examination is as follows: (1) The peritoneal cavity, especially the left upper quadrant and pelvis, is examined. (2) The liver is inspected as described earlier (see Fig. 2–3). (3) The stomach is then visualized. Particular attention is paid to the site of the primary tumor and its local extent. (4) The examination is completed by exposing the ligament of Trietz and mesocolon. The sequence of examination is shown.

FIGURE 2–9B

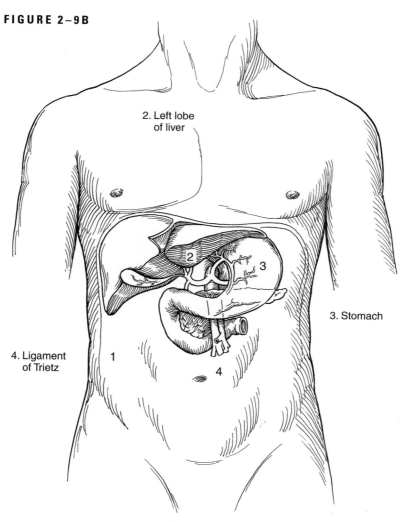

2. Left lobe
of liver

3. Stomach

4. Ligament
of Trietz

1. Peritoneal cavity

FIGURE 2–10. Ultrasound examination of the stomach is demonstrated. The probe is inserted through the right upper quadrant port. The sequence of examination is shown in Figure 2–10B. Visualization of the layers of the gastric wall is facilitated by distending the stomach with 500 ml of warm saline.

X. Postoperative Medications

Oral analgesics (i.e., acetaminophen with codeine or oxycodone) are given to be taken as required.

XI. Advancement of Diet

    A. On completion of the procedure the oro-gastric tube that was placed following induction of anesthesia is removed.

    B. When recovery from anesthesia is complete, diet is resumed and advanced as tolerated.

XII. Determinants of Discharge

Patients are discharged home when they have met the discharge criteria of the department of anesthesia at our hospital.

XIII. Return to Normal Activity

The majority of patients return to full activity within 2 to 4 days following the procedure. No restrictions are applied.

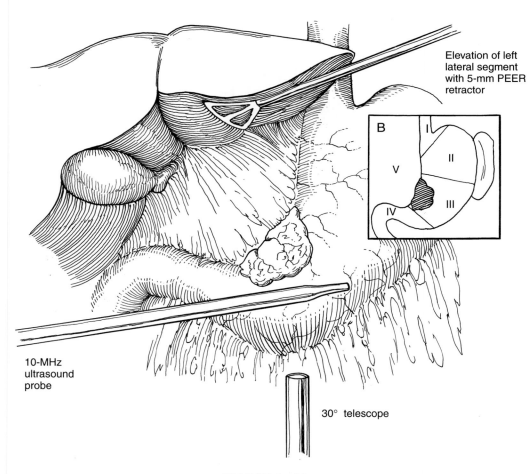

Elevation of left lateral segment with 5-mm PEER retractor

10-MHz ultrasound probe

30° telescope

FIGURE 2–10

Chapter 3

Laparoscopic Staging of Lymphomas

FREDERICK L. GREENE, M.D.

I. Indications

Patients with Hodgkin's disease and non-Hodgkin's lymphoma in whom findings disclosed by staging will alter the approach to therapy.

II. Contraindications

A. Absolute contraindications
1. Lymphoma patients with limited disease in one area, such as an isolated lymph node region in the neck. These patients are best treated with localized radiation therapy and have an overall excellent prognosis.
2. Patients with non-Hodgkin's lymphoma who are thought to have a systemic illness from the onset of the disease. These patients are best treated with chemotherapy, and abdominal staging plays little role in their management.
3. Patients with advanced lymphoma. Chemotherapy, utilizing multiple agents, is necessary in these patients because of the systemic nature of the disease.

B. Relative contraindications
1. Patients with significant pulmonary or cardiac disease
2. Patients with severe coagulopathy
3. Patients with previous abdominal operations

III. Factors Important in Patient Selection

Patients recommended for abdominal staging of lymphoma have already had a diagnosis that is generally based on lymph node biopsy of peripheral lymphadenopathy. The two main groups of lymphoma patients are those with Hodgkin's disease and those with non-Hodgkin's disease. Patients with non-Hodgkin's disease have an extremely diverse group of reticuloendothelial maladies and have a variety of clinical courses. Patients with non-Hodgkin's lymphoma rarely need abdominal staging because it is assumed that they have a systemic illness early in their course and need chemotherapy for overall management. Recent classifications of non-Hodgkin's lymphoma comprise low-, intermediate- and high-grade groups and may, in fact, be characterized by a variety of clinical courses. While some of these patients may benefit from localized therapy using radiation, staging techniques, except under protocol situations, are not routinely performed for patients with non-Hodgkin's disease. Selected patients with lymphoma of the gastrointestinal tract may benefit from laparoscopy because localization of the process may lead to more definitive surgical resection. Non-Hodgkin's lymphomas represent 1 to 4 per cent of all gastrointestinal malignancies and involve primarily the stomach, small bowel, and colon. Patient selection may be based on prior imaging studies that delineate gastrointestinal masses or retroperitoneal involvement that requires directed biopsy. Laparoscopic examination may be very helpful in directing biopsy for patients with non-Hodgkin's lymphoma.

The most important group of patients with lymphoma who undergo laparoscopic staging are those with Hodgkin's disease. This form of lymphoma progresses in a fairly orderly manner, generally from a single focus of disease that spreads peripherally along the lymphatic pathways. Once the diagnosis has been made using node biopsy, a decision about abdominal staging can be made after review of the appropriate imaging studies, which include chest x-ray, chest and abdominal computed tomography (CT) scans, and lower extremity lymphangiography. As mentioned previously, the decision to perform staging laparotomy is based solely on whether the information obtained will alter therapy.

Patients with disseminated disease or extensive extranodal disease (Stages III and IV) require chemotherapy and are not candidates for staging laparoscopy. In addition, patients with a limited focus of Hodgkin's disease (Stage IA) who have no evidence of any other involvement according to imaging studies may be treated with radiation therapy alone and are also not candidates for staging laparoscopy. Patients with bulky mediastinal Hodgkin's disease, which is defined as more than one-third of the greatest transverse diameter of the chest on posterior-anterior chest x-ray, are usually treated with combined therapy using chemotherapy and radiation. None of these patients are candidates for laparoscopic staging. If radiation therapy is to be used as the sole treatment modality, patients with clinical Stage I and IIA disease (those without clinical symptoms of fever, night sweats, and weight loss) may require staging laparoscopy to ensure that no evidence of abdominal disease is present. Patients with pathologic Stage IIB disease may be candidates for nodal radiation as well if disease limited to one side of the diaphragm is found. Generally, patients with clinical Stage IIB disease are treated with chemotherapy because of their systemic symptoms.

IV. Preoperative Preparation

A. Preadmission testing including complete blood count, electrolytes, and coagulation parameters
B. Ambulatory surgery
C. Routine preoperative medications may include vitamin K, platelets, or fresh frozen plasma if coagulation problems are present.
D. Pneumococcal vaccine (Pneumovax) is administered preoperatively.
E. Patients are kept nil per os (NPO) the night prior to the laparoscopic procedure.
F. Full bowel preparation is not indicated, although a cleansing enema is helpful for evacuation of the colon when retroperitoneal evaluation or splenectomy is undertaken.
G. Preoperative antibiotics using a cephalosporin are given in the holding area prior to induction of anesthesia.

V. Choice of Anesthesia

General anesthesia is used for the laparoscopic staging examination because of the time needed to provide all the components of the examination and the need for complete abdominal wall relaxation.

VI. Accessory Devices

A footboard on the operative table is mandatory.

VII. Instruments and Telescopes

A. Standard laparoscopic camera as well as carbon dioxide insufflation
B. Telescopes should be of 30 degree and 0 degree variety
C. Linear stapler to allow for wedge biopsy of liver

D. Vascular linear stapler for use during splenectomy

E. Specimen bag for intra-abdominal use for
collection of lymph nodes or spleen

F. Laparoscopic refractors

VIII. Position of Monitor, Placement and Size of Trocars

FIGURE 3–1A. The operating room is set up
to allow for monitors at both the head and foot
of the table. The surgeon is positioned on the
left side of the patient with the assistant on the
patient's right side. The camera operator stands
adjacent to the assistant, and the scrub nurse
stands adjacent to the surgeon. The patient is
generally placed supine on the operating table,
but alternatively, the patient may be positioned
in a modified lithotomy position, and the camera operator may stand between the patient's
legs. A pneumatic bean bag may be placed to
help change the patient's position during the
procedure.

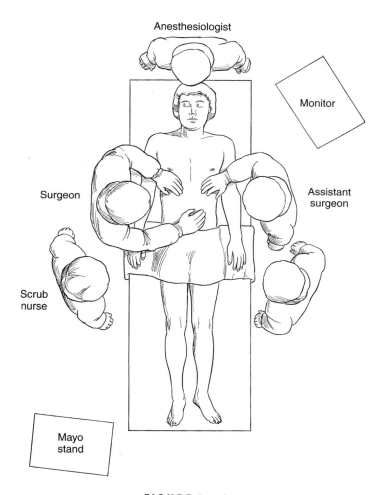

FIGURE 3–1A

FIGURE 3–1B. Only 12-mm ports are used, and these are positioned in the midline as well as the left abdominal area. Insufflation is performed through the umbilical area using an open or Hasson technique. The 10-mm balloon Hasson cannula (Origin) is used. Video taping capability is used routinely to review the operative technique as well as to show any intra-abdominal disease graphically at conferences such as Tumor Board conferences.

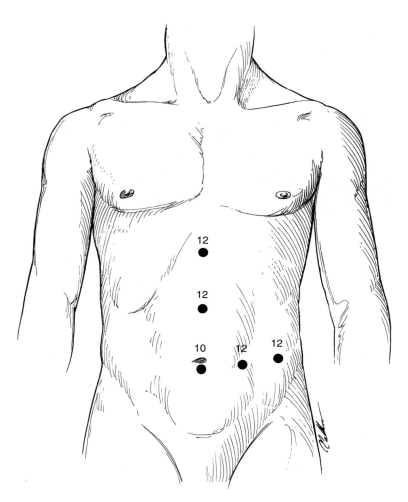

FIGURE 3–1B

IX. Narrative of Surgical Technique

FIGURE 3–2. Laparoscopic staging of abdominal lymphoma is carried out in a fashion similar to that used in traditional "open" celiotomy for staging. The liver biopsy is performed initially, using both a Tru-Cut needle and a linear stapler to facilitate wedge biopsy. Suspicious areas are initially sampled for biopsies, and frozen section is used to confirm the biopsy results. The Tru-Cut needle is used to obtain a deep liver biopsy from both the right and left lobes of the liver. Use of electrocautery to control any bleeding from Glisson's capsule is important. The two midline ports are used for retraction while the lateral ports are used for dissection and introduction of the linear stapler as needed. Placement of ports in the lower abdominal area may facilitate periaortic or peri-iliac artery node biopsy. Wedge biopsy of the left lateral lobe of the liver is performed using a linear stapler. The stapler is fired at right angles using two cartridges of the stapler. It is important to use sharp dissection to remove the wedge rather than electrocautery because this may damage the tissue needed for pathologic evaluation.

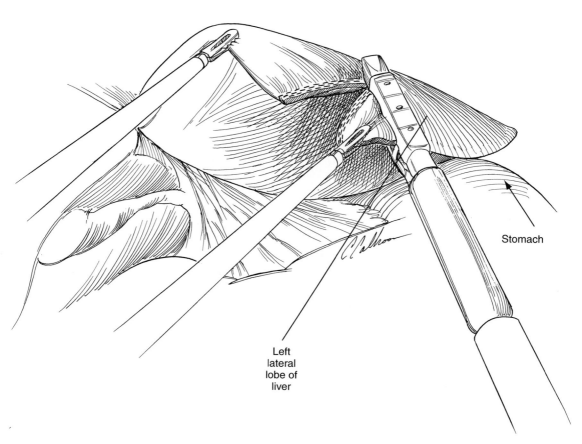

Stomach

Left
lateral
lobe of
liver

FIGURE 3–2

FIGURE 3-3. At this point in the procedure, attention is turned toward evaluation of the spleen. The patient is placed in a reverse Trendelenburg position and a modified right side down decubitus position, using position changes of the operating table. It has been our preference not to perform a splenectomy routinely unless obvious lesions are noted on the splenic capsule or imaging studies have revealed intrasplenic suspicious lesions. If evaluation of the liver confirms the presence of hepatic lymphoma, the spleen is left intact to avoid any additional immunosuppression of the patient. If splenectomy is to be undertaken, dissection is begun from the upper pole, selectively clipping the short gastric vessels in a double fashion. Alternatively, the splenic artery may be initially occluded using a large clip. The vessel is approached through the gastrocolic omentum above the pancreas. The splenic artery and vein are secured with double ties of permanent suture, and the spleen is removed from a small flank incision. The introduction of a tissue bag is helpful to ensure that the spleen does not fracture on withdrawal. Morsellation techniques of the spleen are inappropriate during staging of lymphoma because the organ must be carefully evaluated by the pathologist. In addition, we do not use preoperative embolization prior to splenectomy because of the increased patient discomfort caused by this technique. The final operative dissection procedure is used for lymph node biopsies.

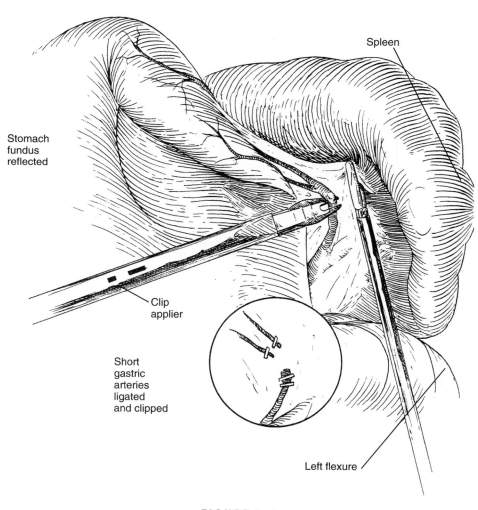

FIGURE 3-3

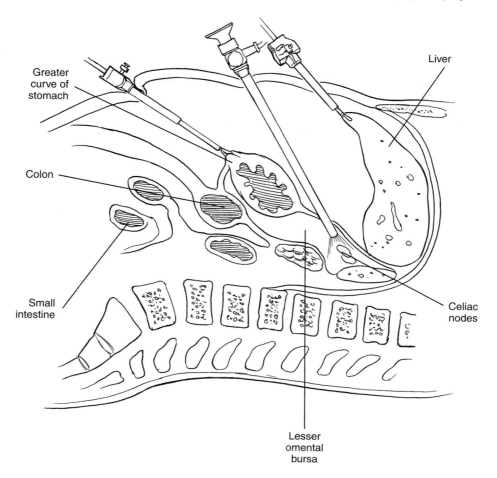

Greater
curve of
stomach

Liver

Colon

Small
intestine

Celiac
nodes

Lesser
omental
bursa

FIGURE 3-4

FIGURE 3-4. Careful identification of pathologic nodes on the lymphangiogram is helpful, and therefore the lymphangiogram should be in the operating room at the time of laparoscopic dissection. As stated previously, additional trocars may be necessary in the lower abdominal area to facilitate the retroperitoneal dissection of the lower aorta as well as the iliac vessels. The monitor placed at the foot of the table is used for visualization of this portion of the procedure. Retractors are inserted through the 12-mm port in the midline to facilitate the approach to the lesser omental bursa and the lesser curve of the stomach. In this manner, the retroperitoneal tissue is dissected to facilitate direct access to the celiac nodes, which can then be sampled. In addition, sampling of the nodes adjacent to the porta hepatis is appropriate if these are thought to be abnormal by direct visualization or CT study. It is important to attempt to remove the lymph nodes in toto because pathologic identification will be easier than if the biopsy sample is fractionated.

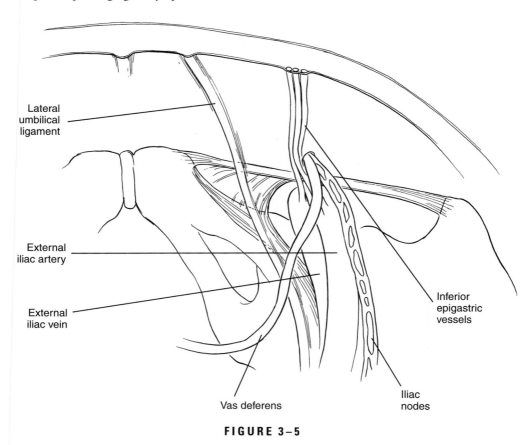

Lateral
umbilical
ligament

External
iliac artery

External
iliac vein

Inferior
epigastric
vessels

Vas deferens

Iliac
nodes

FIGURE 3–5

FIGURE 3–5. Attention then turns to the lower abdominal area and pelvic region for dissection of the periaortic and iliac nodes.

FIGURE 3–6. A small counterincision in the midline, especially in a thin individual, may make this difficult dissection more tolerable. Bilateral nodes from both the iliac areas are biopsied or sampled. An incision is made along the umbilical ligament.

FIGURE 3–7. The vas deferens is transected.

FIGURE 3–6

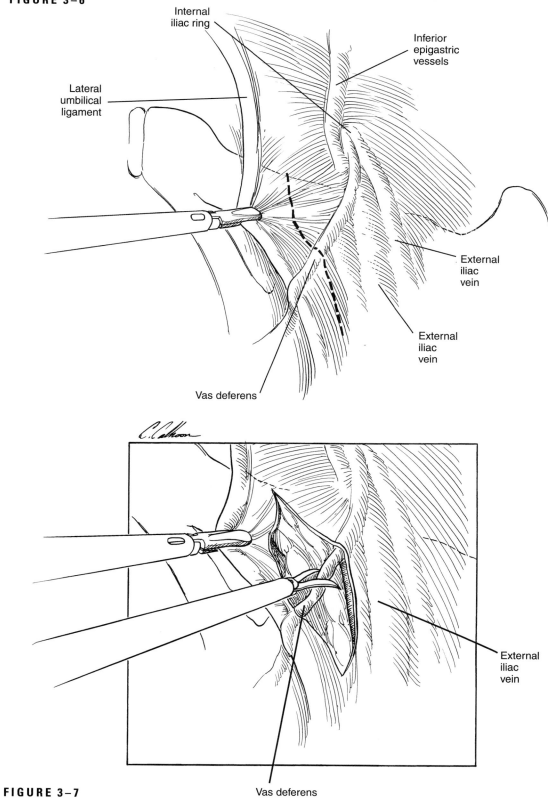

FIGURE 3–7

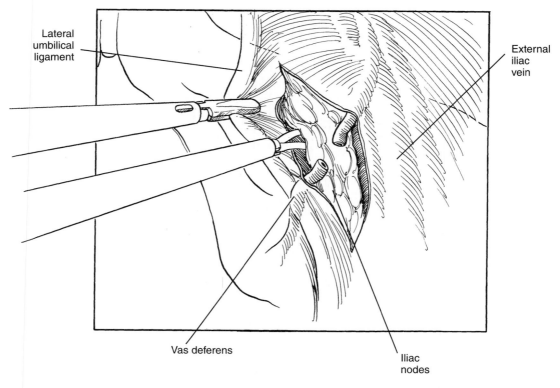

Lateral
umbilical
ligament

External
iliac
vein

Vas deferens

Iliac
nodes

FIGURE 3–8

FIGURE 3–8. The dissection proceeds along the lateral border of the lateral umbilical ligament up to the pubic bone.

FIGURE 3–9. The lymph node–bearing tissue is dissected off the external iliac vein.

FIGURE 3–10. When the dissection is completed the obturator vein and nerve are exposed.

Following lymph node dissection and biopsy, an attempt to mobilize the ovaries should be made in young women if radiation therapy to

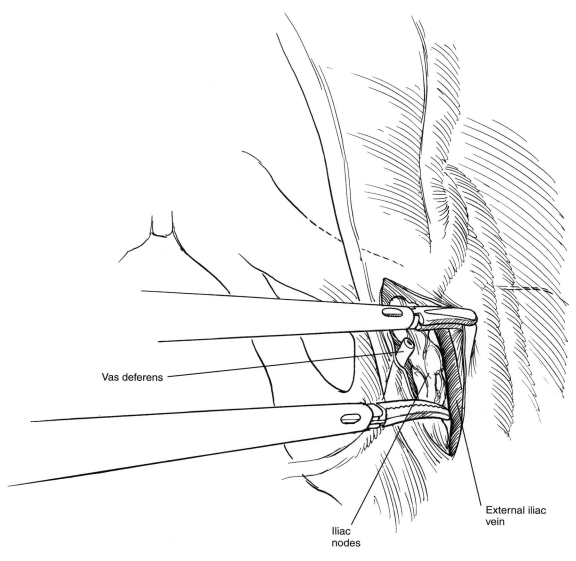

Vas deferens

Iliac
nodes

External iliac
vein

FIGURE 3–9

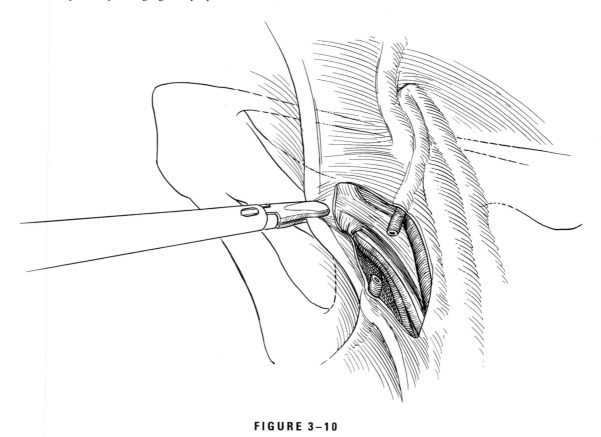

FIGURE 3–10

the pelvis is planned. The ovaries may be moved to the midline behind the uterus, and clips may be placed in proximity to help the radiation oncologist plan the appropriate fields of radiation.

X. Postoperative Medication

A. Oral Tylenol with codeine or meperidine (Demerol) or morphine is used with a patient-controlled analgesia (PCA) device.
B. Use of nonsteroidal anti-inflammatory drugs (NSAIDs) is relatively contraindicated because of the bleeding tendency these agents may cause.

XI. Advancement of Diet

A. Clear liquids are given when the patient is fully awake. A regular diet is ordered on the day following the procedure.

B. Following splenectomy, patients should be kept NPO until the first postoperative day; then a regular diet can be given.

XII. Determinants of Discharge

Patients are discharged once the gastrointestinal tract is functioning well and there is no evidence of any postoperative bleeding process. If a patient has undergone splenectomy, identification of thrombocytosis should be made by observing platelet counts during the first 48 hours. The decision for discharge is made in conjunction with the medical oncologist and the surgeon who has performed the staging procedure.

XIII. Return to Normal Activities

Return to normal activity depends on the decision made about further treatment of the patient's lymphoma and the overall problems created by the underlying lymphomatous process.

Part II

LAPAROSCOPIC HEPATOBILIARY SURGERY

Chapter 4

Laparoscopic Cholecystectomy

AVRAM COOPERMAN, M.D.

I. Indications

A. Symptomatic patients with documented stones or gallbladder disease remain the sole indication.
B. Prophylactic operations for patients "at risk" may include some patients with congenital anemias, but this is a debatable indication because laparoscopic cholecystectomy itself is not without risk, and the natural history of cholecystitis is usually short-lived and benign.

II. Contraindications

Early pregnancy, first trimester.

III. Factors Important in Patient Selection

The patient should be medically capable of tolerating general anesthesia.

IV. Preoperative Preparation

Same day admission.

V. Choice of Anesthesia

General endotracheal anesthesia.

VI. Accessory Devices

Footboard on operating room table.

VII. Instruments and Telescopes

A. 10-mm, 0-degree telescope
B. 5-mm, 0-degree telescope
C. Veress needle
D. Two 5-mm laparoscopic graspers
E. Laparoscopic suction/irrigation device
F. Harmonic scalpel, electrocautery hook, or electrocautery scissors
G. Laparoscopic surgical clips

VIII. Position of Monitors, Placement and Size of Trocars

Technique Position

FIGURE 4–1A. In the United States, the patient is positioned supine with a footboard in place. The alternative position is frog-legged, in which case the surgeon will work between the patient's legs, which are placed in a low lithotomy position. This position is more popular abroad than in the United States. For the supine position, the footboard is essential because the patient's head may be elevated during the procedure to facilitate exposure of the gallbladder and prevent having it obscured by the transverse colon.

Trocar and Port Position

In the absence of previous abdominal surgery, closed laparoscopy (needle puncture) is used.

When previous abdominal surgery has been performed or two needle passes do not allow easy insufflation, a transverse incision is made in the midline fascia below the umbilicus, and the abdominal cavity is entered directly. Access to the peritoneal cavity may be difficult, particularly in patients with previous abdominal surgery or in obese patients. An adherent loop of bowel may be entered even with direct laparoscopy. After the fascia has been incised, the peritoneal cavity is entered and explored digitally to be certain that no loops of bowel are adherent to the abdominal wall. The sheath of a 10-mm trocar is then placed directly in the abdomen, and a towel clip or suture is placed around the skin edge to prevent leakage of gas around the cannula. An alternative method is to use an optical cannula, a Hasson cannula, or one of the newer balloon catheters to seal the opening. The abdomen is then insufflated with carbon dioxide.

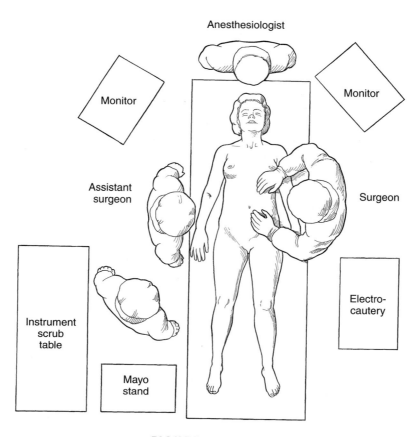

FIGURE 4–1A

Placement of Ports

FIGURE 4–1B. Two to four ports are then placed—two lateral to the rectus muscle and one in the midline epigastrium to the right or left of the falciform ligament. Despite the best aim, this port frequently is found to be placed in or through the ligament itself. If this happens, bleeding should be checked when the port is withdrawn, since the epigastric artery or ligamentum teres may be punctured. It is important to place the "retracting" 5-mm sheaths far enough away from the gallbladder fossa so the jaws of the instruments will not be impeded by the sheath. One way to determine accurate positioning is to locate the gallbladder by putting pressure on the abdominal wall and measuring one and a half sheath lengths from the gallbladder before puncturing the abdominal wall, directing the puncture to the gallbladder. This method maintains the sheath position during instrument transfer and avoids the need to track the ports by the camera when instruments are changed. The decision to use a fifth port depends on the need for additional exposure.

FIGURE 4–2. Difficulties with exposure can be caused by a large gallbladder, a large left lobe of the liver, or adhesions. When the gallbladder is contracted, 5-mm clamps with short teeth often provide ineffective traction on the

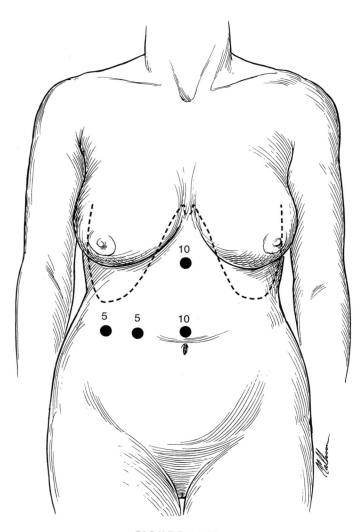

FIGURE 4–1B

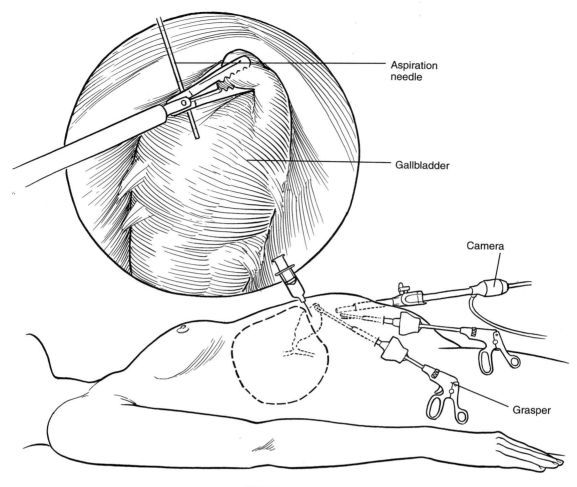

FIGURE 4-2

gallbladder, and slippage is common. One 10-mm lateral port and a 10-mm grasping clamp provide traction and allow exposure of vital structures. When the gallbladder is distended, decompression may be necessary to secure the gallbladder wall. When a tensely distended gallbladder is present, traction cannot be provided until the gallbladder is decompressed. This may be done percutaneously by a syringe or "cauterizing" an opening in the fundus and suctioning luminal contents.

IX. Narrative of Surgical Technique

Collateral Exploration

Limited depth perception and lack of tactile sensation limit collateral exploration, but a thorough look at the solid viscera, including the liver, spleen, ovary, uterus (when present), and whatever loops of bowel are visualized, is advisable. The occasional serendipitous finding justifies this exploration.

FIGURE 4-3. Identification of the common duct above and below the cystic duct has been an unchallenged principle of open biliary surgery and may account for the lower incidence of common duct injury associated with the open technique. With laparoscopic surgery, several changes jeopardize this principle:

1. The surgeon's eye (the laparoscope) is parallel, not perpendicular, to the common duct when the camera is placed in the umbilicus.
2. The lower common duct is often identified laparoscopically as an extension of the cystic duct, particularly with upward traction on the gallbladder.

3. The hepatic duct is less commonly seen at laparoscopy unless it is sought by blunt exposure of the hilar structures or by moving the camera to the right upper quadrant where the view is the more common one perpendicular to the common duct.

Downward traction on the infundulum (to the pelvis) exposes the cystic triangle and frequently exposes the common duct. The common duct above and below the cystic duct must be visualized.

Exposure

Providing exposure of the gallbladder is the initial step. Whatever energy is required to ac-complish this is worthwhile because it facilitates the dissection. In most cases, the two 5-mm laterally placed clamps control and manipulate the fundus and the infundibulum. They are interchangeable with other ports and may be used for suction, irrigation, dissection, or cautery.

Chronic Cholecystitis

Most cholecystectomies are performed as elective procedures. Minimal inflammation is present, and once the hilar structures have been identified, the dissection and control of the cystic artery and cystic duct can be accurately secured. In nearly all instances antegrade dissection from the infundibulum to the fundus can be accomplished.

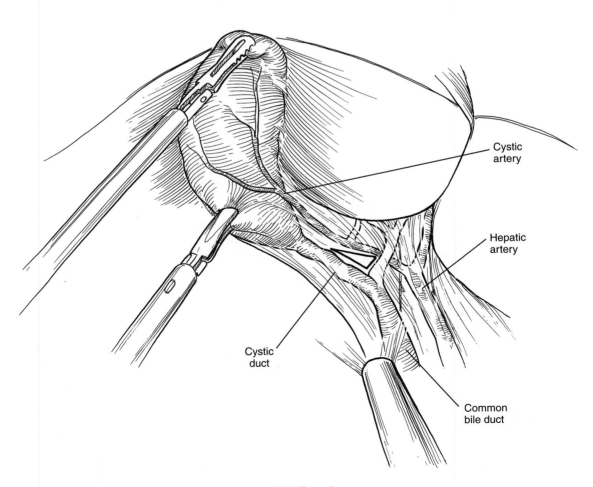

Cystic artery

Hepatic artery

Cystic duct

Common bile duct

FIGURE 4–3

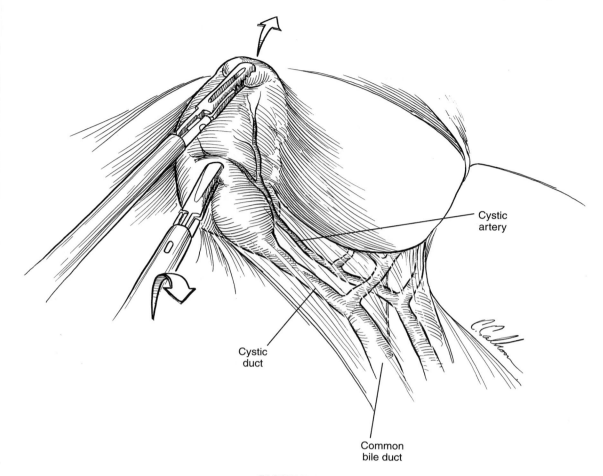

Cystic
artery

Cystic
duct

Common
bile duct

FIGURE 4–4

FIGURE 4–4. The fundic clamp elevates the gallbladder out of its fossa. The infundibular clamp applies upward and pelvic traction on the lower gallbladder to expose the hilar structures. This places traction on the cystic duct and lower common duct and can distort exposure of the upper hepatic duct.

FIGURE 4–5. The peritoneum over the cystic duct is incised with a cautery attached to a scissors, hook, or spatula or with the harmonic scalpel. The peritoneum is retracted downward to expose the cystic duct. The peritoneum over the medial or lateral lower third of the gallbladder is incised. This adds mobility to the liver and gallbladder and length to the cystic duct. The entrance of the cystic duct to the common duct and the common duct above the site of cystic duct entry is more easily and accurately identified by this maneuver.

FIGURE 4–5

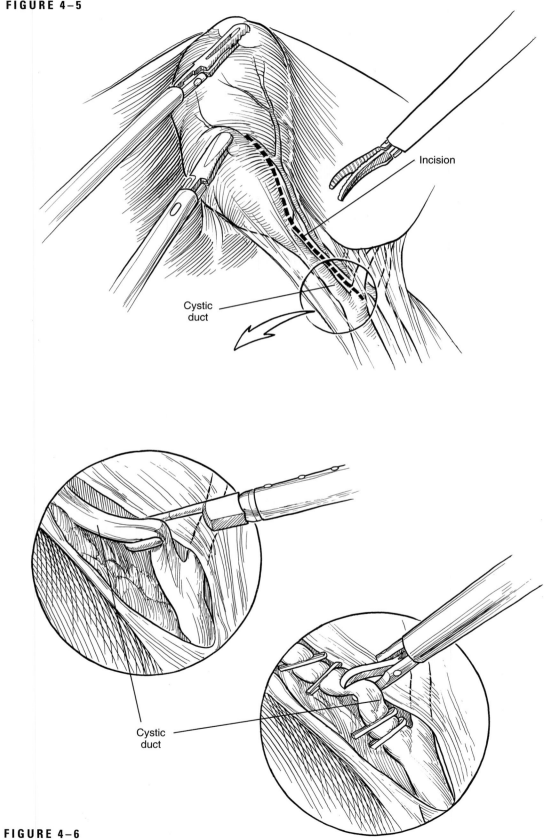

Incision

Cystic
duct

Cystic
duct

FIGURE 4–6

FIGURE 4-6. The cystic duct is encircled, tied, or clipped (singly or doubly) and divided. The lumen of the transected cystic duct should be inspected for a bile leak, since the clips do not always appose securely. A collapsed lumen without a bile leak is the goal.

FIGURE 4-7. Upward and outward traction on the gallbladder facilitates exposure of the cystic artery—either a single large trunk or a small branch (the posterior divisional artery)—will be seen. If a small divisional branch is encountered, it can be clipped or cauterized. If two branches are encountered (the posterior divisional branch runs in the gallbladder fossa along the posterior wall of the gallbladder), both should be dissected, ligated, and controlled by clip. A single artery can be clipped before it is divided.

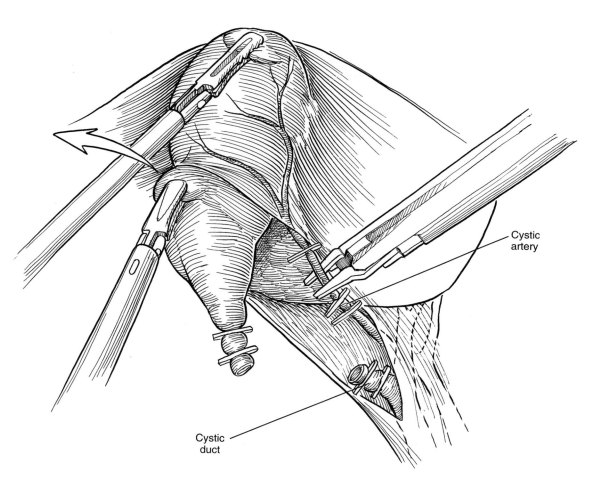

FIGURE 4-7

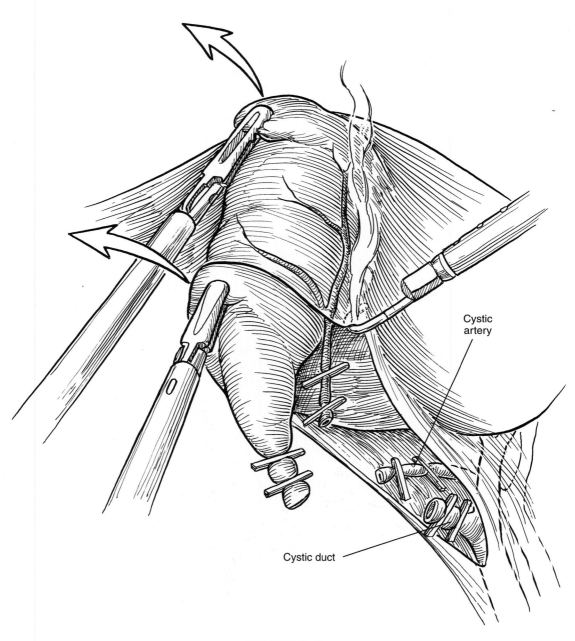

Cystic artery

Cystic duct

FIGURE 4–8

FIGURE 4-8. The peritoneum between the gallbladder and the liver bed is cut, cauterized, treated with the laser, or separated with the Harmonic scalpel. Changing the position of the infundibular clamp to provide the necessary traction and exposure facilitates dissection.

FIGURE 4-9. The gallbladder is freed completely and placed between the lateral abdominal wall and the liver. It is left secured by the fundic clamp so that it can be retrieved easily.

The gallbladder fossa is exposed just as easily with the gallbladder detached as with it attached. A suction irrigation probe and cautery or Harmonic scalpel is placed through the epigastric port and one of the lateral ports to irrigate, suction, and coagulate the liver bed. The gallbladder is removed through the epigastric port. Both 10-mm fascial incisions are closed, but only the subcutaneous 5-mm incision is closed with subcuticular catgut.

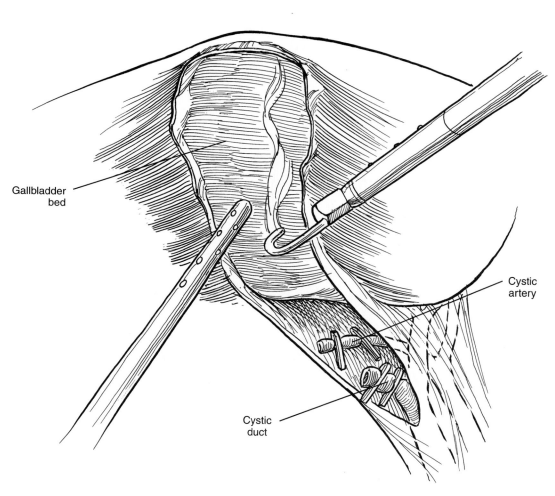

Gallbladder bed

Cystic artery

Cystic duct

FIGURE 4-9

The Difficult Gallbladder

FIGURE 4–10. Any gallbladder that is embedded, is associated with a cystic duct–common duct junction that is difficult to identify, has a thick wall, or is contracted can be technically difficult to dissect. Multiple technical approaches to these situations can be used, but the principles remain unchanged—namely, accurate identification of the common duct above and below the cystic duct before any structure is clipped or divided.

If exposure of the hilar structure is difficult or precarious, dissection should be started on the lateral lower aspect of the gallbladder. This frees the lateral lower third of the gallbladder and exposes the cystic duct–common duct junction. If this does not provide the necessary exposure, the gallbladder is freed from the liver bed on the medial side by using a similar method of dissection. By freeing the gallbladder completely from the lower third of the liver, any ducts that enter the gallbladder from the liver will be identified. If the cystic duct and common duct cannot be seen, then the remaining peritoneal attachments to the gallbladder can be freed, leaving only the cystic duct and artery to be dissected and secured last.

Retrograde Dissection

FIGURE 4–11. The final method that ensures the integrity of the ducts when the hilar anatomy is obscure is retrograde dissection. This is facilitated by emptying the gallbladder of its bile, which is accomplished most easily by aspirating the gallbladder percutaneously through a syringe and attached needle or cauterizing a

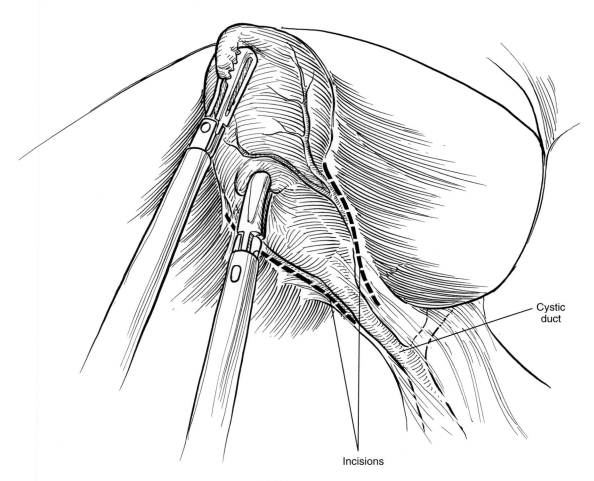

Cystic
duct

Incisions

FIGURE 4–10

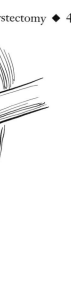

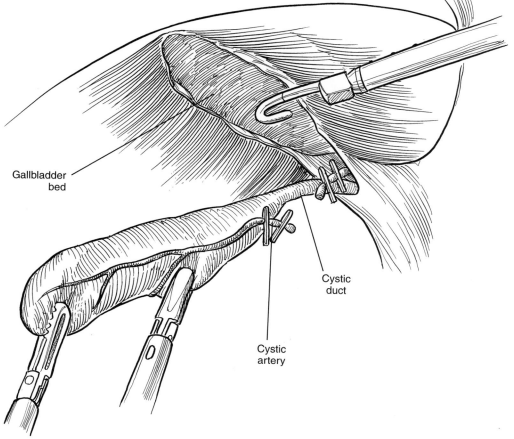

Gallbladder bed

Cystic duct

Cystic artery

FIGURE 4–11

small opening in the fundus and introducing a suction probe into the gallbladder. Traction and countertraction are placed on the gallbladder and liver, and the gallbladder is dissected from the fundus to the infundibulum using the electrosurgical unit or the Harmonic scalpel. Upward traction on the liver and downward traction on the gallbladder provide the necessary exposure. This leaves the cystic duct and the cystic artery as the last two structures remaining to be identified and secured.

Use of Drains

In patients with acute cholecystitis or when there has been bleeding or oozing from the liver bed some surgeons prefer to use drains. A suction drain (Blake or Jackson-Pratt drain) is placed through the epigastric port or the lateral 5-mm port. It should be placed in the subhepatic space or between the liver and the abdominal wall in a posterior and dependent position and is left on suction until drainage is minimal.

When to Abandon the Procedure

The purpose of laparoscopic cholecystectomy is to hasten convalescence and cause less pain than with open surgery. These goals must not substitute for safety. If intraoperative progress is slow and dubious and a feeling of uneasiness settles in, a laparotomy incision is in order.

X. Postoperative Medications

Analgesics are started in the recovery room with one dose of parenteral medicine.

XI. Advancement of Diet

Patients are started on clear liquids in the recovery room and advanced to a regular diet as requested and tolerated.

XII. Determinants of Discharge

Patients are discharged when they are:
1. Comfortable
2. Able to drink and eat
3. Voiding

XIII. Return to Normal Activity

Patients are permitted to return to normal activity as tolerated.

Laparoscopic Cholecystectomy for Acute Cholecystitis

KARL A. ZUCKER, M.D.

I. Indications

Acute cholecystitis

II. Contraindications

A. Patients who cannot tolerate general anesthesia.
B. Patients who cannot tolerate a carbon dioxide pneumoperitoneum because of severe restrictive pulmonary disease.

III. Factors Important in Patient Selection

A. The diagnosis of acute cholecystitis is reserved for patients presenting with all or most of the following characteristics: acute abdominal pain, fever, leukocytosis, abnormal biliary ultrasound or scintillation studies, and unplanned admission to the hospital.
B. The finding of common bile duct stones in patients presenting with acute cholecystitis is extremely uncommon, and, in most individuals, these stones are readily diagnosed prior to operative intervention. If choledocholithiasis is suspected, a decision must be made about whether to attempt preoperative endoscopic retrograde cholangiopancreatography (ERCP) or proceed directly to cholecystectomy and possible common bile duct exploration.

C. If the episode of acute inflammation is mild and responds rapidly to medical management, we will offer the patient a preoperative ERCP. Often the stone or stones will have already passed through the ampulla.
D. Only individuals with strong indications of persistent choledocholithiasis such as common bile duct dilation (e.g., based on ultrasonography), continued abnormalities of liver function tests (e.g., alkaline phosphatase, hepatic transaminases, or bilirubin), or elevated pancreatic enzymes (e.g., amylase or lipase) undergo preoperative biliary endoscopy.
E. If the clinical signs of acute inflammation continue or even progress, a laparoscopic cholecystectomy and intraoperative cholangiogram are performed.
F. If common bile duct stones are visualized on the radiographic study, a laparoscopic common bile duct exploration is performed.

IV. Preoperative Preparation

A. Patients are administered intravenous fluids for rehydration and correction of electrolyte imbalances
B. Patients are started on broad-spectrum antibiotics (usually a first- or second-generation cephalosporin.
C. Patients are kept NPO.
D. A nasogastric tube is used if there are indications of an accompanying ileus.

FIGURE 5–1

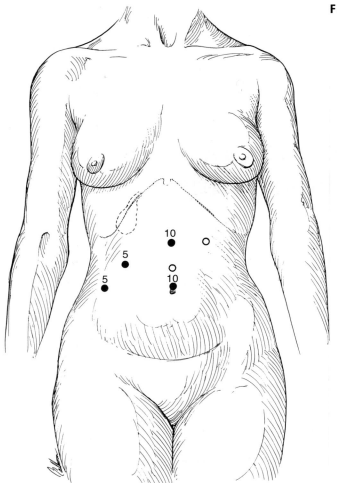

E. A thorough explanation of the diagnosis and the various therapeutic alternatives is conducted with the patient; the options discussed include continued medical management, laparoscopic surgery, and the possibility of conversion to an open laparotomy.

V. Choice of Anesthesia

General endotracheal anesthesia is used.

VI. Accessory Devices

A. Nasogastric tube
B. Urinary catheter
C. Pneumatic stockings

VII. Instruments and Telescopes

A. 10-mm, 0-degree laparoscope
B. 10-mm, 30- (or 45-) degree laparoscope
C. Veress needle or Hasson cannula
D. Atraumatic grasping forceps
E. Grasping forceps with teeth
F. Fan retractor
G. Pre-tied laparoscopic sutures
H. Laparoscopic surgical clips
I. Laparoscopic aspiration/irrigation cannula
J. Laparoscopic impermeable specimen bag
K. Electrocautery scissors
L. Laparoscopic Maryland dissector
M. Laparoscopic Kittners
N. Laparoscopic cholangiography catheter

VIII. Placement and Size of Trocars

FIGURE 5-1. Pneumoperitoneum is established using either a percutaneous approach or an open (e.g., Hasson) technique or significant abdominal distention (i.e., ileus). In patients with prior upper abdominal surgery we prefer the open technique for insufflation and use one of the specially designed cannulas developed for this approach. The three accessory trocars and cannulas are then inserted through the abdominal wall under laparoscopic guidance. In patients with acute cholecystitis it is often necessary to insert a fourth or even a fifth cannula to obtain adequate exposure. The location of these additional punctures varies depending on the operative findings. The most common sites are in the midline halfway between the umbilical and subxiphoid sheaths or in the left subcostal space. Additional instruments such as fanlike retractors or grasping forceps introduced through an extra port often improve the exposure and allow a procedure to be completed that otherwise might have been necessary to convert to an open laparotomy. In our experience the placement of a fifth or even a sixth cannula results in little or no additional postoperative discomfort or cosmetic deformity.

IX. Narrative of Surgical Technique

FIGURE 5-2. In patients operated on for acute cholecystitis the gallbladder is grasped and retracted cephalad toward the right shoulder in a manner similar to that employed for elective procedures. This maneuver, combined with elevation of the head of the operating table 20 to 30 degrees, facilitates exposure of the cystic duct

FIGURE 5-2

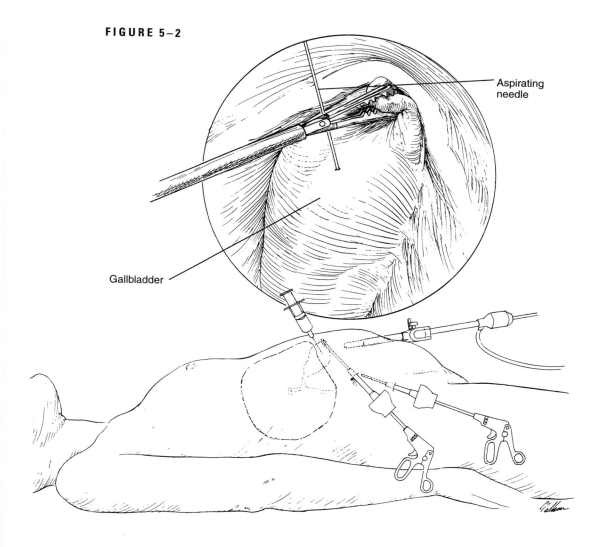

Aspirating needle

Gallbladder

and artery. Unfortunately, the inflamed gallbladder often proves difficult to grasp and hold.
This may occur because the tissues are too
edematous and necrotic, or the gallbladder may
simply be too distended to allow the forceps
to obtain an adequate bite. A tense, distended
gallbladder or hydrops should be partially decompressed before an attempt is made to retract
it with either sharp or atraumatic forceps. Decompression can be accomplished with a cyst
aspiration needle (with a 5-mm upper shaft)
inserted through one of the laparoscopic cannulas or with an 18-gauge (or larger) long needle
guided percutaneously into the dome of the
gallbladder.

FIGURE 5-3. The gallbladder should be decompressed enough to allow the forceps to
grasp and retract it cephalad. Partial decompression of a distended gallbladder also aids in
exposure of the cystic and common bile ducts.
The gallbladder should not be completely
drained because an empty, flaccid gallbladder is
more difficult to dissect away from the underlying liver bed. The puncture site is then occluded
by applying the grasping forceps over the opening or using a pre-tied laparoscopic suture.

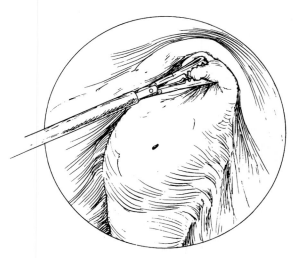

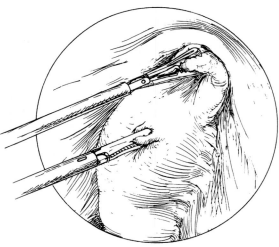

FIGURE 5-3

FIGURE 5-4. A large number of laparoscopic forceps have been designed specifically to retract an inflamed or necrotic gallbladder. The choice of which instrument to use of course depends on the intra-abdominal findings, but for an edematous and inflamed gallbladder, a sharp, penetrating forceps is often the best instrument to grasp and retract such tissues. These sharp forceps are readily available in both 5- and 10-mm diameter sizes; however, we prefer to use the larger versions. To introduce these larger forceps the most lateral 5-mm cannula is replaced with a larger sheath. Another method of providing adequate retraction is to place one or more large suture ligatures through the fundus of the gallbladder and lift upward. Although a pre-tied laparoscopic suture may occasionally be used for this purpose, we prefer a deep, penetrating suture using a curved or straight needle. The suture may be pulled out through the abdominal wall or held with a grasping forceps.

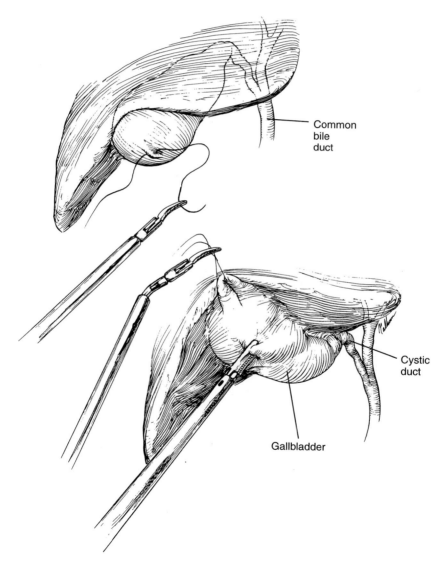

Common
bile
duct

Cystic
duct

Gallbladder

FIGURE 5-4

FIGURE 5-5

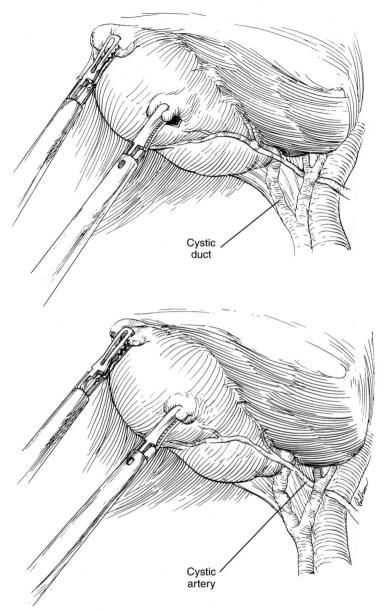

Cystic
duct

Cystic
artery

FIGURE 5-5. In addition to being difficult to grasp and retract, the acutely inflamed gallbladder is also more easily torn, resulting in bile or stone spillage. These injuries usually occur at the site where the grasping forceps have been applied for retraction. A tear into the gallbladder should be controlled as rapidly as possible. If the opening is small it may be controlled by simply reapplying the same or larger forceps over the puncture site.

FIGURE 5-6. Larger tears generally require closure with either a suture ligature or a pre-tied laparoscopic suture. Once again, the gallbladder should not be allowed to drain completely empty. If bile or purulent fluid has escaped, the peritoneal cavity should be copiously irrigated. Both 5- and 10-mm suction/irrigation devices are now available. Many incorporate a pool-tip configuration, which facilitates complete re-

moval of the fluid. Stones that may have dropped into the peritoneal cavity should also be retrieved if possible.

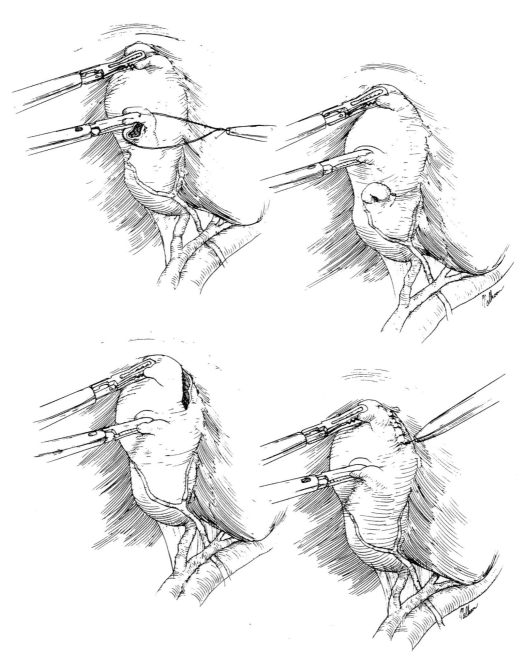

FIGURE 5–6

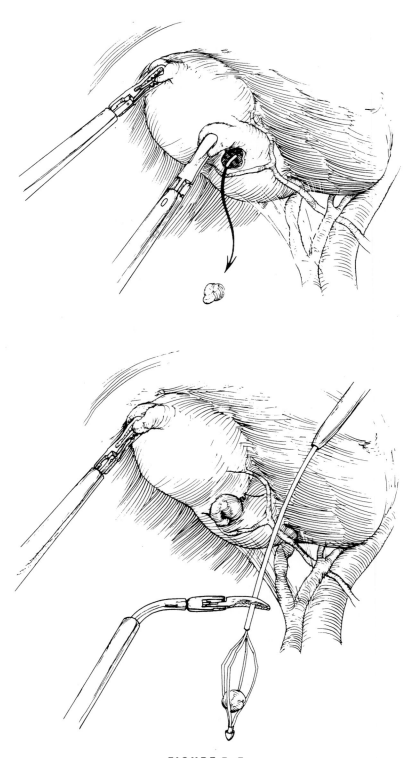

FIGURE 5–7

FIGURE 5-7. Small stones may be aspirated with irrigation/suction cannulas, but most require extraction using forceps or balloon baskets. If there are many stones or very large stones it may be easier and faster to insert a sterile "bag" into the abdomen, placing the calculi within it. This pouch minimizes the need to remove the grasping forceps repeatedly and then reorient the video camera and laparoscope. Initially, surgeons used gas-sterilized condoms or operating room gloves (one finger of a large glove) to contain spilled stones, but now commercially available bags are available (Endo-Catch, United States Surgical Corporation, Norwalk, CT), which are easier to use. The bag and calculi may be removed through the larger, upper midline cannula, or, if it is too distended, it can be extracted at the end of the procedure through an enlarged umbilical fascial defect.

FIGURE 5-8. Meticulous dissection of the gallbladder and surrounding tissues is important in both emergency and elective laparoscopic biliary tract surgery. The inflammation and edema of the porta hepatis that accompany acute cholecystitis often severely distort the ductal and vascular anatomy. As in the elective procedure, the operative dissection begins high, near the fundus of the gallbladder, and proceeds distally toward the cystic and common bile ducts. The dissection is continued close to the wall of the gallbladder with careful attention paid at all times to hemostasis. Adhesive attachments to the gallbladder from the surrounding omentum, transverse colon, or duodenum are carefully exposed and divided. Often these inflammatory attachments can be removed with blunt dissection. Dense adhesions require sharp dissection using scissors or electrocautery. Many dissecting instruments are now designed to be used with monopolar electrocautery, and this has facilitated the maintenance of a bloodless operating field.

In addition to the acute inflammation and edema characteristic of acute cholecystitis, the cephalad retraction of the gallbladder and right lobe of the liver also distort the normal anatomy of the cystic and common bile duct junction. It should be recognized that the common bile duct may be tented upward several centimeters from its normal position within the porta hepatis. The cystic and common bile duct juncture may therefore prove especially difficult to recognize when it is surrounded by dense and highly vascularized inflammatory adhesions. Occasionally the edematous reaction may mimic an enlarged cystic duct when in fact the ducts are of normal

FIGURE 5-8

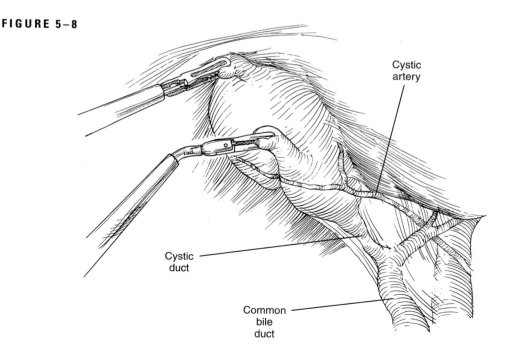

Cystic artery

Cystic duct

Common bile duct

caliber. Operative dissection should continue distally until the complete course of the cystic duct as well as its junction with the common bile duct is readily apparent, either by direct visualization or by means of intraoperative cholangiography. Small cotton sponges or Kittners (Endoscopic Kittner, OR Concepts, Roanoke, TX) may prove especially useful in dissecting edematous structures within the triangle of Calot. A stroking or twisting motion with this cotton-tipped device will help to separate and expose the tissue planes surrounding the cystic duct and artery. On more than one occasion a completely mobilized cystic duct has been shown on further dissection to be the common bile duct. No presumed ductal or vascular structure should be divided until the anatomy has been completely demonstrated. If the cystic duct and artery are not easily dissected free

from the surrounding tissues, some authors advocate performing a retrograde dissection beginning at the fundus of the gallbladder. This is not practiced by our group, and it is our impression that if the ductal and vascular structures are so obscured by dense inflammation that a safe antegrade dissection is precluded, then the procedure should be converted to an open laparotomy.

It is our policy to perform intraoperative cholangiography in *all* patients undergoing laparoscopic cholecystectomy. This is done not only to determine the presence of common bile duct stones but also to provide a road map of the ductal anatomy. Unusual or aberrant ductal anatomy is often difficult to demonstrate in the presence of acute inflammation and edema. Intraoperative cholangiography supplies the surgeon with accurate details about the junction of

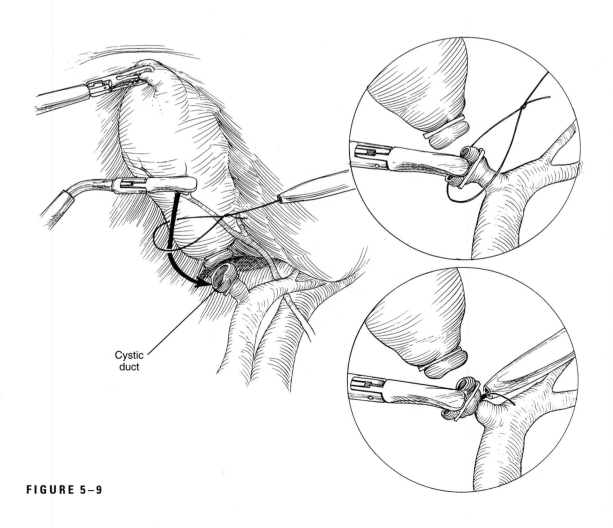

Cystic duct

FIGURE 5–9

the cystic and common bile ducts as well as the presence of any accessary ducts that may be injured during the operative dissection. It should be noted, however, that performing an intraoperative cholangiogram does not eliminate the risk of a bile duct injury.

Occasionally one or more stones may be identified within the distal cystic duct. These stones should be removed because they may later pass into the common bile duct and cause symptoms. An atraumatic forceps can be used to "milk" them back into the gallbladder or out through the cystic duct opening. Rarely, a stone impacted at the common bile duct juncture requires the cystic duct to be opened down to this point to allow direct removal.

FIGURE 5-9. After confirming the status of the ductal anatomy with intraoperative cholangiography, the cystic duct may be ligated. During elective cholecystectomy the cystic duct is usually secured with multiple titanium staples and divided with laparoscopic scissors. If the tissues are severely edematous, the standard clips may not be large enough to completely occlude the cystic duct. Also, if the inflammation should resolve rapidly following gallbladder removal, the clips might loosen and become dislodged. This may, in fact, be a factor in some cases of postoperative bile leak. Therefore, if the cystic duct appears edematous or inflamed we prefer to use both surgical clips and pre-tied laparoscopic sutures. A laparoscopic clip applier is introduced through the upper midline cannula and used to ligate the cystic duct. The duct is divided between the clips, and a pre-tied laparoscopic suture is introduced through the upper midline cannula and placed around the cystic duct stump.

FIGURE 5-10. The clips or sutures must be carefully positioned on the cystic duct to avoid occluding the juncture with the common bile duct.

FIGURE 5-10

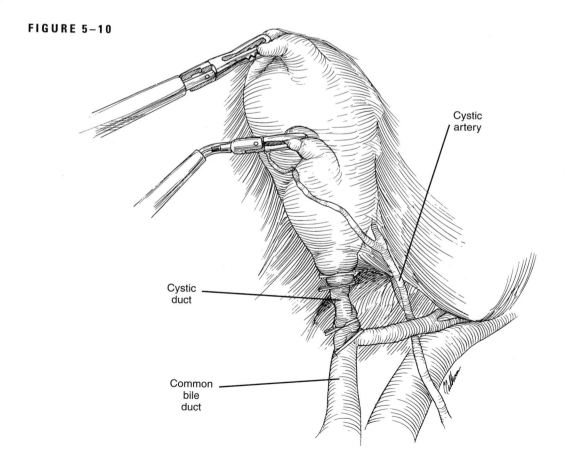

Cystic artery

Cystic duct

Common bile duct

FIGURE 5–11. Before the cystic duct is divided, the blood supply to the gallbladder should be identified and controlled. Consequently, if the cystic artery should be torn during the course of its dissection, the intact ductal structures may keep the vessel from retracting back into the porta hepatis. However, in some cases, the cystic artery may not be visible because of its close proximity to the cystic duct. In such cases, it may be necessary to divide the cystic duct before gaining control of the artery. The cystic artery is usually found medial and slightly posterior to the cystic duct. It should be carefully dissected free from the surrounding tissues using the same care in demonstrating the anatomy as used with the ductal structures. Acute and chronic inflammation occurring within the angle of Calot may render identification of the blood supply difficult. One of the most common causes of significant intraoperative bleeding during elective or emergent cholecystectomy is failure to identify the posterior branch of the cystic artery. Often the anterior branch is readily visualized coursing along the exposed surface of the gallbladder. The magnification of the video system as well as the direction of the image (from the umbilicus) can lead the surgeon to assume wrongly that this represents the main cystic artery trunk. If only the anterior branch is ligated and divided, the posterior branch may later be torn or avulsed as the gallbladder is being dissected from the underlying liver bed. The cephalad retraction of the gallbladder combined with acute or chronic inflammation in the porta hepatis may also lead to inadvertent injury of the right hepatic artery. To avoid such injuries it is important to carefully dissect and identify both branches of the cystic duct as well as the main trunk before any supposed vascular structures are divided. After the cystic duct and artery have been transected, the next step is to dissect the gallbladder from the underlying liver bed. This dissection has also been described in the presence of acute inflammation using either electrocautery or the Harmonic scalpel.

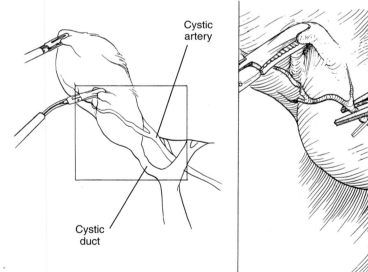
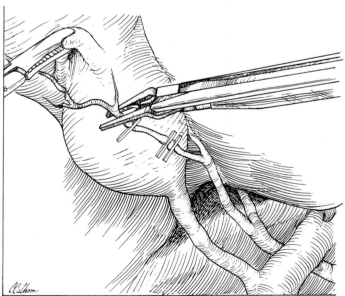

Cystic artery

Cystic duct

FIGURE 5–11

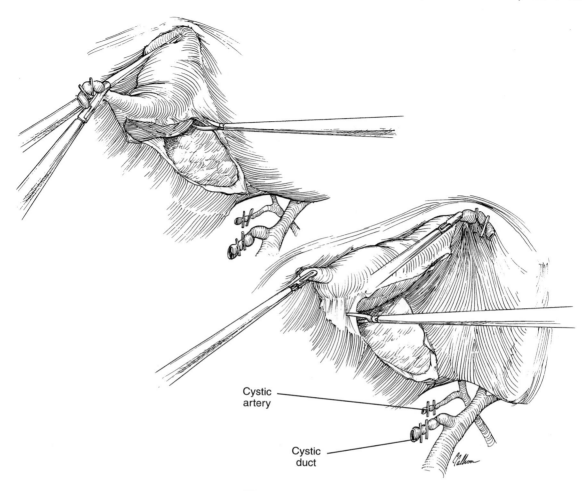

Cystic
artery

Cystic
duct

FIGURE 5-12

FIGURE 5-12. To minimize the risk of gall-bladder perforation or liver injury it is important to maintain adequate exposure of the operative field. The most useful maneuver in our experience has been the "right-left twist." This is performed by having the first assistant manipulate the two grasping forceps holding the gallbladder. The "right twist" exposes the medial aspect of the gallbladder and is accomplished by pushing the fundus toward the patient's left side while at the same time retracting the gallbladder neck to the patient's left. The "left twist" exposes the lateral attachments of the gallbladder to the liver and is performed by reversing the direction of each forceps. Successive right-left retractions of the gallbladder afford maximum exposure of the plane of dissection, thus avoiding inadvertent gallbladder or liver injury.

FIGURE 5-13

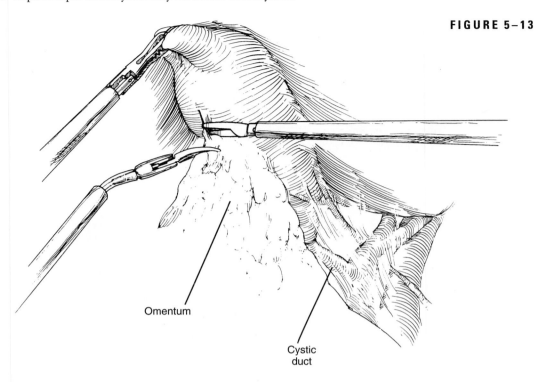

Omentum

Cystic
duct

FIGURE 5-13. In addition to cystic artery in-juries, other possible sources of intraoperative blood loss include torn omental or mesenteric vessels, liver capsular tears, or bleeding from the liver bed. Torn mesenteric or omental ves-sels may occur during dissection of inflamma-tory adhesions away from the gallbladder and ductal structures. These adhesive bands should be carefully removed using a combination of blunt and sharp dissection. Generally, we use

FIGURE 5-14

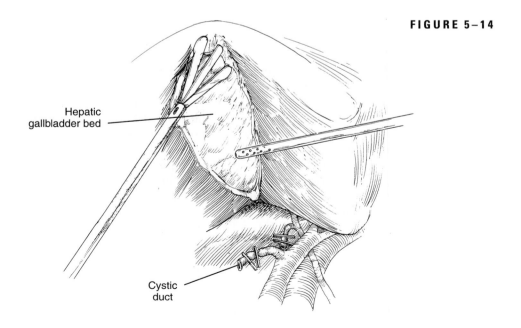

Hepatic
gallbladder bed

Cystic
duct

blunt dissection to separate these tissues from the anterior wall of the gallbladder. Dense or vascular adhesions are controlled with short bursts of monopolar cautery energy and then sharply dissected.

FIGURE 5–14. Prior to complete dissection of the gallbladder from the liver the peritoneal cavity should be copiously irrigated with saline and the operative field examined for any signs of persistent bleeding or bile leaks. While the gallbladder is still attached to the liver the surgeon can easily maintain the proper exposure to inspect the gallbladder fossa and ensure that the clips or sutures securing the duct and artery remain in place. If the gallbladder has already been freed from the liver a fanlike retractor should be used to expose the operative field. A careful examination of the abdomen should be conducted to exclude other possible sources of

bleeding or previously unrecognized bowel injuries.

FIGURE 5–15. We have rarely placed closed suction drains following elective laparoscopic cholecystectomy but have used them more often when operating on patients with acute cholecystitis. Indications for placing drainage catheters include bile spillage, persistent bile leakage, or bleeding from the liver bed. Smaller, closed suction drainage catheters may be introduced through the lateral 5-mm cannula. The tip of the catheter is then held in place along the liver bed while the cannula is removed. Larger drains can be introduced through the upper midline 10/11-mm cannula. After pneumoperitoneum has been reestablished, the distal portion of the catheter is appropriately positioned. The opposite end is then brought out through the lateral 5-mm sheaths and secured to the skin.

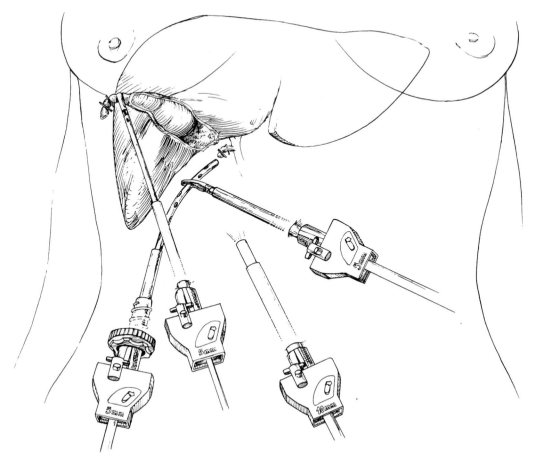

FIGURE 5–15

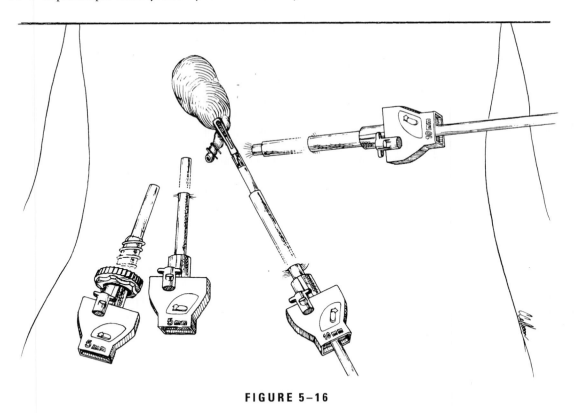

FIGURE 5-16

FIGURE 5-16. After the gallbladder has been completely detached from the liver, the video laparoscope is removed and replaced through the upper 10/11-mm cannula. This allows the surgeon to remove the gallbladder through the umbilical fascial defect. The neck of the gallbladder is grasped with a larger (10/11 mm) penetrating forceps introduced through the umbilical cannula. As the gallbladder is pulled through the umbilical fascial defect, the entire sheath and forceps are removed from the abdomen. The neck of the gallbladder is then secured with a Kelly or Kocher clamp and pulled from the abdomen.

FIGURE 5-17. In many patients who are operated on for acute cholecystitis, the gallbladder may not be easy to remove through the standard umbilical fascial defect. This is especially true if the tissues are edematous and inflamed or if the gallbladder contains very large stones. In such circumstances the periumbilical skin incision should be extended and the fascial opening dilated. If the adjacent rectus muscles are not

incised, such a maneuver will result in minimal additional postoperative pain or cosmetic disfigurement. If the gallbladder has been torn and there is a possibility of further spillage during extraction, the gallbladder should first be placed in a sterile "bag" or glove. This will allow the gallbladder to be removed without the risk of additional stones, bile, or purulent fluid escaping into the peritoneal cavity.

Following gallbladder removal, the remaining carbon dioxide is expelled from the abdomen, and the umbilical fascial opening is closed with one or more large, absorbable sutures. This fascial defect is often distended beyond the initial 10 or 11 mm during gallbladder removal, and failure to close this opening may lead to future formation of a hernia. The other 10/11-mm fascial openings are not routinely sutured unless the fascial defects are easily visualized. We do not advocate extending the skin incisions further to close these accessary punctures because the likelihood of any subsequent problems is extremely low.

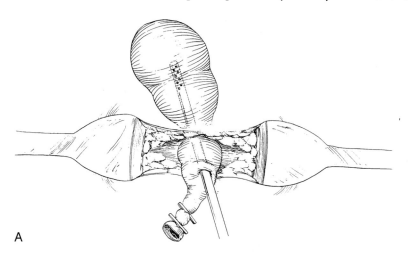

A

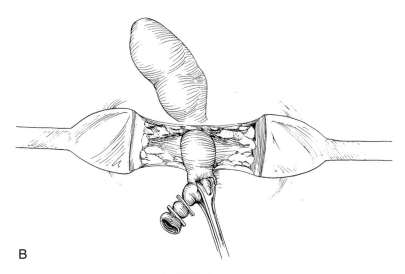

B

FIGURE 5-17

X. Postoperative Medications

A. Intravenous antibiotics are continued post-operatively until the patient is afebrile and the white blood cell count returns to normal.
B. Oral antibiotics are then continued for a total of 7 to 10 days.

XI. Advancement of Diet

A. The nasogastric tube is not routinely removed at this time because many patients operated on for acute cholecystitis manifest signs of postoperative ileus. Usually this resolves within 24 to 48 hours.

B. Once the ileus resolves, diet is advanced as tolerated.

XII. Determinants of Discharge

Patients are discharged when they are tolerating a regular diet and their pain can be adequately controlled with oral agents.

XIII. Return to Normal Activity

Patients are allowed to return to their normal activities as tolerated.

Chapter 6

Laparoscopic Transcystic Common Duct Exploration

STEPHEN J. SHAPIRO, M.D.

I. Indications

A. Common duct stones noted during intraoperative cholangiography
B. Common duct stones noted during preoperative evaluation
C. Biliary pancreatitis with common bile duct stones
D. Suitable cystic duct anatomy

II. Contraindications

A. Inappropriate cystic duct anatomy (e.g., cystic duct inserting in the distal common duct close to the ampulla of Vater)
B. Primary common duct stones (e.g., earthen stones)
C. Hepatic duct stones (relative contraindication)
D. All contraindications applying to laparoscopic cholecystectomy (e.g., severe cirrhosis, bleeding dyscrasia, etc.)
E. Unskilled team unfamiliar with instrumentation
F. Hospital operating room without image amplification

III. Factors Important in Patient Selection

Same as those for laparoscopic cholecystectomy (see Chapter 5)

IV. Preoperative Preparation

A. Patient is admitted on the day of surgery.
B. One dose of antibiotic, usually cefotetan, given intravenously (IV) 1 hour prior to surgery.
C. Patient is kept nil per os (NPO) after midnight.
D. If bilirubin level is above 14, an osmotic diuresis is started prior to the surgical procedure. We usually use mannitol.

V. Choice of Anesthesia

A. Endotracheal intubation
B. Anesthetic agents: Desflurane, narcotic, and muscle relaxant

VI. Accessory Devices

A. Orogastric tube
B. Urinary catheter
C. Pneumatic compression stockings

VII. Instruments and Telescopes

A. Image amplifier
B. Hydrophilic gel–coated .035-inch angled guide wire
C. Torque device for both the choledochoscope and the wire
D. Phantom 5 dilating catheter

E. LeVeen syringe

F. 3 French Segura wire baskets, both radial and straight

G. 3 French three- and four-pronged retrieving graspers

H. Flexible, 9 French two-way, fiberoptic endoscope with a 1.2-mm working channel and a deflecting capacity of 90 to 120 degrees

I. Two cameras and two 300-watt xenon light sources

J. Image splitter

K. Irrigating system

L. Touhy-Borst adapter

M. Pulse dye laser or electrohydraulic lithotripter

N. Skilled team

VIII. Position of Monitors and Placement and Size of Trocars

FIGURE 6–1. A. Two monitors are placed at the head of the table in the routine manner for laparoscopic cholecystectomy. B. Trocar placement is the same as that of laparoscopic cholecystectomy. We use one subumbilical 5-mm trocar, one 10-mm subxyphoid trocar, and two lateral 5-mm trocars. The most lateral trocar is placed at the anterior axillary line. The more medial trocar is placed as lateral as possible and as high as possible toward the costal margin to facilitate transcystic laparoscopic common duct exploration. The patient is placed in a supine position, head up at 20 degrees, and right side up at approximately 15 degrees.

FIGURE 6–1

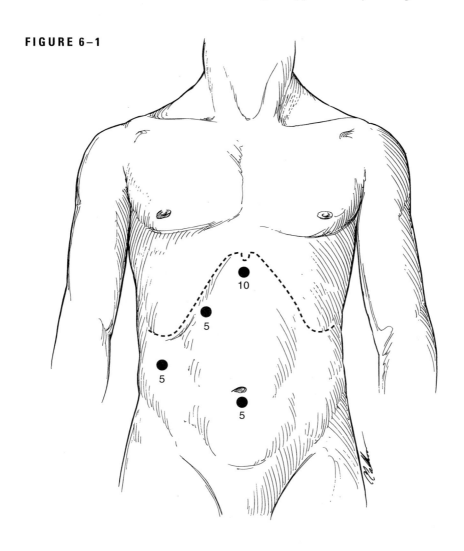

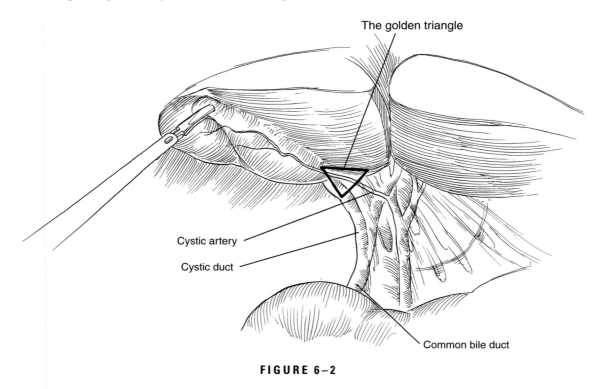

FIGURE 6-2

IX. Narrative of Surgical Technique

FIGURE 6-2. Laparoscopic cholecystectomy is performed using the usual technique. In addition, the critical dissection of Calot's triangle (the "golden" triangle) is carried out medially and superiorly, freeing the whole neck of the gallbladder from the liver bed. The cystic artery and the cystic duct should be well defined prior to placement of any clip. The cystic duct is dissected up to the neck of the gallbladder.

FIGURE 6-3. At this point, a clip is placed at the junction of the neck of the gallbladder and the cystic duct. A lateral ductotomy is made using a microscissors. An intraoperative cholangiogram is obtained using a 4 French ureteral catheter and an Olsen clamp. If we have difficulty in intubating the cystic duct, a .035-inch hydrophilic-coated guide wire is placed in a 5 French ureteral catheter. The guide wire navigates the spiral valves of Hyster and is inserted into the common bile duct. The catheter is then placed over the guide wire into the cystic duct and the wire is then removed. We have been able to complete cholangiography in 97 per cent of over 700 laparoscopic cholecystectomies during the past 5 years.

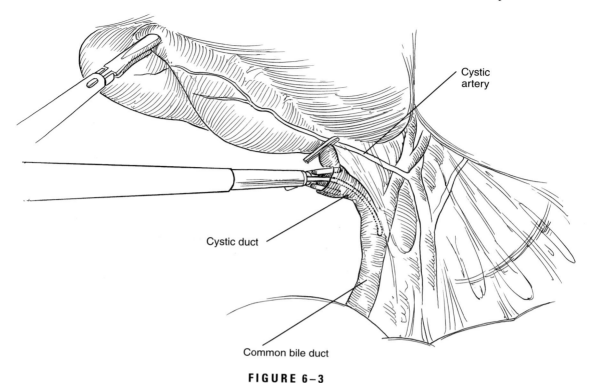

Cystic
artery

Cystic duct

Common bile duct

FIGURE 6–3

Cholangiography can be accomplished using a fixed overhead image amplifier or the OEC 9600, a portable unit that gives excellent real time or fixed imaging. The cholangiogram is then evaluated, looking at two major points:

1. Is the cystic duct anatomy appropriate for the transcystic approach? If the cystic duct enters at the distal common duct, the transcystic approach is abandoned.

2. The visualized biliary system is evaluated, looking for filling defects. If stones are seen in the distal duct, we then proceed with transcystic common duct exploration. If there are stones in either the right or left hepatic duct, we proceed with direct choledochotomy.

Using these two criteria, we have been able to perform 85 to 90 per cent of our duct explorations through the cystic duct. If stones are seen in the distal common duct and the cystic duct has suitable anatomy, we dissect the cystic duct down to its junction with the common duct. This facilitates angling the choledochoscope and the balloon catheter. If the initial lateral incision in the cystic duct is more than 2 cm away from its junction with the common duct, an additional ductotomy is made so that we are 1.5 cm from the common duct.

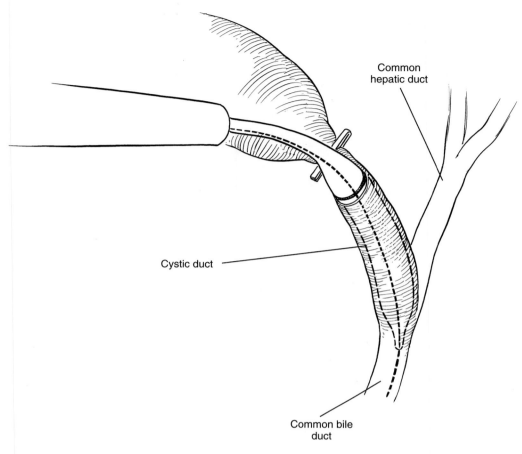

Common
hepatic duct

Cystic duct

Common bile
duct

FIGURE 6-4

FIGURE 6-4. A .035-inch hydrophilic-coated guide wire is then preloaded into a Phantom 5 balloon dilating catheter balloon (Microvasive). The dilating catheter balloon has an outside diameter of 7 mm and a length of 4 cm. The guide wire balloon catheter is loaded into a 5-mm reducer and is placed through the midclavicular 5-mm trocar. Under direct vision, the balloon catheter engages the opening of the cystic ductotomy. The operator then gently places the guide wire in the cystic duct and, using a torquing device and the image amplifier, extends the guide wire through the cystic duct well into the common duct. The position of the guide wire should be verified by image amplification. The balloon catheter is then placed along the guide wire in the cystic duct, the second mark just showing at the exit site. Depending on the catheter, the balloon is dilated with saline to 6 to 12 atmospheres of pressure. If the cystic duct is very short and we are less than 6 mm from the common duct, the dilation should be performed using visual cues. Not infrequently, with a short cystic duct, 6 to 12 atmospheres of pressure may split the duct and injure the common duct. The cystic duct is dilated for 3 to 5 minutes. At this point, a second assistant (we frequently use our scrub nurse) is placed on the patient's right.

FIGURE 6-5. The balloon is deflated, and the balloon catheter is removed, leaving the guide wire in the common duct.

FIGURE 6-6. The 9 French choledochoscope is then brought into the field and is connected to the second camera. The split image is seen on both monitors. While the first assistant holds the laparoscope and the intra-abdominal image is maintained, the surgeon and the second assistant backload the guide wire into the choledochoscope. A Tuohy-Borst adapter is placed on the channel of the coledochoscope, and an irrigation device is attached to the scope.

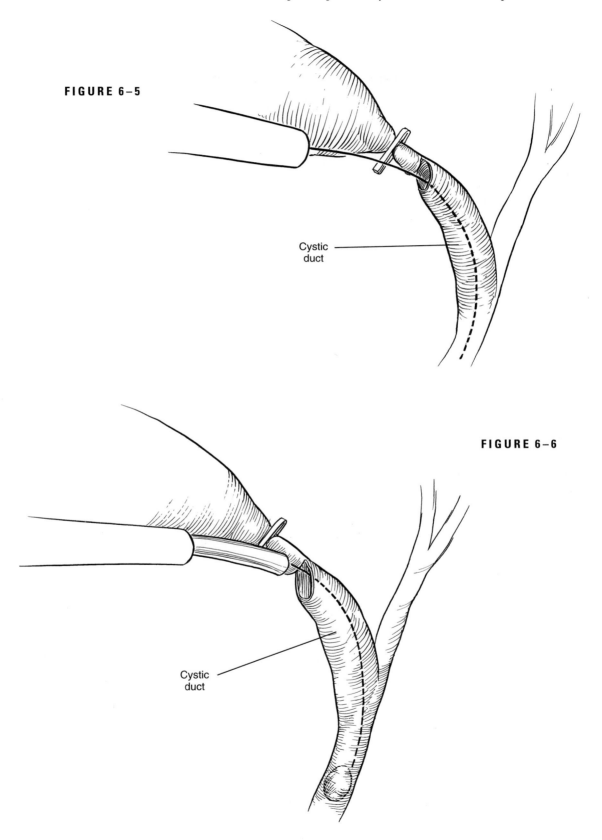

FIGURE 6−5

Cystic
duct

FIGURE 6−6

Cystic
duct

FIGURE 6–7. The choledochoscope is then inserted through the 5-mm reducer and follows the guide wire into the cystic duct. The irrigation device is turned on, and once the choledochoscope engages the cystic duct, the surgeon's focus remains on the choledochoscopic image. The choledochoscope is not moved until the lumen of the ductal system is seen. The 5-mm reducer is kept as close to the ductotomy as possible, so that all movements of the choledochoscope can be transmitted to the distal tip of the scope. Navigating the choledochoscope through the common duct toward the ampulla requires two major movements. The first and most important is a torquing movement of the choledochoscope. This is accomplished by rolling the scope between the index finger and the thumb or by using a torquing device placed on the scope. The second movement is flexing the scope so that the choledochus is always kept in the middle of the field. The scope is then inserted deep into the duct, and the ampulla of Vater is visualized.

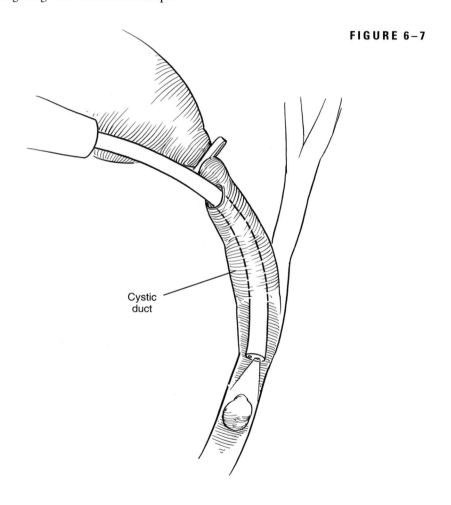

FIGURE 6–7

Cystic duct

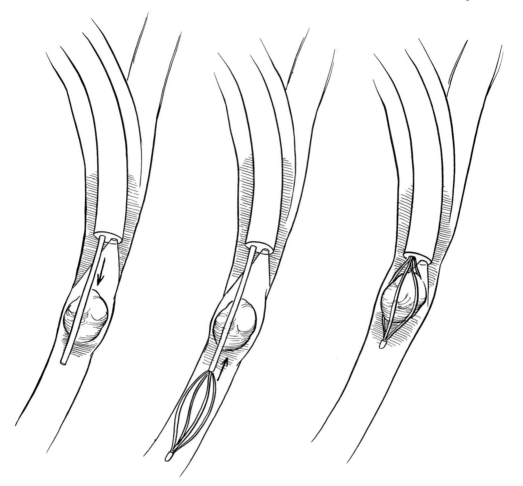

FIGURE 6–8

FIGURE 6–8. If stones are present in the distal duct, irrigation is decreased, which decreases the movement of free-floating stones. The guide wire is removed, and if the stone is 6 mm in diameter or less, a straight 3 French Segura basket is inserted through the channel of the endoscope until it is located beyond the stone. The second assistant opens the Segura basket and engages the stone. Usually a rapid back and forth motion of the basket will capture the stone.

FIGURE 6–9. Once the stone is seen within the basket, the basket is closed and withdrawn to the end of the scope. The scope is then removed from the ductal system, and the Segura basket is opened. The stone is deposited in the pouch of Morrison to be retrieved at a later time. If there are additional stones, the scope is inserted back into the cystic duct, and the maneuver is repeated.

If a small stone is impacted at the distal duct, two additional tools can be helpful. One is the radial Segura basket, and the other is a three-pronged grasper. Both tools can be used to dislodge the stone. If the stone is impacted in the distal duct and cannot be removed using either of these methods, the operator can perform lithotripsy. The electrohydraulic lithotripter is frequently found in most urologic suites and can fragment stones very rapidly. One must be careful to make certain that the wire of the lithotripter engages the stone. If it touches the common duct wall, it will perforate the duct. Another method of stone lithotripsy involves use of the pulse dye laser used at 504 ng. The pulse dye laser effectively fractures both soft and hard stones, and the laser fiber does not injure the common duct wall. This is a safer device, especially in patients with a small common duct.

In patients with multiple small stones in the common duct, several other techniques are available to the surgeon. One can use glucagon to dilate the ampulla of Vater and irrigate it with saline, flushing smaller stones through the ampulla. Another technique is balloon dilation of the ampulla of Vater. This technique uses the same instruments as transcystic duct dilation (e.g., the preloaded Phantom 5 catheter placed in the common duct). The guide wire is inserted through the ampulla of Vater using the image amplifier. The choledochus is filled with dye, so that the end of the common duct is visualized. The balloon catheter is then inserted through the ampulla of Vater, using the proximal and distal opaque markers as guides. The catheter is slowly dilated to 6 atmospheres of pressure for approximately 3 minutes, and the balloon is then withdrawn, leaving the catheter in the proximal common duct. Using irrigating techniques, stones as large as 4 mm have been successfully flushed out of the distal duct. This can be corroborated both by x-ray and direct choledochoscopy.

We have performed ampullary dilation more

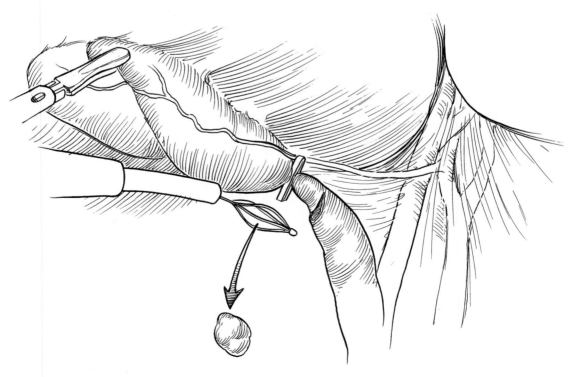

FIGURE 6–9

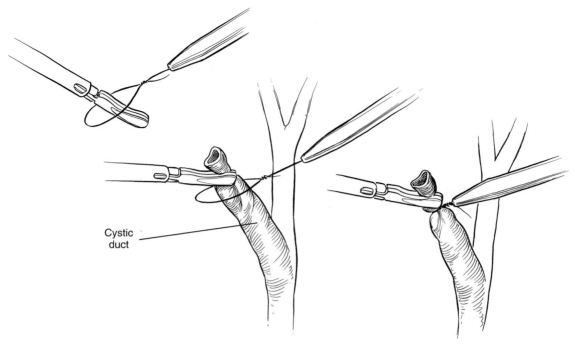

Cystic
duct

FIGURE 6-10

than 45 times in the past 4 years and have noted three cases of transient hyperamylasemia without clinical pancreatitis. In a number of our patients, some of the smaller stones have migrated to the proximal common hepatic duct during transcystic laparoscopic common duct exploration. In only 5 to 10 per cent of patients can we place the choledochoscope in the common hepatic duct using the transcystic duct approach. When we cannot visualize the common hepatic duct, the patient is placed in steep reverse Trendelenburg position for 5 to 10 minutes. Glucagon is given for ampullary drainage, and the choledochoscope is removed from the cystic duct. In three of four such cases, the stones migrated down to the distal duct and could then be retrieved in the usual fashion.

Once the duct has been cleared of all calculi, the choledoschoscope is removed. A postexploration cholangiogram is then performed to make sure that no additional stones are present. In addition, it is important to make sure that the exploration has caused no damage to the duct. We have seen no injury in the 92 patients we have treated during the past 4 years.

FIGURE 6-10. The cystic duct is then ligated using a PDS endoloop. The gallbladder is removed in the usual fashion. Using this technique, we have successfully removed common duct stones in 85 per cent of patients via the transcystic duct approach.

X. Postoperative Medications

A. Vicodin, one tablet every 3 to 4 hours as needed for pain
B. Ativan, 1 to 2 mg sublingually for sleep

XI. Advancement of Diet

The patient is started on clear liquids 6 hours after surgery and is given a regular diet on the second postoperative day. If the patient is afebrile and has only mild pain and stable vital signs, he is discharged on the first postoperative day. We use the same discharge criteria for transcystic duct laparoscopic common duct exploration as we do for laparoscopic cholecystectomy. Most frequently, the patient can return to work in 8 to 10 days.

Chapter 7

Laparoscopic Choledochoduodenostomy

MICHAEL EDYE, M.B., B.S., F.R.A.C.S., F.A.C.S.

I. Indications

A. Gross common bile duct dilation (>15 mm internal diameter) with:
1. Biliary stasis and/or choledocholithiasis
2. Recurrent cholangitis
3. Failed endoscopic retrograde cholangio-pancreatography (ERCP) stone clearance due to duodenal diverticulum or other technical difficulties
4. Postcholecystectomy choledocholithiasis

II. Contraindications

A. Duct wall thickening and internal diameter of the bile duct less than 15 mm
B. Portal hypertension

III. Factors Important in Patient Selection

A. Patients must be as fit as for laparoscopic cholecystectomy.
B. Previous cholecystectomy creates adhesions between the liver, duodenum, and colon. Time must be allowed for careful dissection of the subhepatic space in these patients.
C. Patients with a duct smaller than 15 mm are better suited to surgical sphincteroplasty if endoscopic sphincterotomy has proved impossible.
D. Surgical drainage of malignant bile duct stricture is usually achieved by performing a bili-enteric anastomosis using jejunum because of the risk of tumor encroachment at a choledochoduodenostomy.

IV. Preoperative Preparation

A. Most patients will have had ERCP, and surgery should be performed no earlier than the following day to avoid gaseous distention of the intestine.
B. A transpapillary stent should be placed if possible to allow drainage if ERCP failed to clear the duct.
C. Preoperative medications include broad-spectrum antibiotics.
D. Bowel preparation: none.

V. Anesthesia

General anesthesia in all patients

VI. Accessory Devices

A. Nasogastric tube, inserted after induction of general anesthesia
B. Urinary catheter for all patients
C. Pneumatic compression stockings for all patients

VII. Instrumentation

A. 45-degree laparoscope (5-mm telescope reduces number of 10-mm cannulas)

76

B. 4 × 5 mm and 1 × 10 mm cannulas
C. Thick suture material (e.g., 2-nylon (to elevate the round ligament)
D. Dyed and undyed 3–0 polyglactin sutures on a tapered needle (half circle preferred)
E. Two laparoscopic needle holders
F. Two-handed operative technique and advanced endoscopic stitch and knot skills are essential to make acceptable progress during the anastomosis.

VIII. Operating Room Set-Up and Trocar Positions

FIGURE 7–1. Position: modified lithotomy with thighs parallel to trunk. The monitor is sited above the patient's head.

Cannula 1: Umbilicus (scope)
Cannula 2: Left pararectal (10 mm)
Cannula 3: Epigastric (5 mm)
Cannula 4: Mid right subcostal (5 mm)
Cannula 5: Lateral right subcostal (5 mm)

IX. Technique

The decision to perform choledochoduodenostomy is made prior to commencing surgery. The usual indication is failure of ERCP to adequately clear the duct. The aim of the procedure is to clear the common duct of calculi to avoid a sump syndrome and to provide permanent decompression of the dilated system by performing a bili-enteric anastomosis.

Operative Steps

1. Insertion of cannulas, insufflation, elevation of the liver
2. Limited kocherization of the duodenum and exposure of the anterior aspect of the common duct
3. Choledochotomy, duct clearance, and choledochoscopy

FIGURE 7–1

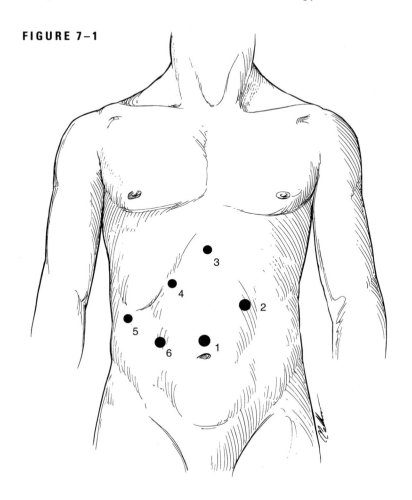

4. Duodenotomy

5. Side-to-side choledochoduodenal anastomosis constructed with a posterior and anterior row of interrupted absorbable sutures

6. Methylene blue test through cystic duct

7. Cholecystectomy and placement of drain

The operation begins as for cholecystectomy. STEP 1: Five cannulas are inserted from the outset. Elevation of the liver by suspending the round ligament with a strong stitch inserted through the skin may avoid the need for an extra cannula.

The gallbladder, if present, is retracted over the liver. If previous cholecystectomy has been performed, the edge of the liver is defined, a grasper is attached to it to elevate it, and the undersurface is sharply dissected from the subhepatic structures. The dilated common duct is deceptively anterior. A good landmark is the outer edge of the duodenum. Dissecting from lateral to medial facilitates access to the correct tissue plane.

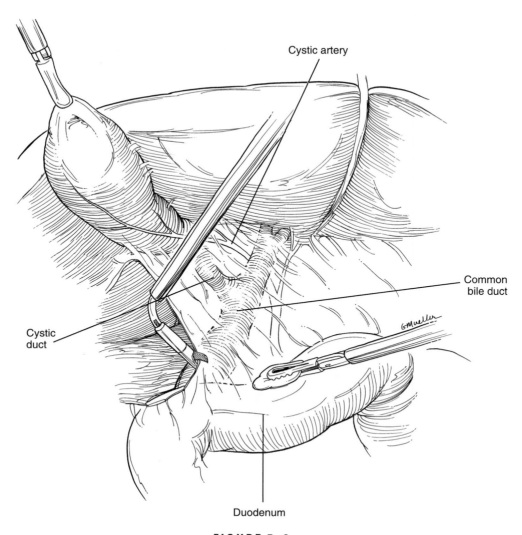

Cystic artery

Common bile duct

Cystic duct

Duodenum

FIGURE 7–2

FIGURE 7-2. STEP 2: Complete kocherization of the duodenum is not necessary, but mobilization of the junction of the first and second parts from lateral to medial will help keep the anastomosis tension-free. Downward lateral traction on the duodenum to the left is provided by a cotton pledget locked in a toothed grasper inserted through cannula 2. The peritoneal reflection of the duodenum is incised with scissors inserted through cannula 3 towards the hepato-duodenal ligament. The incision is carried over the anterior aspect of the common bile duct to open the plane between it and the duodenum.

FIGURE 7-3. The peritoneum over the anterior aspect of the duct is pushed away with a cotton pledget to thin out the tissues through which the choledochotomy is to be made. Superficial bleeders are coagulated with brisk precise cautery applied to each vessel. All available duct is exposed for a length of 25 mm on its anterior aspect below the cystic duct and behind the first part of the duodenum. The suction cannula inserted through cannula 2 depresses the duodenum and allows constant evacuation of smoke, bile, and blood.

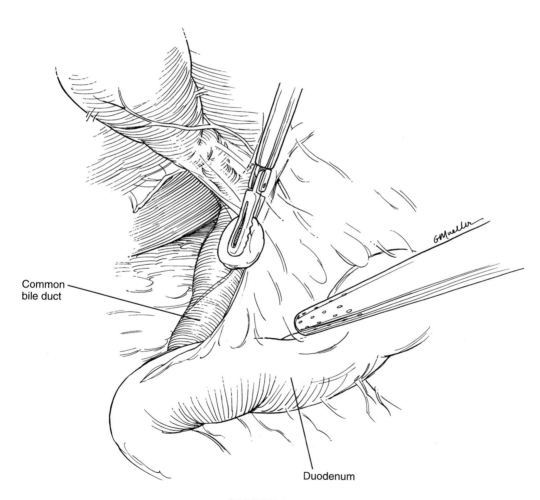

Common bile duct

Duodenum

FIGURE 7-3

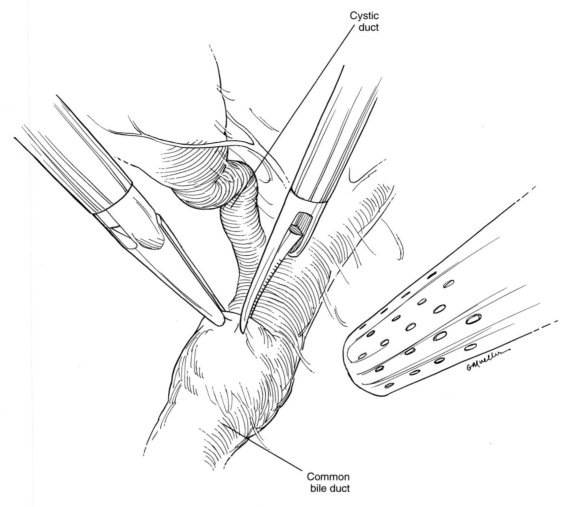

Cystic
duct

Common
bile duct

FIGURE 7-4

FIGURE 7-4. STEP 3: Prior to making the incision, superficial blood vessels along the line of the choledochotomy are briskly cauterized to reduce bleeding. A fine grasper is inserted through cannula 5, and the part of the duct that will be the midpoint of the choledochotomy (about 15 mm from where the duct passes behind the duodenum) is seized gently with the tip. Cutting directly through the fold created, close to the grasper, with scissors inserted through cannula 3, makes a longitudinal choledochotomy of about 5 mm. Suction cannula 2 aspirates the flood of bile to clear the field.

FIGURE 7-5. Two 3–0 polyglactin sutures, trimmed to 13 cm in length, are inserted outside-in on each side of the choledochotomy. These are used as stay sutures but are later tied as the corner stitches at the lateral extremity of the choledochoduodenal anastomosis.

FIGURE 7-6. The choledochotomy is extended proximally and distally at this point using the stay sutures for traction. Total length should be 25 mm.

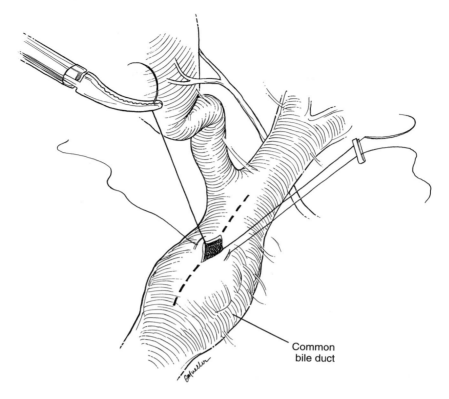

Common
bile duct

FIGURE 7–5

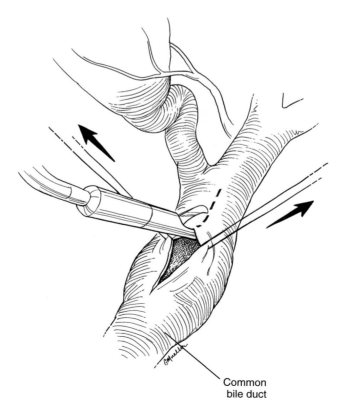

Common
bile duct

FIGURE 7–6

FIGURE 7–7. The stay sutures are laid to each side of the duct in the soft tissues. A 7 French Fogarty balloon catheter on a suitable reducer inserted through cannula 3 or 4 is the easiest way to clear the common duct of large stones. The catheter is swept cephalad through the bile duct and caudad through the common hepatic duct. Choledochoscopy is performed to ensure that all gross calculous debris has been removed. Gentle traction on the stay sutures crossed over the choledochotomy helps to reduce irrigant leak and improves the quality of the choledochoscopy.

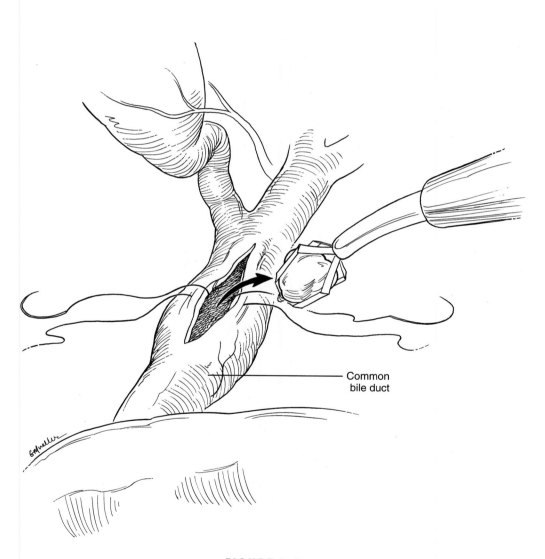

Common bile duct

FIGURE 7–7

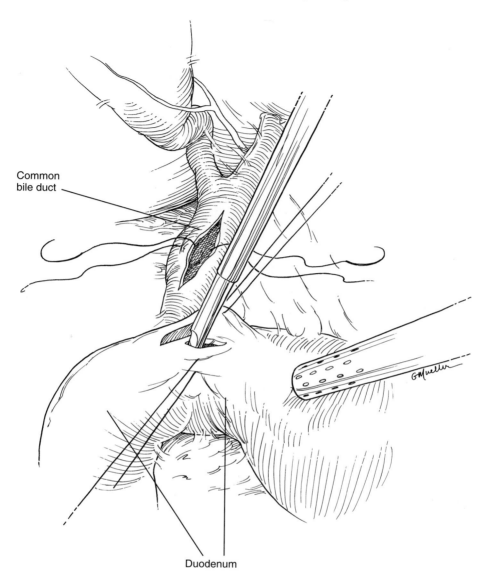

Common
bile duct

Duodenum

FIGURE 7–8

FIGURE 7–8. STEP 4: The superior border of the duodenum just distal to the pylorus is scored for a distance of 20 mm with electrocautery. Using a single scissor blade and cutting electrocautery, a full-thickness hole is made through the midpoint of the score line, and extended 10 mm proximally and distally. Inside-out stay stitches may facilitate the duodenotomy.

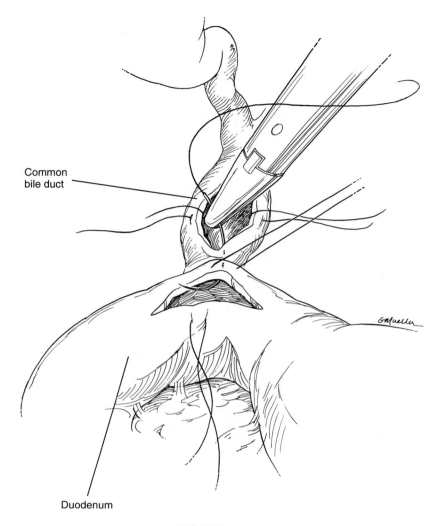

Common
bile duct

Duodenum

FIGURE 7–9

FIGURE 7–9. STEP 5: Posterior row: A central stitch is inserted inside-out from the inferior angle of the choledochotomy to outside-in at the midpoint of the upper edge of the duodenotomy. If suitably sited the upper duodenotomy stay can be used. This is knotted intracorporeally and cut long for traction.

FIGURE 7–10. The needle of each common duct stay suture is passed inside-out at its respective end of the duodenotomy and left untied (these are the corner stitches). Depending on the length of the anastomosis, one or two evenly spaced stitches are inserted and tied in the lumen working from the center toward each cor-

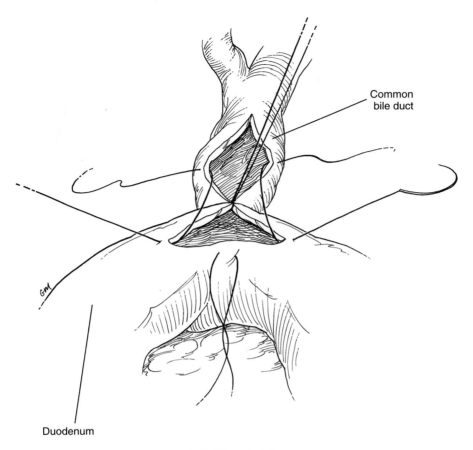

Common
bile duct

Duodenum

FIGURE 7–10

ner stitch to approximate the duct wall to the duodenum. Because of the fixed angles imposed on the instruments by their fulcrum in the abdominal wall, the optimal needle path is achieved more comfortably by using a combination of (1) traction on the central stitch to align the next stitch site perpendicular to the needle, and (2) using two needle holders through cannulas 2 and 5, switching the needle between the right and left holders, depending on the

alignment. The corner stitches are tied and cut long, and the central stitch is trimmed, completing the back row of the anastomosis.

Anterior row: Three evenly spaced anterior row sutures are now inserted (for outside knots) but left untied: one for the apex at the midpoint (dark thread), and one on each side (undyed thread), placed between the apex and each corner.

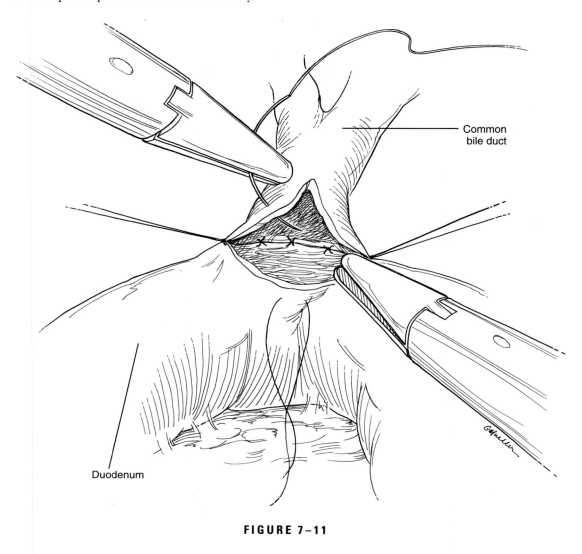

Common
bile duct

Duodenum

FIGURE 7–11

FIGURE 7–11. The needle holder in cannula 5 is used to start the right anterior stitch, but having passed through the duct, the needle is switched to the holder in cannula 2 for the duodenal side.

FIGURE 7–12. Inadvertent tangling of each stitch by passing it through a loop of its neigh-bor must be avoided. Alternating dark and light colored suture material reduces confusion later when one is picking up each thread to tie.

FIGURE 7–13. Traction aligns tissue to needle rather than needle to tissue.

FIGURE 7–12

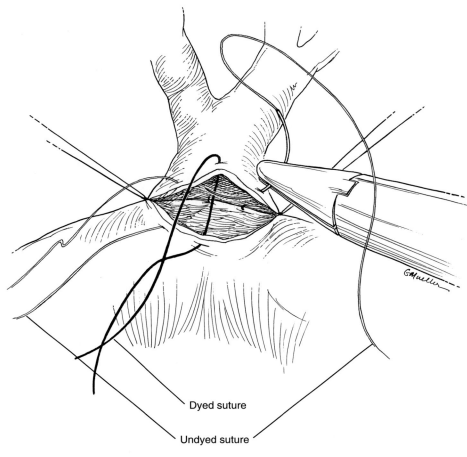

Dyed suture

Undyed suture

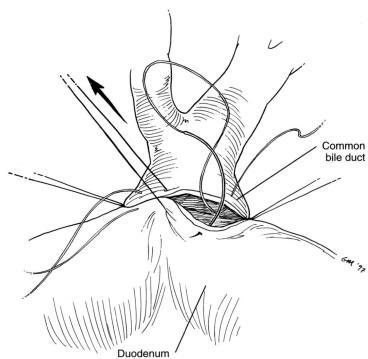

Common
bile duct

Duodenum

FIGURE 7–13

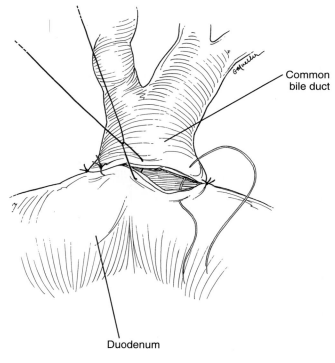

Common
bile duct

Duodenum

FIGURE 7–14

FIGURE 7-14. The anterior row stitches are tied and cut starting at the right side and working to the left.

FIGURE 7-15. STEP 6: To test for leaks, the common duct is filled with methylene blue/saline solution injected into the cystic duct through a catheter secured with a pre-tied loop. A clean rolled gauze is tucked behind the anastomosis and checked for blue staining.

STEP 7: Cholecystectomy is completed in the usual way, and a soft silicone drain (e.g., Jackson-Pratt drain) is laid in the subhepatic space, its tip adjacent to, but not in contact with, the anastomosis. It is brought out through the most lateral 5-mm puncture on the right.

X. Postoperative Medications

No specific postoperative medication or antibiotics are necessary.

XI. Advancement of Diet

A. An optional nasogastric tube is left in overnight and then removed, as is the drain if there is no bile in it, the following morning.
B. The patient starts on a liquid diet and is rapidly advanced to solids as tolerated.

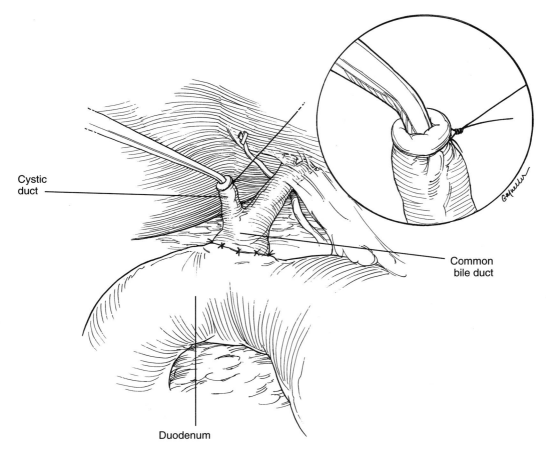

Cystic duct

Common bile duct

Duodenum

FIGURE 7–15

XII. Determination of Discharge

In the absence of ileus, the patient can be discharged on the second or third postoperative day.

XIII. Return to Normal Activity or Work

Return to normal activity is similar to that characteristic of laparoscopic cholecystectomy.

Liver chemistry test results are evaluated within 2 to 3 weeks to ensure that cholestasis is resolving. It is normal to see an air cholangiogram on abdominal radiographs. The anastomosis can be evaluated endoscopically, but adequacy of drainage is best gauged by performing a barium contrast study with 24-hour delayed films looking for residual barium in the ductal system.

Part III

LAPAROSCOPIC SURGERY OF THE ESOPHAGUS

Chapter 8

Laparoscopic Nissen Fundoplication

BERNARD DALLEMAGNE, M.D.

I. Indications

A. Failure of medical therapy (at least 6 months of medical, diet, and/or postural treatment)
   1. Recurrence of symptoms when treatment is stopped
   2. Persistence of symptoms despite maximum therapy
   3. Persistent esophagitis despite maximum therapy
B. Complications of gastroesophageal reflux
   1. Esophageal stricture
   2. Barrett's esophagus
C. Obstructive symptoms from a large hiatal hernia or a small hiatal hernia in combination with a Schatzki ring

II. Contraindications

A. Patients who cannot tolerate general anesthesia
B. Patients with Barrett's esophagus in whom a biopsy discloses severe dysplasia or intramucosal carcinoma. These patients are best treated with an esophageal resection.
C. Previous gastric or hiatal surgery may represent a relative contraindication.

III. Preoperative Preparation

A. The decision to proceed with an antireflux operation is based on the presence of objective findings of gastroesophageal reflux disease. Evaluation may include:
   1. Upper endoscopy with esophageal biopsy
   2. Barium swallow or video esophagram
   3. Esophageal manometry
   4. 24-hour pH monitoring
   5. Gastric emptying study
B. Patients are admitted on the day of surgery.

IV. Factors Important in Patient Selection

Candidates for Nissen fundoplication suffer from documented pathologic gastroesophageal reflux, with or without hiatal hernia. All patients have had at least 6 months of medical, diet, and/or postural therapy. They either have recurrence of symptoms when treatment is stopped or experience no relief of symptoms or esophageal lesions despite treatment. In these circumstances, an esophageal function study is carried out. This study includes endoscopy and biopsy, barium studies, esophageal manometry, and 24-hour pH monitoring.

The indications to proceed with antireflux surgery are documentation of a mechanically defective lower esophageal sphincter (LES) and increased exposure to gastric juice. Patients with Barrett's esophagus are candidates for antireflux surgery. If biopsy reveals severe dysplasia or intramucosal carcinoma, esophageal resection should be done. Patients with a manometrically normal LES, patients not responding to medical therapy, and patients with atypical symptoms must be studied by 24-hour pH monitoring to assess the increased esophageal exposure to gastric juice. This increment can be related to a gastric or esophageal cause. On the one hand, if pH monitoring of a patient is normal despite a defective LES, the possibility of alkaline, drug-induced, or retention esophagitis must be considered. On the other hand, some patients do have large paraesophageal hiatal hernias or small hiatal hernias with a Schatzki ring. They complain mainly of dysphagia, chest pain, and sometimes heartburn. The LES is often normal. Surgical repair will relieve the symptoms but must be associated with an antireflux procedure because of the potential destruction of the competency of the cardioesophageal junction during reduction of the hernia.

V. Choice of Anesthesia

All patients undergo general anesthesia.

VI. Accessory Device

A. Large-bore (36 to 60) French gastric tube

VII. Instruments and Telescopes

A. 10-mm, wide angle view, 0- to 30-degree telescope
B. Laparoscopic dissecting scissors
C. Laparoscopic ultrasonic scissors
D. Laparoscopic atraumatic grasping forceps
E. Laparoscopic surgical clip applier
F. Laparoscopic needle holder

VIII. Position of Monitors and Placement of Trocars

FIGURE 8–1. The patient is placed in a modified lithotomy position. The surgeon stands between the legs of the patient with the surgical assistant on his right and the scrub nurse or another assistant on his left. The video-laparoscopy column is placed either on the right or the left of the surgeon. At the beginning of the

FIGURE 8–1

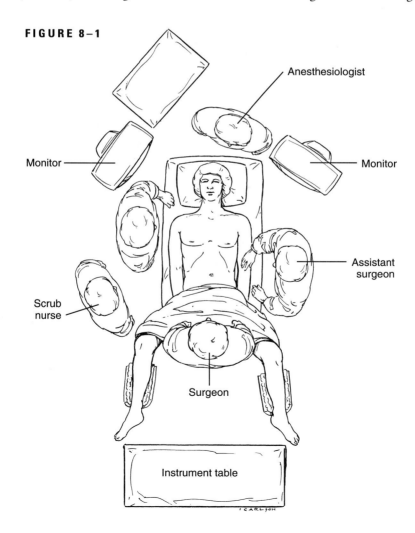

Anesthesiologist

Monitor

Monitor

Assistant surgeon

Scrub nurse

Surgeon

Instrument table

procedure a large-bore (36 to 60 French) gastric tube is placed in the proximal esophagus, above the cardioesophageal junction. As the surgeon gains experience, use of the large gastric tube for sizing the wrap becomes unnecessary. Indeed, passing this sizer is the most common cause of esophageal perforation during laparoscopic fundoplication, and as a result I now rarely use one.

FIGURE 8–2. Pneumoperitoneum is established in the normal fashion, with the usual precautions. A maximum intraperitoneal pressure of 15 mm Hg is obtained. The first trocar,

10 mm, is placed in the supraumbilical midline at the junction of the upper two-thirds and the lower one-third of the esophagus between the umbilicus and the xyphoid process. The laparoscope is introduced through this port. Visual inspection of the entire peritoneal cavity is carried out. Under direct vision, four other trocars are inserted: one 5-mm trocar in the midline under the xyphoid process and a 10-mm trocar in the left upper quadrant at the midclavicular line at a left paraumbilical position. Two 5-mm trocars are also used: one is placed under the right costal margin in the midclavicular line, and the other is positioned laterally under the left costal margin on the anterior axillary line.

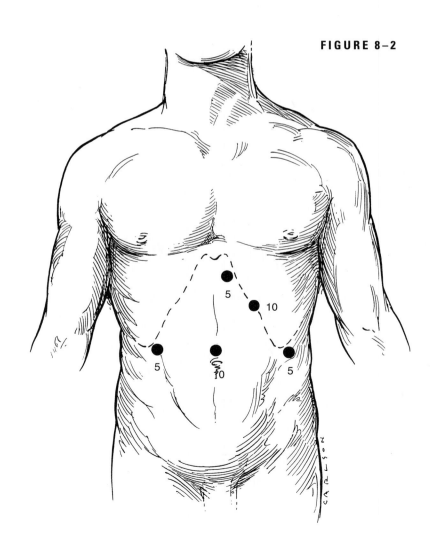

FIGURE 8–2

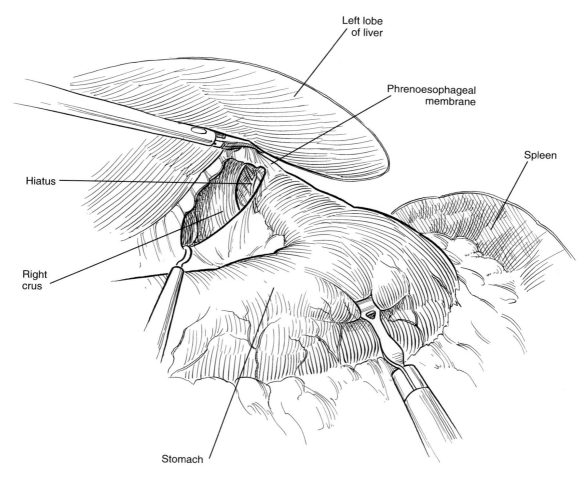

Left lobe of liver

Phrenoesophageal membrane

Spleen

Hiatus

Right crus

Stomach

FIGURE 8–3

IX. Narrative of Surgical Techniques

FIGURE 8–3. The operation begins with retraction of the left lobe of the liver using either an atraumatic forceps or a liver retractor introduced through the 5-mm right trocar. This forceps is fixed to the suprahiatal diaphragm and lifts the left lobe, allowing access to the hiatus. The remainder of the procedure follows the classic sequence of the operation performed through laparotomy.

The phrenoesophageal membrane is divided on the anterior aspect of the hiatal orifice. This incision is extended to the right to allow identification of the right crus. Then, along the inner side of this crus, the right esophageal wall is freed by dissecting the cleavage plane. This dissection is carried out using scissors.

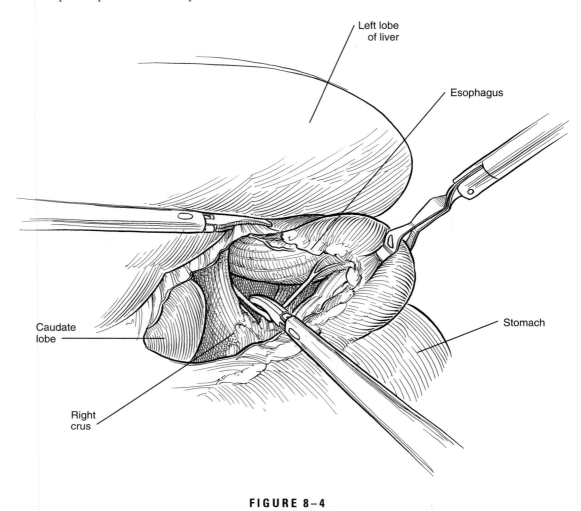

FIGURE 8-4

FIGURE 8-4. The liberation of the posterior aspect of the esophagus is started by extending the dissection the length of the right diaphragmatic crus. The pars flaccida of the lesser omentum is opened, preserving the hepatic branches of the vagus nerve. This allows access to the crura, left and right, the right posterior aspect of the esophagus, and the posterior vagus nerve.

FIGURE 8-5. Attention is turned next to the left anterolateral aspect of the esophagus: at its left border, the left crus is identified. The cleavage plane between it and the left aspect of the esophagus is freed. The gastrophrenic ligament

is incised, beginning the mobilization of the gastric pouch.

At this point, with the intramediastinal dissection of the esophagus, one obtains an elongation of the intra-abdominal segment of the esophagus and a reduction of the hiatal hernia if one exists.

FIGURE 8-6. The next step involves repair of the hiatal orifice: two or three interrupted sutures, using nonabsorbable material, are placed on the diaphragmatic crura to close the orifice. A distance of approximately 1 cm must be maintained between the highest suture and the esophagus.

FIGURE 8–5

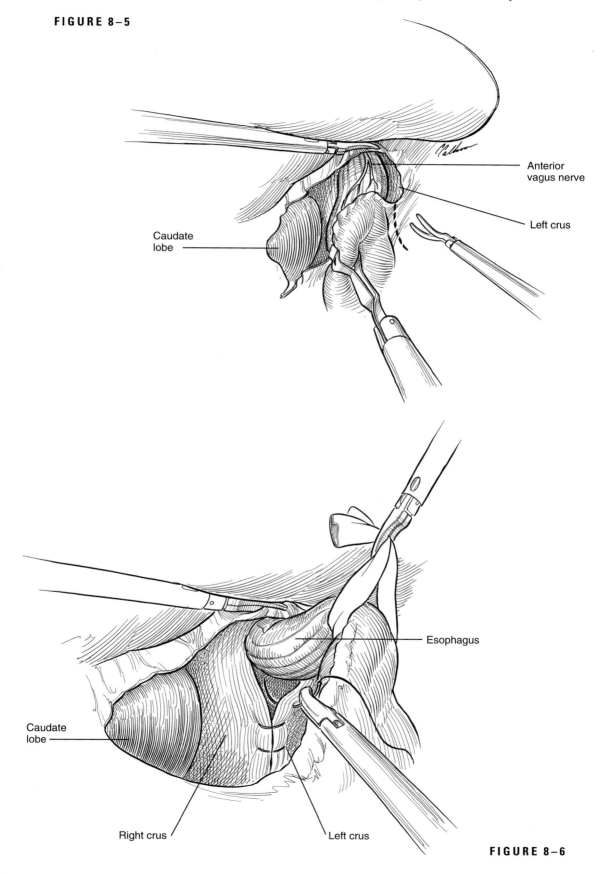

FIGURE 8–6

FIGURE 8–7. The following step consists of the mobilization of the gastric pouch. This requires ligation and division of the gastrosplenic ligament and several short gastric vessels; two or three are clipped and divided as required by the size of the fundus. This dissection starts on the stomach at the point where the vessels of the great curvature turn toward the spleen away from the gastroepiploic arcade.

One now turns to the retroesophageal hiatal orifice. The esophagus is lifted by a forceps inserted through the left upper quadrant port. Careful dissection of the mesoesophagus and the left crus reveals a cleavage plane between this crus and the posterior gastric wall. Confirmation of opening the correct plane is obtained by visualizing the fatty tissue of the gastrosplenic ligament or the spleen itself, when looking behind the esophagus. This retroesophageal channel is enlarged to allow easy passage of the antireflux valve.

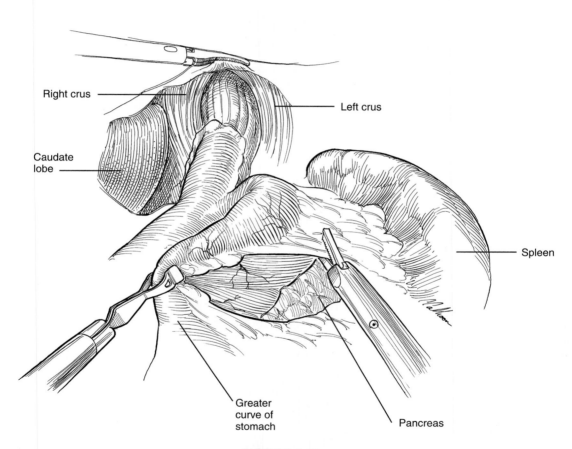

FIGURE 8–7

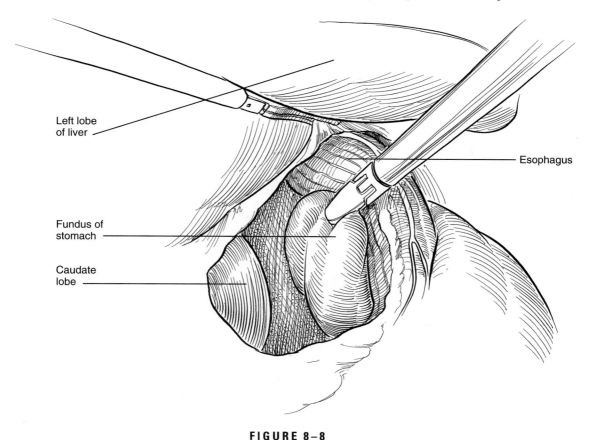

Left lobe
of liver

Esophagus

Fundus of
stomach

Caudate
lobe

FIGURE 8–8

FIGURE 8–8. The last part of the operation consists of the passage and fixation of the antireflux valve. An atraumatic forceps is passed behind the esophagus from right to left. It is used to grab the gastric pouch to the left of the esophagus and pull it behind, forming the wrap. Both the anterior and posterior walls of the stomach fundus are passed to the right of the esophagus. At this point, the gastric tube placed at the beginning of the operation is passed down the cardia. It is used to calibrate the fundoplication. Three interrupted stitches form and secure the sleeve. They are passed into the seromuscular layer of the anterior wall of the gastric pouch to the left of the esophagus, through the seromuscular layer of the anterior esophagus, and finally, to the right of the esophagus, through the seromuscular layer of the stomach, which had been passed behind the esophagus.

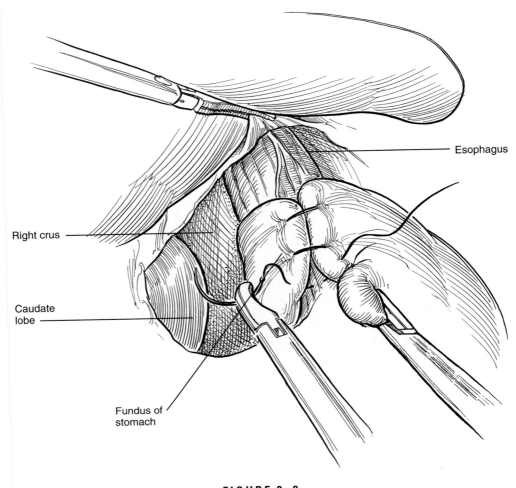

Esophagus

Right crus

Caudate
lobe

Fundus of
stomach

FIGURE 8-9

FIGURE 8-9. A 2-cm sleeve is thus constructed. Passage of a forceps through the sleeve
ensures that the valve does not create a stenosis.

Closure

The large gastric tube (if used) is removed.
No nasogastric tube is used. The peritoneum is
rinsed with warm normal saline. No drains are
placed. The trocars are removed, and the
wounds are stapled closed.

X. Postoperative Medications

A. Patients receive parenteral analgesics as required.

B. Patients are given oral analgesic agents
when taking liquids by mouth.

XI. Advancement of Diet

A. An intravenous line is left in place until the
morning of the first postoperative day at
the latest.
B. The patient is then allowed to eat and drink.
C. On the second postoperative day, a barium
study of the esophagus, stomach, and duodenum is carried out to verify the position
and function of the antireflux valve and to
confirm the absence of significant stenosis.

XII. Determinants of Discharge

The patient is discharged after the barium examination. Dietary instructions are given to avoid the risk of impaction at the sleeve in the early postoperative period. The patient is seen after 1 month; a history allows evaluation of the result and assessment of any secondary effects. At the end of 3 months, patients who accept it undergo a full evaluation including endoscopy, esophageal manometry, and pH studies. A new clinical history concerning the results of the operation is taken.

XIII. Return to Normal Activities

Patients return to normal activities as tolerated.

Chapter 9

Laparoscopic Nissen Fundoplication with Laparosonic Coagulating Shears

JOSEPH F. AMARAL, M.D.

I. Indications

A. Patients must have documented reflux on a 24-hour pH monitoring study, esophageal manometry documenting a normal or low lower esophageal pressure, normal gastric emptying, and one of the following additional indications:
B. Recurrent peptic esophageal stricture
C. Failed attempts at medical therapy
D. Barrett's esophagus
E. Recurrent pneumonia
F. Severe asthma
G. Need for long term medical therapy
H. Large hiatal hernia
I. Paraesophageal hernia

II. Contraindications

A. Intolerance of general anesthesia
B. Severe coagulopathy

III. Factors Important in Patient Selection

Prior to attempting this procedure the surgeon should have gained extensive experience in laparoscopic surgery (more than 100 laparoscopic cases) and be familiar with open antireflux surgery. The initial patients should have small or no hiatal hernias and should be thin.

IV. Preoperative Preparation

A. Same day admission
B. Preoperative medications: metoclopramide hydrochloride intravenously (IV), 1 g cefazolin IV, 5000 units heparin subcutaneously (SQ)
C. Bowel preparation: none

V. Choice of Anesthesia

A. General endotracheal anesthesia
B. Nondepolarizing muscle relaxant: Diprivan
C. Small dose of meperidine

VI. Accessory Devices

A. Nasogastric tube
B. Urinary catheter
C. Pneumatic compression stockings
D. 60 French blunt bougie

VII. Instruments and Telescopes

A. 10 mm, 0-degree laparoscope
B. One curved dissector
C. Two tissue graspers
D. One Babcock forceps
E. One curved grasper or dissector (roticulating grasper, [United States Surgical Corporation])

F. Ultrasonically activated scalpel, laparosonic coagulating shears (LCS) (Harmonic scalpel [EndoEthicon, Cincinnati, OH])
G. Suction irrigation device
H. Pressurized irrigation system (EndoFlow, [Davol, Inc])
I. Nonabsorbable sutures, size 0 for laparoscopic use
J. Two laparoscopic needle holders
K. Open laparoscopy cannula
L. Three 10-mm cannulas
M. One 5-mm cannula

VIII. Operating Room Set-Up and Trocar Positions

FIGURE 9–1A. The patient is placed in the supine position on the operating table. Alternatively, the lithotomy position can be used to make suturing easier, especially if the surgeon is not experienced in laparoscopic suturing. Two monitors are used, located at the patient's right and left sides at about the level of the shoulders. The surgeon stands on the patient's right side, and the camera operator stands on the patient's left side. A second assistant also stands on the patient's right side. The surgeon uses a two-handed technique. The procedure is performed with the patient in the reverse Trendelenburg position. An orogastric tube is present during the entire dissection but is removed when the bougie is passed at the end of the procedure for calibration of the wrap.

Laparoscopy is initiated using an open (Hasson) technique. The procedure is performed by making a 10- to 12-mm vertical incision approximately midway between the xiphoid and the umbilicus and spreading the subcutaneous tissue to the fascia with a hemostat. The fascia is then grasped on either side of the midline with Kocher clamps, and the midline fascia is divided with a scalpel. Heavy sutures, such as 0 silk or polyglycolic acid, are placed on either side of the midline incision for traction and for later closure of the defect. Under direct vision, the preperitoneal fat and posterior sheath are identified and divided, and the peritoneum is identified and incised. Confirmation of entrance into the abdominal cavity is achieved either by visualization of the bowel or omentum or by the ability to pass a blunt instrument freely into the abdominal cavity. A blunt trocar-cannula system designed for open laparoscopy is then placed in the abdomen. Prior to insufflation, the cavity is visually explored with the laparoscope to ensure

FIGURE 9–1A

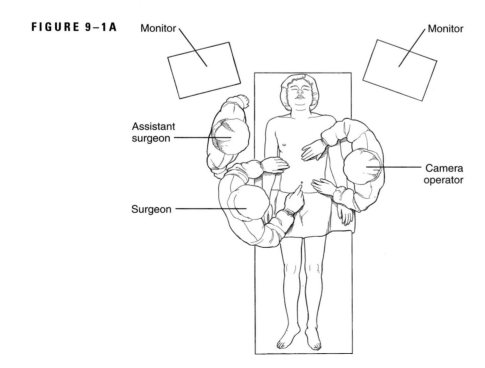

Monitor

Monitor

Assistant surgeon

Camera operator

Surgeon

appropriate location and absence of visceral or vessel injury.

FIGURE 9–1B. Five cannulas are used for the procedure, four 10-mm cannulas and one 5-mm cannula. Their location is shown in this figure. They include a 5-mm subxiphoid cannula that enters the abdomen to the left of the patient's falciform ligament, a 10-mm right midclavicular cannula, a 10-mm left midclavicular cannula, and a 10-mm cannula midway between the xiphoid and the 10-mm cannula used for open laparoscopy in the midline. The surgeon manipulates the subxiphoid and the left midclavicular cannulas for most of the procedure. The camera operator controls the open laparoscopy cannula and the lower left 10-mm cannula. The second assistant controls the right midclavicular 10-mm cannula.

IX. Narrative of Surgical Technique

FIGURE 9–2. Once the cannulas are inserted, the liver is elevated with a retractor through the right midclavicular cannula. We prefer not to use an open fan-type retractor because the limbs tend to cut into the liver. This is especially true in patients with an enlarged fatty liver. Lacerations of the liver at this point lead to bleeding, which obscures dissection in the crural area. To avoid lacerations, we use a 10-mm flat retractor or a closed fan-type retractor. This can be hooked under the liver in the bare space and against the diaphragm.

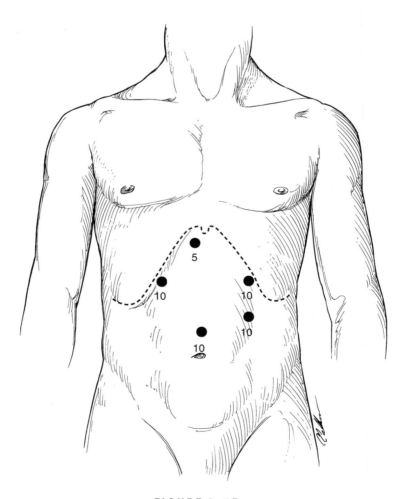

FIGURE 9–1B

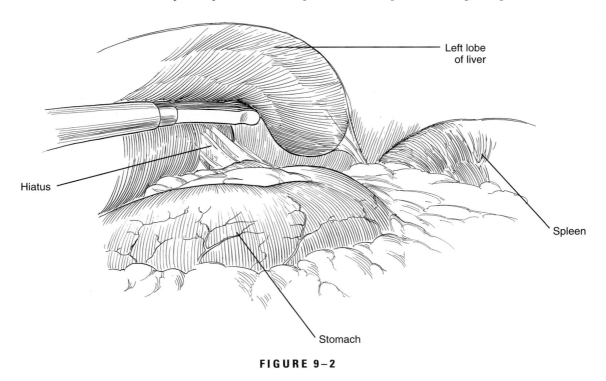

FIGURE 9–2

FIGURE 9–3. The stomach is then grasped with a 10-mm Babcock-type forceps through the lower 10-mm cannula, and traction is exerted on the stomach toward the pelvis. This forceps should not be twisted during traction because it can tear the stomach. Additionally, the instrument used should not be traumatic.

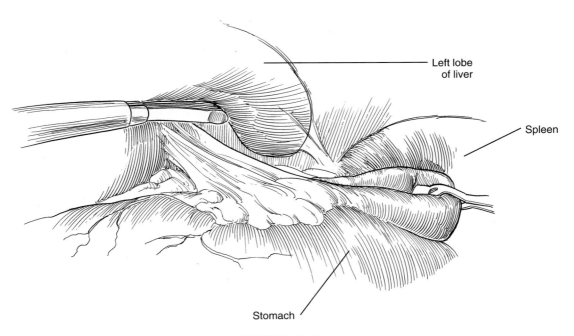

FIGURE 9–3

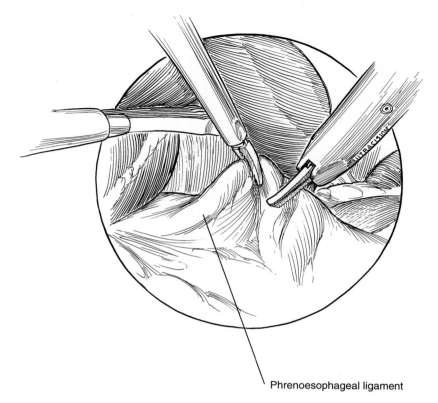

Phrenoesophageal ligament

FIGURE 9-4

FIGURE 9-4. Surgical dissection is started with the surgeon using a two-handed technique through the 5-mm subxiphoid and 10-mm left midclavicular cannulas. The phrenoesophageal ligament is grasped with a dissector and divided using the sharp side of the LCS if the area is avascular. Bleeding is stopped using the blunt side of the LCS by grasping the bleeding site with it and activating it for 3 to 5 seconds. This dissection not only opens the phrenoesophageal ligament across the crura and esophagus but also opens a window in the gastrohepatic ligament.

Care must be taken to avoid injury to the esophagus. If there is no hiatal hernia the crura may be closely applied to the esophagus and may be mistaken for the esophagus itself. If there is difficulty in identifying the esophagus a lighted bougie may help. No energized dissection is used here until these structures are clearly visualized. To facilitate this dissection, we stay between the posterior vagus nerve and the esophagus. There is less adipose tissue in this region than beneath the vagus nerve. The blunt side of the LCS is used to divide small periesophageal blood vessels.

FIGURE 9-5. Blunt dissection using an endo peanut or the suction irrigation device is used to identify the right crura and the esophagus.

FIGURE 9-6. Complete dissection of the crural area requires identification and clearing of the left crura as well as the right.

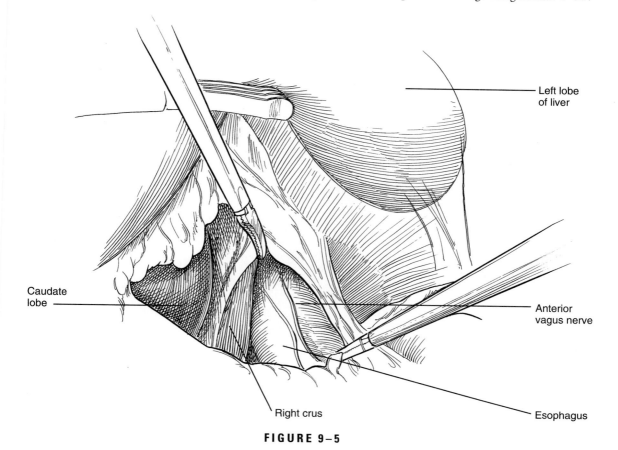

Left lobe
of liver

Caudate
lobe

Anterior
vagus nerve

Right crus

Esophagus

FIGURE 9–5

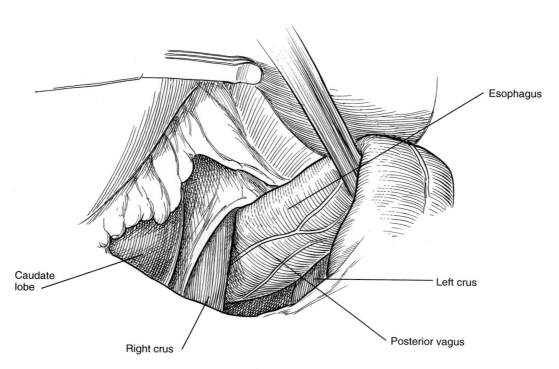

Esophagus

Caudate
lobe

Left crus

Right crus

Posterior vagus

FIGURE 9–6

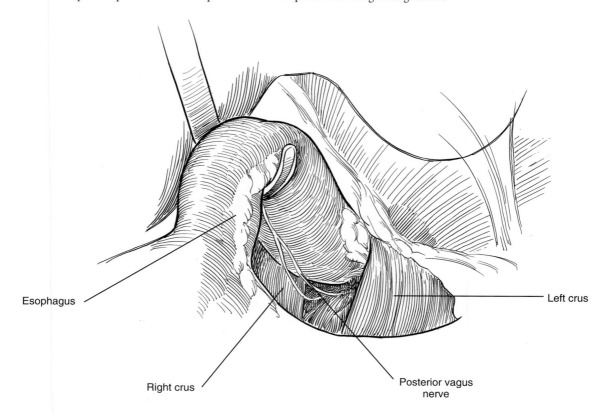

Esophagus

Right crus

Posterior vagus
nerve

Left crus

FIGURE 9-7

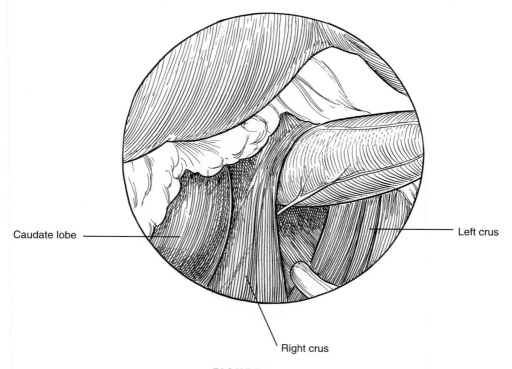

Caudate lobe

Right crus

Left crus

FIGURE 9-8

FIGURE 9–7. Complete dissection of the crura is required to create a large infraesophageal window that allows the esophagus to be encircled with a Penrose drain. A reticulating instrument or curved instrument is helpful to get around the esophagus once a window has been created. Getting around the esophagus is a critical step during which the esophagus may be perforated or the left pleural cavity entered.

FIGURE 9–8. To avoid these complications, this dissection must be performed under direct vision, not by blind puncture. To avoid entering the left pleural cavity, the window must be created between the left crura and the stomach. Once we see the left diaphragm through this space, we place a roticulating instrument through it and enlarge the space by spreading it.

FIGURE 9–9. Once the esophagus has been encircled with an instrument, the crura are cleared and a large space has been created. The crura are then closed. One or two interrupted nonabsorbable 0 sutures are used and are tied extracorporeally.

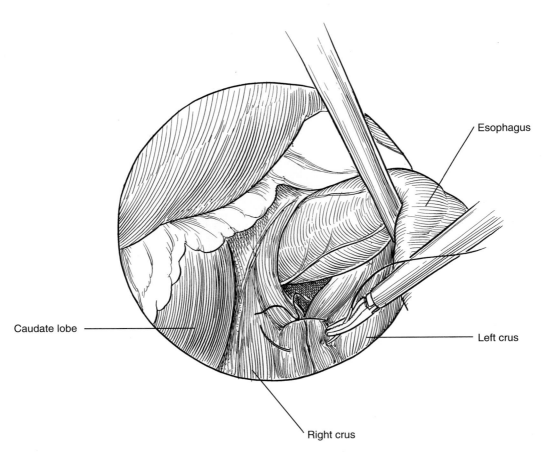

FIGURE 9–9

FIGURE 9-10. It is important not to tie the crural closure too tightly. If it is, it can make passing the bougie later in the procedure difficult and can lead to postoperative dysphagia. To ensure that the closure is not too tight, the space between the last stitch and the esophagus is checked with a 10-mm instrument, which should pass easily through the space. During this dissection we avoid irrigation, which tends to obliterate landmarks and makes the dissection more difficult. We generally dissect the esophagus from the surrounding tissue between the esophagus and the posterior vagus nerve. This tissue plane is easier to dissect than that beneath the posterior vagus nerve, which frequently contains a lot of associated fatty tissue.

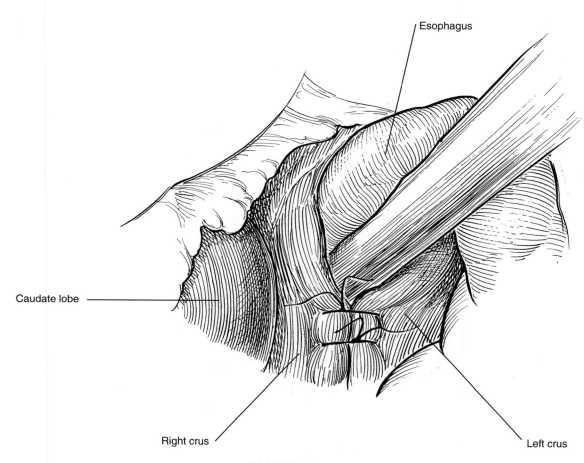

FIGURE 9-10

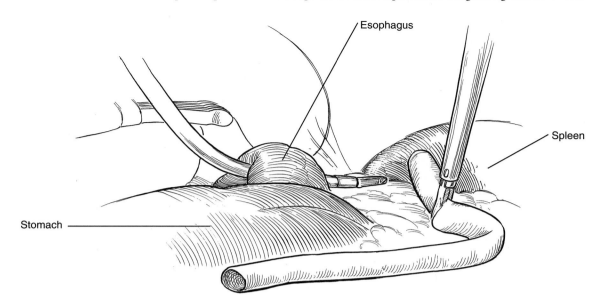

Esophagus

Spleen

Stomach

FIGURE 9–11

FIGURE 9–11. Once the crura are closed, the esophagus is encircled with a Penrose drain. The ¼-inch Penrose drain is cut to approximately 6 inches and passed down the left midclavicular 10-mm cannula. An instrument is passed down the same cannula and is used to feed the end of the drain to the curved instrument that has been passed through the 5-mm subxiphoid cannula underneath the esophagus to the left upper quadrant.

The gastroesophageal fat pad is also removed using the LCS. The sharp edge of the LCS is used to remove the pad until the one or two vessels feeding it are found. These are coagulated with the dull side of the blade.

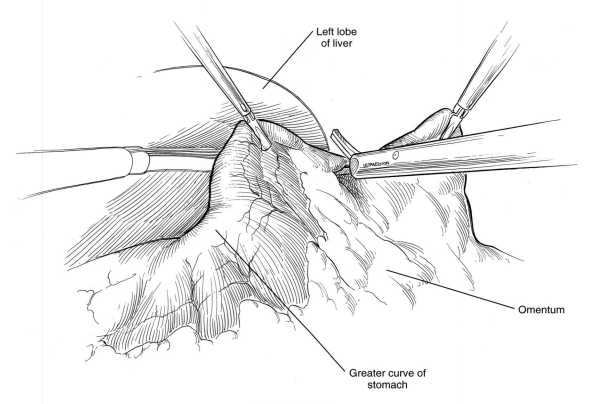

FIGURE 9–12

FIGURE 9-12. Attention is next directed to the greater curve of the stomach at the level of the inferior pole of the spleen. Dissection is aimed at dividing all the vessels to the entire greater curvature as far as the esophageal hiatus. This is done using the LCS. No clips or electrosurgery are used. Since only one instrument is used to coagulate and cut the vessels and tissues, there are no instrument changes. For most of this dissection, the blunt side of the LCS is used.

The stomach is grasped with a grasper through the 5-mm subxiphoid port, and the gastrosplenic ligament is grasped with a 5-mm grasper through the left midclavicular port. The LCS is brought into the abdomen through the lower 10-mm port, where it grasps the tissue and is activated. Coagulation with the LCS is inversely proportional to the tension placed on the tissue, the grip strength on the tissue, and the blade displacement. The tissue is coagulated and cut by varying these factors. Generally, we use level 3 for coagulating (less displacement) and level 5 for cutting (maximum displacement). Once we see the tissue blanching, we pull the LCS off the tissue axially while it is closed, which usually results in cutting.

FIGURE 9-13. Once a space has been created into the lesser sac, the vessels in the gastrosplenic ligament are divided using the LCS. This includes division of the short gastric vessels. As the dissection continues, the graspers are continuously moved cephalad to maintain traction and exposure.

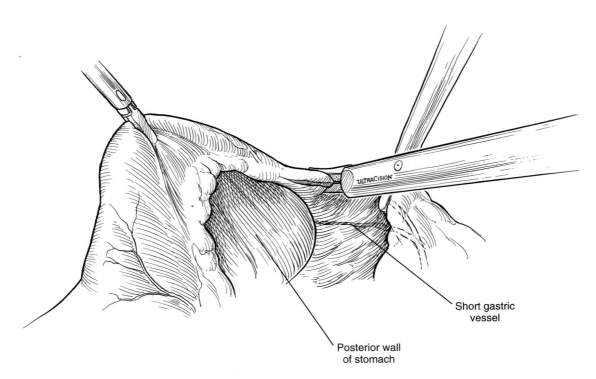

Short gastric vessel

Posterior wall of stomach

FIGURE 9-13

FIGURE 9-14. The difficult part of this dissection is the most important part—namely, division of the first few short gastric blood vessels and division of the reflection of the phrenoesophageal ligament onto the fundus of the stomach. This most superior portion of the dissection may require additional traction on the stomach by means of a grasper brought through the 10-mm right upper quadrant cannula. The liver is therefore no longer retracted. However, this does not interfere with the dissection. It may be occasionally necessary to bring the LCS through the 10-mm left midclavicular port and the camera through the lower 10-mm cannula. The gastrosplenic ligament is then grasped through the 10-mm midline port. This provides a better view of this area, which can facilitate dissection.

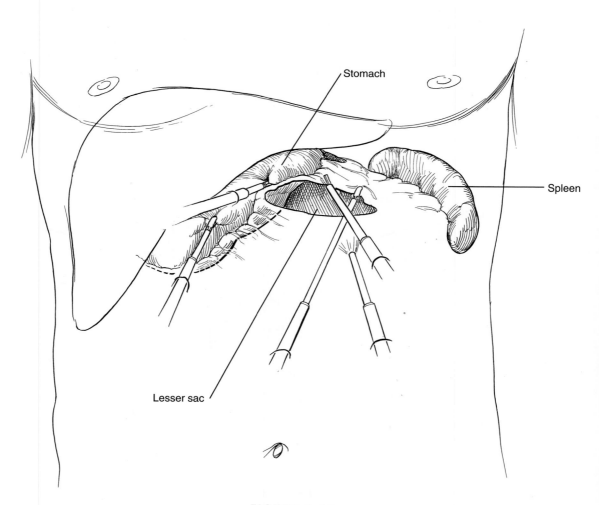

FIGURE 9-14

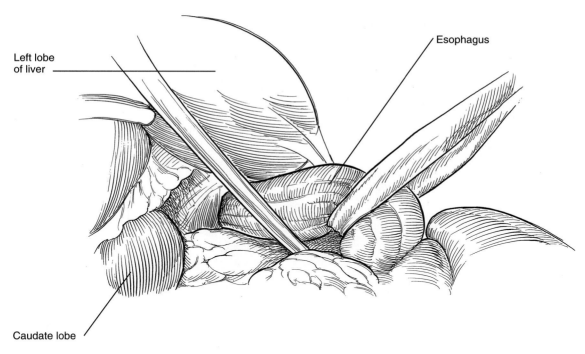

Left lobe
of liver

Esophagus

Caudate lobe

FIGURE 9–15

FIGURE 9–15. The wrap is performed once complete division of the short gastric vessels and clearance of the phrenoesophageal ligament has been completed. A reticulated instrument is passed through the 5-mm cannula into the abdomen and beneath the esophagus into the left upper quadrant. To ease this maneuver, both ends of the Penrose drain are grasped first, and the drain is then elevated toward the anterior abdominal wall. This opens the infraesophageal space and allows the reticulated dissector to be placed under direct vision to avoid perforation of the esophagus.

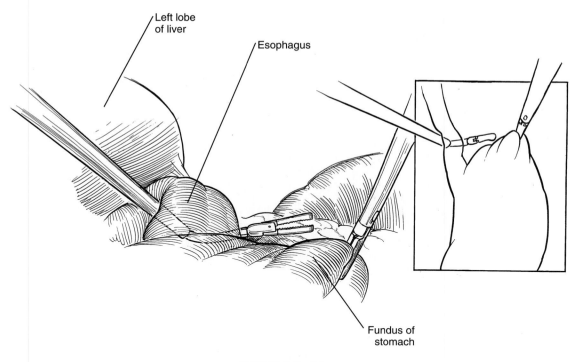

Left lobe
of liver

Esophagus

Fundus of
stomach

FIGURE 9–16

FIGURE 9–16. The fundus of the stomach is grasped with the reticulated grasper by bringing the fundus on the greater curvature edge to the instrument. A firm purchase on the fundus is established, and the fundus is dragged beneath the esophagus. We prefer to push the esophagus toward the left side of the patient while gently pulling the fundus to the patient's right side.

FIGURE 9–17. Once the fundus has been pulled through to the left side, we affirm the absence of tension by letting it go. It should stay where it is. If it retracts, either the fundus has not been fully mobilized or the retroesophageal window is too small.

The next step, placing the 60 French bougie in the stomach, is critical to the procedure and to the avoidance of complications. The bougie may be caught up as it comes through the crura or as it comes into the stomach. This step must be performed under direct vision and requires

great care on the part of the anesthesiologist. A pointed dilator such as a Maloney dilator should not be used because the tip can easily perforate the esophagus. Prior to passing the bougie, we grasp the fundus with a Babcock clamp because the fundus will pull back to the left side as the bougie comes down. The orogastric tube is also removed before the bougie is passed. The use of the orogastric tube together with a smaller bougie (such as a 48 French) should be avoided because it is very difficult to tell if both are in the stomach.

FIGURE 9–18. The final steps of the procedure are the suturing of the wrap. Three 0 nonabsorbable sutures are used over a distance of 2 cm. These are tied extracorporeally but can be tied intracorporeally. Large bites approximately 1 cm deep that are transmural are taken on the stomach. The first two sutures catch the esophagus to the (patient's) right of the anterior vagus nerve.

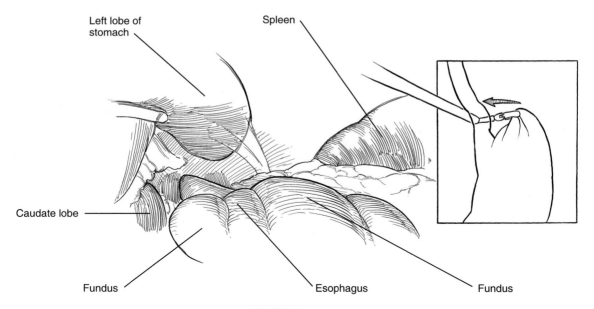

Left lobe of stomach

Spleen

Caudate lobe

Fundus

Esophagus

Fundus

FIGURE 9–17

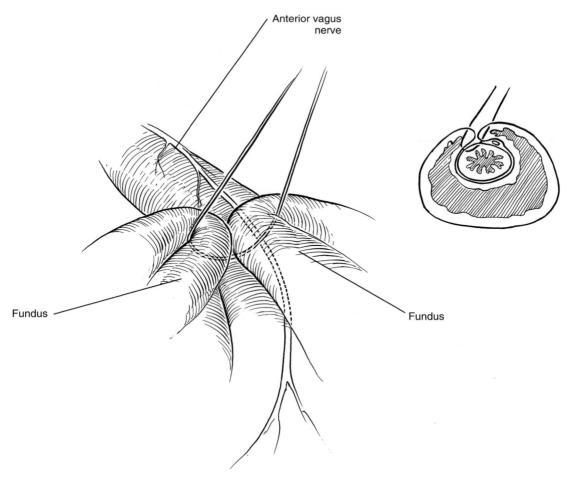

Anterior vagus nerve

Fundus

Fundus

FIGURE 9–18

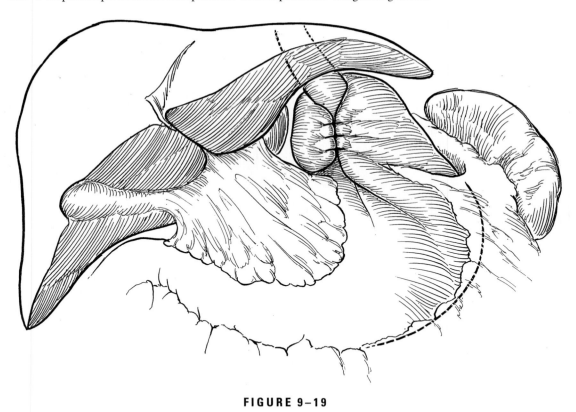

FIGURE 9–19

FIGURE 9–19. Once the wrap is complete, the operative area is irrigated with saline and aspirated to ensure hemostasis. The 10-mm cannulas are removed under direct vision and closed with absorbable suture. The skin is closed at all cannula sites with 4–0 nonabsorbable sutures, and the skin and subcutaneous tissues are infiltrated with bupivacaine.

X. Postoperative Medications

Patients are given intramuscular meperidine according to body weight in the recovery room. They then receive oral acetaminophen-codeine or oxycodone as needed. They also receive an additional dose of cefazolin 1 g in the recovery room.

XI. Advancement of Diet

Patients are given clear liquids for the next 24 hours. They are then allowed to eat soft foods but no red meats or bread products, which may get stuck at an edematous gastroesophageal junction. Patients are advised to continue this diet for the first two postoperative weeks.

XII. Determinants of Discharge

Patients are discharged when they can manage their pain with oral analgesics, are ambulatory, have no fever or tachycardia, and have eaten a soft diet. Typically this is 48 hours after surgery.

XIII. Return to Normal Activity/Work

Patients are allowed to return to their normal activities as tolerated immediately after surgery. The only restriction is that they should not drive for 3 to 4 days and while taking analgesics. They are usually able to return to work in 2 to 3 weeks.

Chapter 10

Laparoscopic Toupet Partial Fundoplication

LEE L. SWANSTROM, M.D.

I. Indications

A. Patients with primary esophageal motility disorder and gastroesophageal reflux disease
B. Patients with secondary esophageal motility disorder and gastroesophageal reflux disease
C. Patients with severe aerophagia and gastroesophageal reflux disease
D. Patients with gastroesophageal reflux disease who have insufficient cardia or fundus to construct a 360-degree fundoplication
E. Patients who are unwilling or unable to tolerate the potential side effects of a 360-fundoplication such as the inability to belch, presence of intestinal gas, transient dysphagia, and early satiety

II. Contraindications

A. Inability to tolerate general anesthesia
B. Severe gastroesophageal reflux disease with a DeMeester score greater than 100
C. Inability to tolerate carbon dioxide pneumoperitoneum due to severe chronic obstructive pulmonary disease
D. Morbid obesity (relative)
E. Multiple previous upper abdominal operations (relative)
F. Shortened esophagus (relative)
G. Dysplastic Barrett's epithelium (relative)

III. Factors Important in Patient Selection

A. Upper endoscopy
B. Esophageal manometry
C. 24-hour pH monitoring
D. Barium swallow

IV. Preoperative Preparation

A. Admission to short-stay unit 2 hours before surgery
B. Discharge instructions are given to the patient preoperatively and are reviewed with the admitting nurse.
C. Preoperative medications: third-generation cephalosporin antibiotic
D. Preoperative sedation before the patient is transferred to the operating room
E. No bowel preparation is required.

V. Choice of Anesthesia

A. General endotracheal anesthesia performed by an anesthesiologist who is familiar with both reflux patients and laparoscopic surgery
B. Preemptive analgesia is obtained by infiltrating all trocar sites with long-acting local anesthetic before the trocar is inserted.

C. Toradol is given intravenously (IV) 30 minutes before the completion of the operation.
D. No invasive monitoring devices are required.
E. End-tidal CO_2 and O_2 saturation monitors are used.

VI. Accessory Devices

A. A Foley catheter is not used unless the operation is expected to last more than 2 hours. Patients are asked to void before they leave the short stay area.
B. Pneumatic compression stockings
C. Orogastric tube
D. 56 French esophageal dilator

VII. Instruments and Telescopes

A. High-quality video camera and two large video monitors.
B. 45-degree laparoscope
C. Bipolar scissors
D. Atraumatic liver retractor, preferably 5 mm
E. Table rail mounted holding device for the liver retractor
F. Short atraumatic grasper such as 5-mm Glassman grasper
G. Monopolar Maryland dissector
H. Good curved-tip, axial-grip laparoscopic needle holders
I. 5-mm atraumatic Babcock grasper
J. Multiple clip appliers or the laparoscopic coagulating shears (UltraCision, Smithfield, RI)

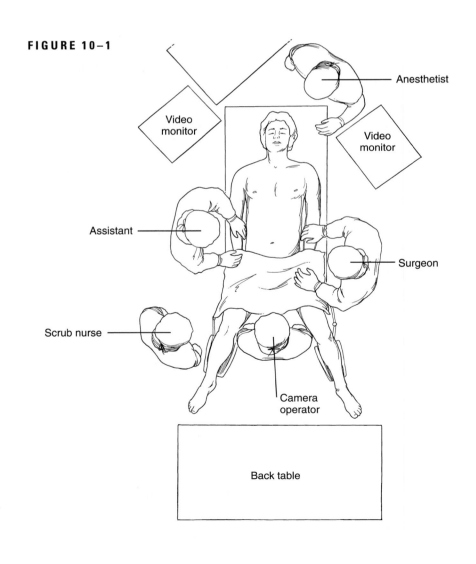

FIGURE 10–1

Anesthetist

Video monitor

Video monitor

Assistant

Surgeon

Scrub nurse

Camera operator

Back table

VIII. Position of Monitors and Placement of Trocars

FIGURE 10-1. The patient is placed in a modified Lloyd-Davies position using Allen stirrups. Both arms are tucked in at the patient's side when possible. The two monitors are placed near either shoulder. The surgeon stands at the patient's left side with the assistant surgeon on the other side. The camera operator stands or sits between the patient's legs.

FIGURE 10-2. Five trocars are used. The initial 10-mm trocar is placed just to the left of the midline and 15 cm from the xyphoid. A second 10-mm trocar is inserted in the left upper quadrant. Three 5-mm trocars are placed in the right upper quadrant: one near the xyphoid, one to the right of the umbilicus, and one on the midclavicular line.

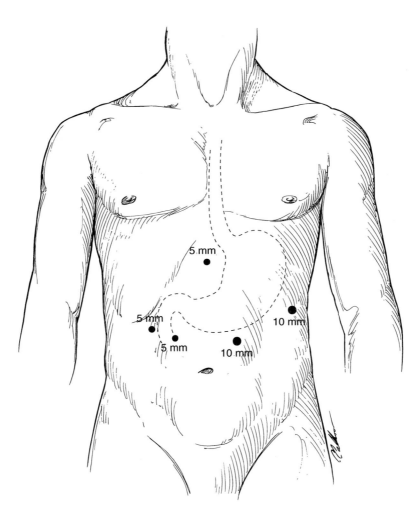

FIGURE 10-2

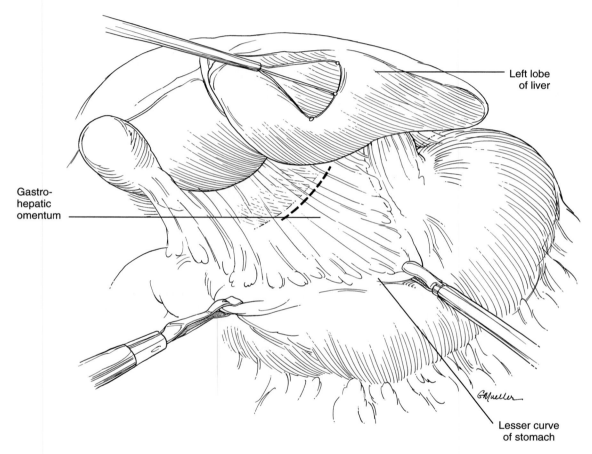

Left lobe
of liver

Gastro-
hepatic
omentum

Lesser curve
of stomach

FIGURE 10–3

IX. Narrative of Surgical Technique

FIGURE 10-3. Once general anesthesia has been induced the patient is placed in a low lithotomy position with arms tucked or out on carefully padded armboards. A Veress needle is used to gain access to the left of the midline in the upper abdomen approximately 15 cm below the xyphoid. The abdomen is then insufflated to the maximum pressure of 15 mm of carbon dioxide. A 10-mm trocar is inserted, and the abdomen is carefully explored. Additional trocars (as illustrated in Fig. 10–2) are placed under direct vision. The patient is then placed in a steep reverse Trendelenburg position, and an atraumatic liver retractor is carefully inserted beneath the left lobe of the liver and lifted upward. This retractor is fastened to a mechanical instrument holder to hold the liver securely in place. The assistant grasps the perigastric fat on the lesser curvature and retracts the stomach laterally.

FIGURE 10-4. The surgeon then uses the bipolar scissors to divide the gastrohepatic ligaments starting in the clear area and following the medial edge of the caudate lobe cephalad. Low-lying hepatic vagal branches are preserved, or, if these branches are high in the gastrohepatic omentum, they can be routinely divided. In 15 per cent of patients a replaced left hepatic artery courses through the gastrohepatic ligament. These arteries should be preserved and left in place.

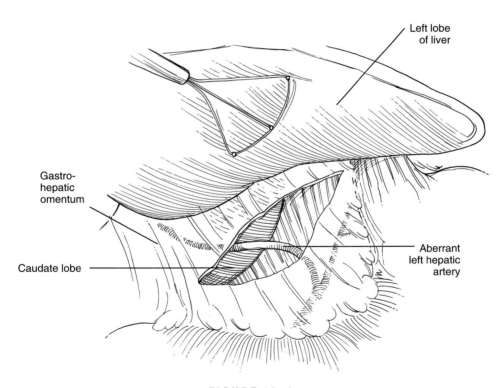

FIGURE 10-4

FIGURE 10-5. The right crus is identified and dissected by dividing the phrenoesophageal ligament medial to the crus and entering the mediastinum. The right crus is dissected down to its junction with the left crus posteriorly.

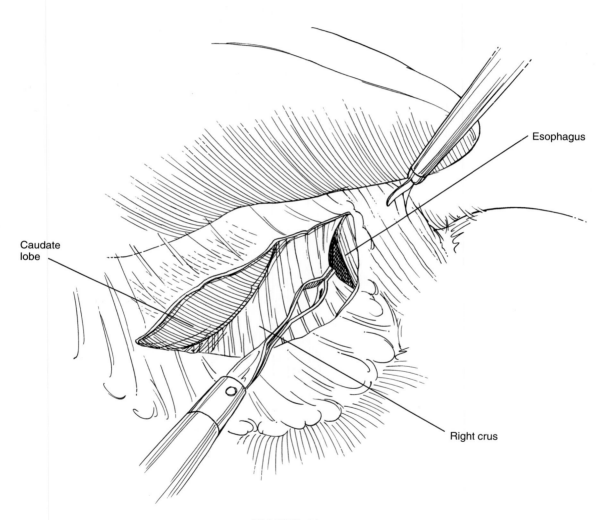

FIGURE 10-5

FIGURE 10-6. The anterior aspect of the mediastinal esophagus is then dissected free using sharp bipolar dissection. The left crus is exposed, and the esophagus is separated from the left crus. The angle of His and the cardia of the stomach are dissected off the left crus and diaphragm.

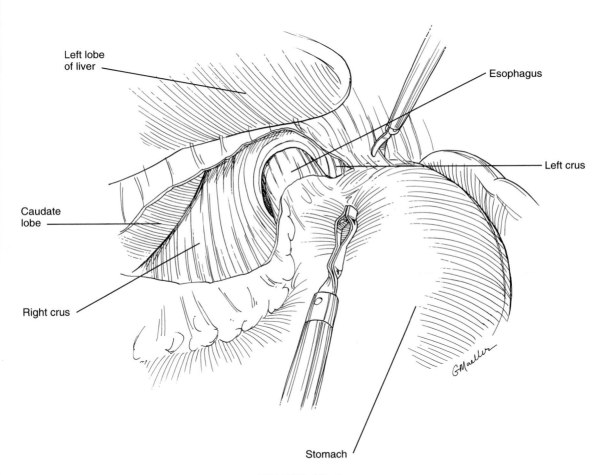

FIGURE 10-6

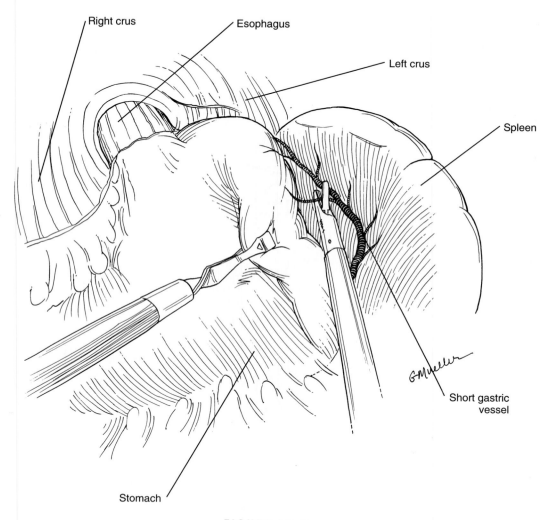

Right crus

Esophagus

Left crus

Spleen

Short gastric
vessel

Stomach

FIGURE 10–7

FIGURE 10–7. Attention is then turned to the short gastric vessels starting at the level of the midsplenic hilum. The omentum is grasped and retracted inferiorly, and the stomach is retracted medially with the surgeon's left hand. The short gastric vessels are divided starting low and working toward the esophagus. The vessels can be divided either by dissecting, clipping, and dividing them or by using the ultrasonic coagulating shears. Thoroughness is critical in this step, and both the anterior leaflet of the short gastric vessels and the posterior leaflet should be divided to allow full mobility of the fundus.

FIGURE 10–8. Attention is then returned to the gastroesophageal junction. Using the 45-degree angled laparoscope, the retroesophageal space is carefully visualized and the posterior mediastinal attachments are taken down using the bipolar scissors. This creates a window beneath the esophagus that can be progressively mobilized down into the abdomen to provide the intra-abdominal length of esophagus needed for the fundoplication. The vagus nerve is left with the esophagus if it is closely adherent, or, if it lies posterior, it is excluded from the wrap (illustrated).

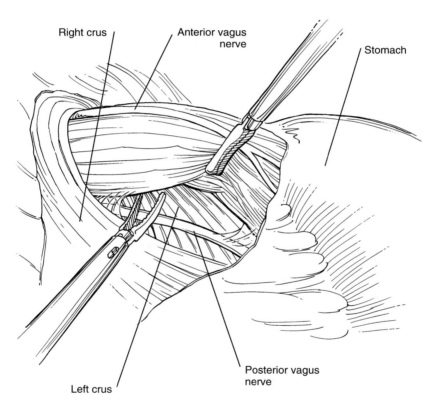

FIGURE 10–8

FIGURE 10-9. The assistant can now reach through the created window and grasp the previously freed fundus to bring it beneath the esophagus. This wrap is used to retract the esophagus laterally, providing adequate exposure of both the posterior aspect of the wrap and the right and left crura beneath the esophagus. Interrupted intracorporeally tied or extracorporeally tied sutures can then be placed from the posterior aspect of this wrap first to the left crus and then to the right crus. After the posterior fixation suture has been placed, one or two additional sutures are placed from the posterior wrap to both the right and left crura beneath the esophagus, and an additional suture is placed from the upper portion of the wrap to the upper right and left crura. This should line the wrap up appropriately to allow performance of the final two esophageal suture rows.

FIGURE 10-10. Before placing the anterior sutures the bougie is carefully advanced back into the esophagus. The wrap should be gauged to be a minimum of 270 degrees. Interrupted intracorporeally tied sutures of nonabsorbable suture material are then placed between the left and right wraps to the corresponding portion of the anterior esophagus. Care must be taken not to entrap the anterior vagus nerve with these suture rows. The wrap should be approximately 3 cm long, and this usually requires two to three sutures on each side. At the completion of this step the bougie is withdrawn, and the area is irrigated with saline to remove all blood from the upper abdomen. The liver retractor is carefully withdrawn, and the abdomen is deinsufflated after the two 10-mm trocar sites have been closed with transfascial sutures. The skin is then closed with interrupted subcuticular sutures, and waterproof dressings are applied.

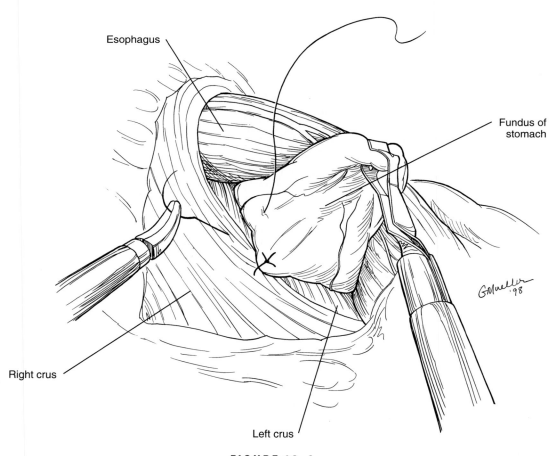

Esophagus

Fundus of stomach

Right crus

Left crus

FIGURE 10-9

X. Postoperative Medications

A. Morphine sulfate IV as needed
B. Hydrocodone elixir given orally as needed
C. Ondansetron 4 mg IV every 6 hours as needed
D. Additional medications as required by underlying medical problems

XI. Advancement of Diet

The patient is kept nil per os (NPO) for the first 6 hours. Then he or she is started on clear liquids and advanced to a soft diet as tolerated. At discharge the patient is sent home with instructions to remain on a soft diet for 10 days postoperatively. In addition, the patient is warned to avoid extremes of hot and cold liquids and to avoid carbonated beverages for the first 2 weeks.

XII. Determinants of Discharge

The majority of patients are able to go home on postoperative day 1. Patients must demonstrate an ability to tolerate a soft diet, be afebrile, and have good pain control with oral narcotics. It is critical for these patients not to be discharged home if they are nauseated; they should be kept in the hospital until the nausea is under control.

XIII. Return to Normal Activity/Work

After discharge from the hospital patients are encouraged to be as active as possible. Workers are encouraged to return to work at 1 week. They are requested, however, to perform only light duty with no lifting of more than 25 pounds for a total of 3 weeks following surgery. In our experience a week at home is long enough to allow adequate recuperation. Weight-lifting restrictions may be essential because some reports have described a higher rate of wrap disruptions following an immediate return to heavy lifting.

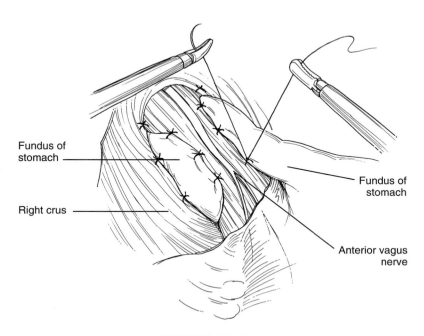

Fundus of stomach

Right crus

Fundus of stomach

Anterior vagus nerve

FIGURE 10–10

Laparoscopic Hill Repair

LUCIUS D. HILL, M.D., and DAVID E. MAZZA, M.D.

I. Indications

A. Intractability or failure of medical therapy
B. Desire to avoid lifelong medication
C. Severe esophagitis
D. Esophageal stricture
E. Esophageal ulceration
F. Bleeding from esophagitis or esophageal ulcer
G. Respiratory complications of gastroesophageal reflux (chronic aspiration)
H. Barrett's esophagus
I. Large hiatal hernia that causes cardiorespiratory embarrassment

II. Contraindications

A. Reoperation for a previously performed antireflux surgery (absolute)
B. Medical contraindication for pneumoperitoneum (absolute)
C. Gross obesity (relative)
D. Previous upper abdominal surgery (relative)

III. Factors Important in Patient Selection

A. History of gastroesophageal reflux disease (GERD)
  1. Severity of reflux
  2. Complications of reflux
  3. Medical treatment: duration, result
  4. Documentation of coexisting medical or surgical problems

B. Preoperative evaluation of GERD
  1. Endoscopy for assessment of:
    a. Severity of esophagitis
    b. Ulceration or stricture
    c. Barrett's esophagus
    d. Gastroesophageal flap valve
    e. Dysplasia or cancer
  2. Upper gastrointestinal radiographs (when indicated) for assessment of:
    a. Stenosis
    b. Ulceration
    c. Hiatal hernia
    d. Foregut anatomy
  3. Esophageal manometry (in most patients considered for surgery) for assessment of:
    a. Lower esophageal sphincter pressure
    b. Esophageal motility
  4. 24-hour pH monitoring (when indicated)
  5. Abdominal CT scan or ultrasound (when indicated) to rule out tumors in the retroperitoneal area and pelvis (i.e., areas inaccessible to laparoscopic evaluation)

IV. Preoperative Preparation

A. A modified nasogastric tube (NGT) is inserted prior to surgery.
B. A urinary catheter is placed.
C. Pneumatic compression stockings are used in all patients.

V. Choice of Anesthesia

General anesthesia is used in all cases.

VI. Accessory Devices

A. Esophageal manometer to measure the pressure of the lower esophageal sphincter after construction of the repair.

B. Modified nasogastric tube with a standard sump part and an additional portion with an internal diameter of 1.2 mm and a side built-in pressure port. This NGT is used to decompress the stomach during surgery and to perform intraoperative manometric measurements

C. Video endoscope to assess the newly recreated gastroesophageal valve at the end of the procedure

D. Guide wire and 36 French dilator

VII. Instruments and Telescopes

A. 30-degree telescope

B. 5-mm laparoscopic needle holders

C. Liver retractor attached to self-retaining system to elevate left lobe of liver

D. 5-mm electrocautery scissors

E. 5-mm laparoscopic graspers

F. Laparoscopic Babcock clamp (5 or 10 mm) (optional)

G. Suction/irrigation device

H. Clip applier

I. Fascia-closing device

J. Knot tier (extracorporeal tying)

K. 0 polyester sutures 36 inches long (at least) and color-coded

VIII. Operating Room Set Up and Position of Trocars

FIGURE 11–1. The patient is placed in a modified Lloyd-Davies position with his or her legs in Allen stirrups. The surgeon stands between the legs of the patient. The assistant surgeon is on the patient's left side, and the camera operator is on the patient's right side. The two video monitors are near either shoulder of the patient.

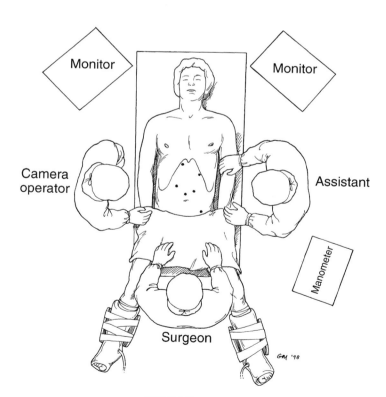

FIGURE 11–1

FIGURE 11-2. This figure shows the positions of the six trocars. The liver retractor is inserted through the L1 trocar (10 mm) and is used to elevate the left lobe of the liver. A second L2 is shown that can be used as an alternative site for the 5-mm flexion liver retractor. The 10-mm 30-degree telescope is inserted through the supraumbilical 11-mm trocar (C). The surgeon operates using a two-handed technique through trocars S1 (5 mm) and S2 (11 mm). The assistant uses trocar A (11 mm) and a second optional port at B (5 or 10 mm) for retraction. A Babcock clamp can be used for retraction through B.

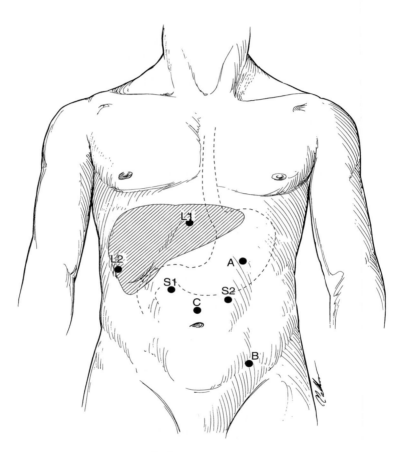

FIGURE 11-2

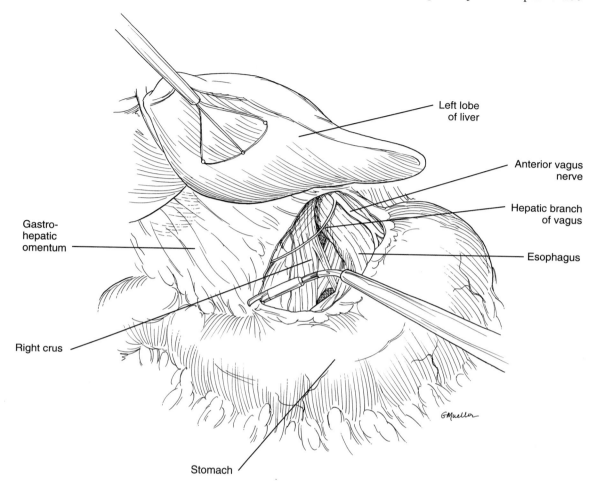

Left lobe
of liver

Anterior vagus
nerve

Hepatic branch
of vagus

Esophagus

Gastro-
hepatic
omentum

Right crus

Stomach

FIGURE 11–3

IX. Narrative of Surgical Technique

Endoscopy is performed once the patient has been anesthetized to introduce a guide wire over which a dilator can be safely passed later when needed. The modified NG tube (with a side pressure port for manometrics) is passed at this time also.

FIGURE 11–3. The left hepatic lobe has been lifted, exposing the esophageal hiatus. Incision of the gastrohepatic omentum follows. The hepatic branch of the vagus nerve must be divided, and an artery that occasionally accompanies it is clipped and severed.

The phrenoesophageal membrane is divided (from the patient's right to left) to expose the anterior esophageal wall. The anterior phrenoesophageal bundle, fibroareolar tissue that surrounds the GEJ, is thus obtained (dissection must be kept close to the diaphragm). Caution must be used not to injure the anterior vagus nerve or the esophagus. To avoid the risk of pneumomediastinum we do not dissect the esophagus up into the mediastinum.

Dissection of the right crus from the esophagus down to its confluence with the left crus is accomplished through an avascular plane.

FIGURE 11–4. Following the left crus superiorly (an artery running parallel to the left crus commonly has to be divided) while diverting the esophagus to the patient's left opens a retroesophageal space that allows exposure of the posterior aspect of the fundus. Because this fundus is going to be employed later for suturing, sufficient dissection must be performed to avoid tension. During this part of the procedure, care must be taken not to injure the left gastric pedicle. The preaortic fascia is now defined from its most superior part (represented by the confluence of both crura) to the most caudal portion at the level of emergence of the celiac axis. Finally, the important anatomic structures are identified, the crura of the diaphragm, the preaortic fascia, and the vagus nerves. Downward traction on the anterior phrenoesophageal bundle allows visualization of the anterior vagus nerve, and retraction to the patient's left allows identification of the posterior vagus nerve. The posterior phrenoesophageal bundle lies immediately lateral and posterior to the nerve. Placement of the "reinforcing" and repair stitches is done while visualizing both vagus nerves to avoid injury to the nerves by including them in the suture.

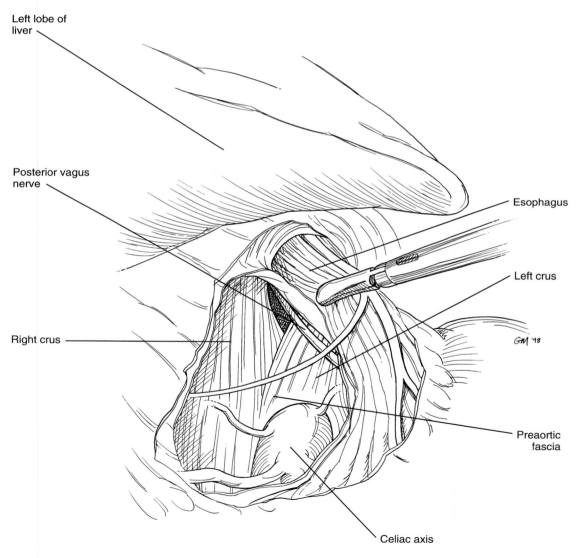

Left lobe of liver

Posterior vagus nerve

Right crus

Esophagus

Left crus

GM '98

Preaortic fascia

Celiac axis

FIGURE 11–4

FIGURE 11-5. Diverting the esophagus to the patient's left allows visualization of both crura. Using 0 nonabsorbable suture material, the esophageal hiatus is closed posteriorly. Usually two sutures suffice. The hiatus is closed securely but not too tightly (an important cause of dysphagia). Tying is extracorporeal. It may be necessary to perform anterior hiatal closure after the repair has been completed.

To further anchor the repair, two or three "reinforcing" seromuscular 0 nonabsorbable stitches are placed from the posterior gastric wall to the left crus and left aspect of the preaortic fascia. Deep penetration into the preaortic fascia is avoided because the aorta lies immediately beneath. The posterior vagus nerve is identified before the stitch is placed.

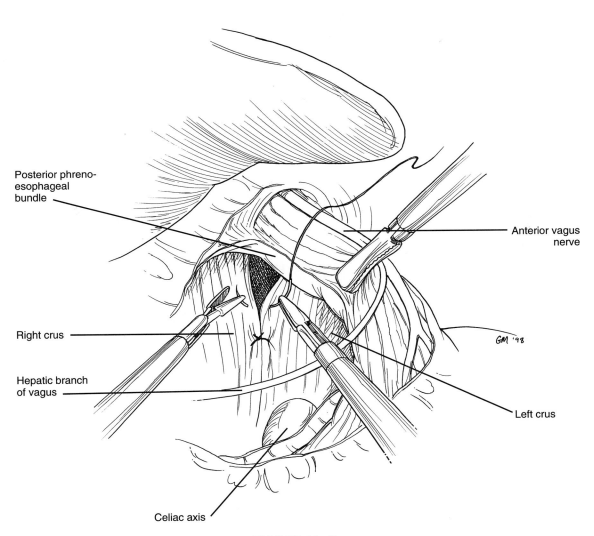

FIGURE 11-5

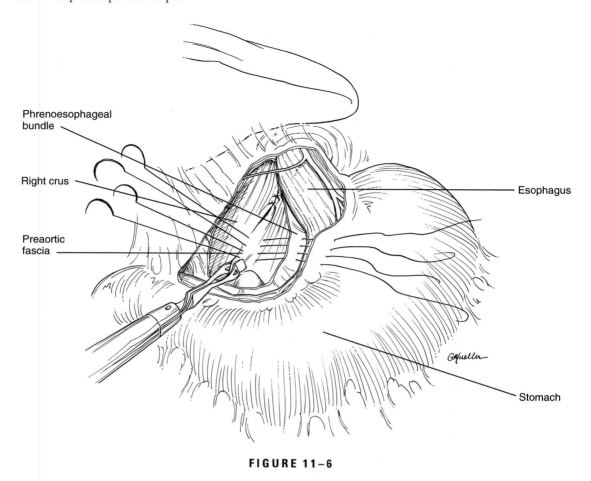

Phrenoesophageal
bundle

Right crus

Preaortic
fascia

Esophagus

Stomach

G.Mueller

FIGURE 11-6

FIGURE 11-6. Placement of the repair sutures follows. In addition to the phrenoesophageal bundle, they all include the seromuscular layer of the stomach (but not entering the gastric or esophageal lumen). The first two sutures are introduced through the surgeon's right-hand port, and the third and fourth through the assistant's port (but these are employed by the surgeon once they are intracorporeal). Using sutures of different colors and adjusting their angle of entry are methods used to avoid crossing them. Employing 0 nonabsorbable suture material, the first and lowermost of four identical sets of sutures is placed; this set includes the anterior bundle and exits just lateral to the anterior vagus nerve. It is aimed in a superior-inferior direction, almost parallel to the vagus nerve.

This same suture passes in front of the esophagus, enters the posterior bundle immediately lateral to the posterior vagus nerve, and exits in the posterior gastric wall. The assistant, by pulling anteriorly on the tissue between the two bundles, greatly enhances exposure.

The preaortic fascia is pulled off the aorta by a Babcock clamp while this suture is passed through the preaortic fascia from the patient's left to right. This lowermost suture must include the most caudal portion of the preaortic fascia while avoiding the celiac artery. Placement of a grasper against the suture while it is being pulled back out of the trocar diverts tension from the tissue and avoids sawing through it.

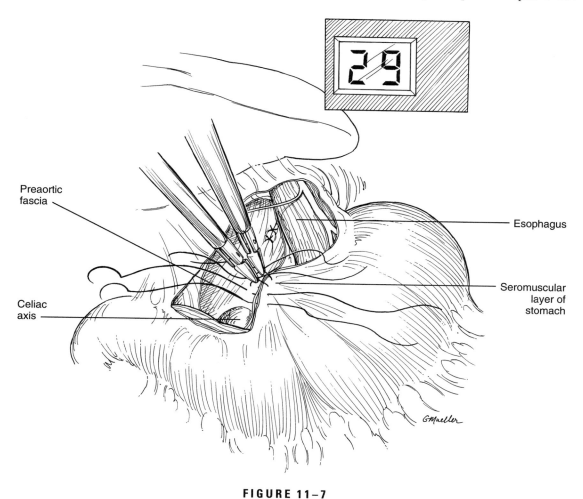

Preaortic
fascia

Esophagus

Celiac
axis

Seromuscular
layer of
stomach

GMueller

FIGURE 11–7

FIGURE 11–7. Three more repair sutures are placed. These are identical but parallel to the first one, advancing superiorly with 3 to 4 mm between each set of stitches. If the sutures are placed too close together, the repair will probably be loose; conversely, if separation is important, the last suture will be too high on the bundle, and the repair may be tight. Both vagus nerves are visualized when placing every suture.

With the four sutures in place, a 36 French dilator is advanced over a guide wire alongside the modified NGT and placed across the GEJ. The top two sutures are tied with a single throw in the knot and clamped. At this time, using the NGT, two or three manometric readings are taken (an average is calculated) but not before withdrawing the dilator. For our system, the ideal pressure is 25 to 35 mm Hg.

Depending on the result and the appearance of the repair, the two top sutures are either tied (over the dilator, which is reinserted), loosened, or tightened. A manometric reading is performed every time these two sutures are adjusted. Once an adequate pressure and appearance have been obtained and all sutures have been tied, a final reading is performed (without the dilator). At this point, if the pressure is still low or the repair seems loose, additional sutures from the anterior bundle to the preaortic fascia can usually be used to increase the pressure. Conversely, pulling the anterior bundle laterally loosens a repair that seems too tight or yields a high lower esophageal sphincter pressure. (For all sutures, the bundles are pulled inferiorly as they are tied.)

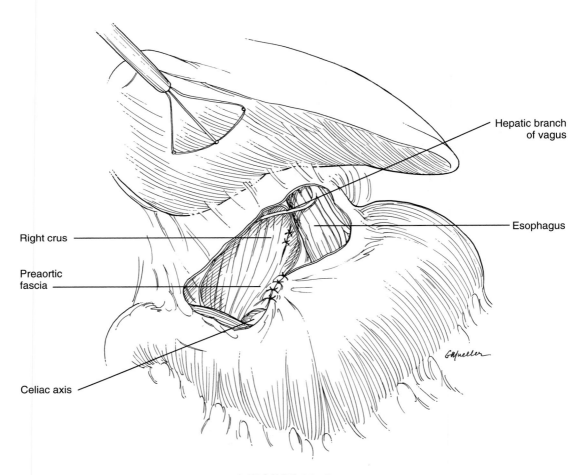

Hepatic branch
of vagus

Esophagus

Right crus

Preaortic
fascia

Celiac axis

FIGURE 11-8

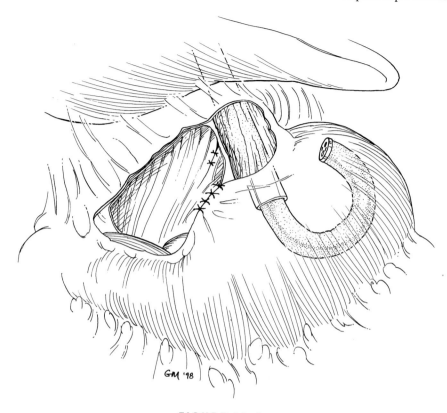

FIGURE 11-9

FIGURE 11-8. If necessary, anterior closure of the hiatus is performed. A suture is also placed from the anterior fundus (using 0 nonabsorbable material) to the diaphragm to prevent a paraesophageal hernia. Finally, a suture is placed from the fundus to the right crus, and two or three are placed from the anterior gastric wall to the right side of the preaortic fascia. These stitches further accentuate the endoscopic appearance of the valve.

FIGURE 11-9. Assessment of a Grade I valve is obtained with endoscopy. This evaluation also rules out an obstruction caused by an overly tight repair. Rarely at this point is there a need for modifications to the repair, but it may be necessary to place some extra stitches or to replace some. A Grade I valve is clearly defined as a musculomucosal fold opposed to the endoscope through all phases of respiration. It is created by the oblique angle of entry of the esophagus into the stomach and extends 3 to 4 cm along the lesser curve.

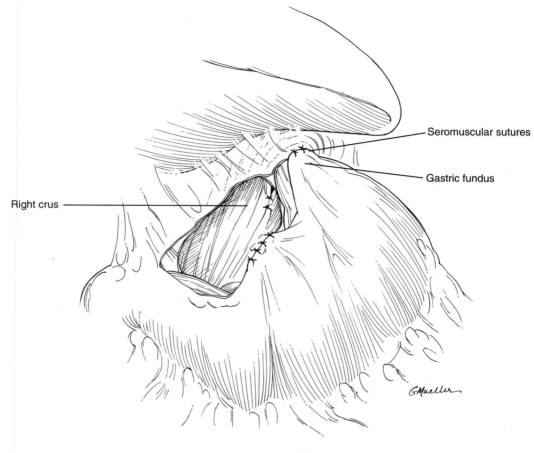

Right crus

Seromuscular sutures

Gastric fundus

FIGURE 11–10

FIGURE 11–10. The final aspect of the repair is shown with the sutures from the seromuscular layer of the gastric fundus to the edge of the diaphragmatic hiatus in place.

The trocars are removed under direct vision, using a fascia-closing device, all 10-mm sites are closed, and subcuticular stitches are used for the skin.

X. Postoperative Medications

A. Continuation of preoperative antibiotic for 24 hours
B. Analgesics as required
C. Metoclopramide in some cases

XI. Advancement of Diet

A. NG tube removed in the operating room
B. When patient is alert, a clear liquid diet is begun—no ice, no carbonated drinks
C. Progression to a bland diet as tolerated
D. Small, frequent meals are advised.

XII. Determinants of Discharge

A. Usually in the first 48 hours
B. Determinants:
   1. Tolerance of diet
   2. Absence of postoperative ileus
   3. Absence of gastric distention
      a. Cause of repair disruption
      b. May require gastric suction

XIII. Return to Normal Activity/Work

A. Return to work in 10 to 15 days
B. No physical activity (other than walking) for 6 weeks
C. Avoid constipation

Chapter 12

Laparoscopic Repair of Paraesophageal Hernias

DAVID C. BROOKS, M.D.

I. Indications

A. Presence of a paraesophageal hernia:
   1. Type 2 hiatal hernia

FIGURE 12–1. Two types of hernias occur at the esophageal hiatus. Type 1, or sliding esophageal hernias, are associated with gastroesophageal (GE) reflux (A). In this hernia, the gastroesophageal junction herniates from its normal position just inferior to the diaphragm into the chest. These hernias may be asymptomatic or may produce symptoms. They should be repaired only for intractable symptoms of reflux or the complications of reflux.

B, Type 2, or paraesophageal hernias, on the other hand, rarely produce symptoms but should be repaired when they are identified because of their well-documented potential to cause serious sequelae such as incarceration or bleeding. Type 2 hernias are differentiated from Type I hernias by the location of the GE junction. In a Type 2 hernia, the GE junction maintains its normal position at the inferior margin of the diaphragm. However, a patulous hiatus is present, and portions of the fundus or the body of the stomach herniate into the chest through the widened hiatus. Previous series that have examined the natural history of paraesophageal hernias have clearly demonstrated serious morbidity and mortality when these hernias are not repaired.

II. Contraindications

A. Inability to tolerate general anesthesia
   1. Inadequate pulmonary reserve
   2. Recent myocardial infarction
   3. Inadequate cardiac reserve
B. Uncorrectable coagulopathy

III. Factors Important in Patient Selection

A. Adequate cardiac and pulmonary reserve
B. Minimal prior upper abdominal surgery
C. Determination of presence or absence of gastroesophageal reflux disease (GERD)
   1. Upper endoscopy
   2. Esophageal manometry
   3. 24-hour esophageal pH monitoring
D. Previous abdominal operations

IV. Preoperative Preparation

A. Preoperative admission
   1. Significant co-morbid disease
      a. Coronary artery disease
      b. Chronic renal failure
      c. Pulmonary insufficiency
      d. Patients on chronic anticoagulation therapy
         i. Anticoagulation therapy stopped 2 days before surgery
         ii. Prothrombin time or Interna-

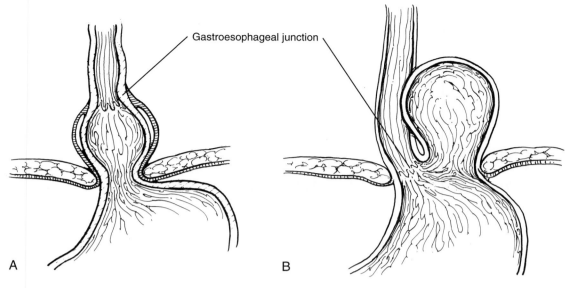

Gastroesophageal junction

A   B

FIGURE 12–1

tional Normalized Ratio (INR) measured
   iii. Intravenous heparin stopped 4 to 6 hours before surgery
   iv. Fresh frozen plasma as needed to adjust prothrombin time
B. Same day admission
  1. All other patients
C. Preoperative medications: none
D. Bowel preparation
  1. No mechanical preparation
  2. Clear liquids for supper the night before surgery

V. Choice of Anesthesia

A. General anesthesia for all patients
  1. Inhalational technique
  2. Avoid nitrous oxide
B. Local anesthesia (bupivacaine 0.5 per cent) in all cannula sites

VI. Accessory Devices

A. Nasogastric tube inserted in all patients and left in place for first postoperative night
B. Large Maloney dilators for sizing of hiatus if fundoplication is constructed
C. Foley catheter inserted in all patients
D. Sequential compression boots on all patients

VII. Instruments and Telescopes (Generic Names)

A. 0-degree and 30-degree laparoscopes
B. CCD camera and processor
C. High-flow CO_2 insufflator
D. Aspiration/irrigation cannula
E. 10-mm cannulas (four)
F. 12-mm cannula (one, optional)
G. Liver retractor
H. 5-mm grasper, atraumatic
I. 5-mm or 10-mm Babcock-type atraumatic grasper (two)
J. Electrified shears
K. Harmonic shears (optional)
L. Endostitch with 0 Dacron sutures (optional)
M. Needle holder

VIII. Patient/Monitor Position and Placement and Size of Trocar

FIGURE 12–2. The patient is placed in a dorsolithotomy position. The legs should be placed in skis rather than hung from stirrups so that there is minimal flexion at the knee. A flatter position of the lower extremity interferes less with camera and instrument manipulation. Furthermore, a flatter position is less likely to cause deep venous thrombosis at the knee. The patient's arms may remain abducted.

A single monitor is placed at the head of the table and slightly toward the left shoulder of the patient, where it can easily be seen by the surgeon and assistants but will not interfere with the anesthesiologist's access to the patient.

A total of five ports is used, corresponding to the set-up for laparoscopic antireflux procedures. In addition to the camera port, accessory ports are placed in the right midclavicular line for liver retraction, in the subxyphoid and left midclavicular position for dissection, and in the left mid to lower abdomen for placement of a Babcock clamp for retraction on the stomach. If the hernia is closed with mesh or reinforced with mesh, a 12-mm cannula is necessary to allow insertion of the endoscopic stapler. Initial access to the abdomen is obtained through a port placed at or slightly above the umbilicus.

A minor variant is to place this cannula slightly to the left of the midline, but I have found that a supraumbilical approach is adequate in all cases.

Recently, I have modified this technique and have found that by placing the camera port slightly below and to the left of the xyphoid process, a 0-degree laparoscope can be placed and provides excellent visualization. A 5-mm left-hand port is placed midway between the xyphoid and the umbilicus, and the right-hand 10-mm port is placed in the left midclavicular region to form an ideal "working triangle." This allows the umbilical port to be used by an assistant to maintain the reduced stomach within the abdomen.

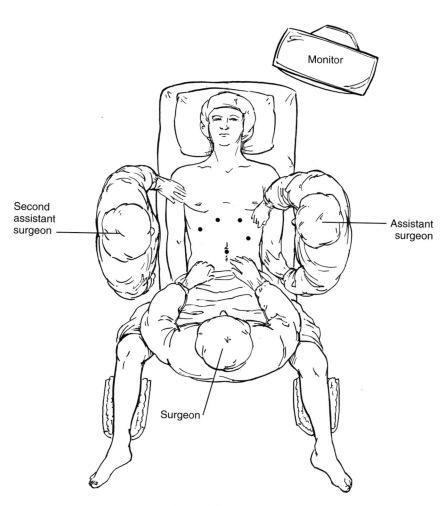

FIGURE 12–2

IX. Narrative of Surgical Technique

The periumbilical port is placed first. An open technique is favored for placement of this cannula because of the ease and speed with which it can be established and the increased margin of safety when it is performed under direct vision. The fascia and peritoneum are incised, and a purse-string suture of 0 Vicryl is placed. The 10-mm cannula is placed in the abdomen, and the purse string is tightened around it with a red rubber catheter tourniquet. This technique ensures a nearly perfect airtight seal. Should any air leak from this port a piece of petrolatum-soaked gauze can be wrapped around the cannula to create an additional seal.

A 0-degree laparoscope is first inserted after pneumoperitoneum has been established. A general exploration of the abdomen is undertaken if possible. Lower abdominal adhesions, if present, are not specifically incised unless there are preoperative indications to do so. After this inspection, the patient is placed in a reverse Trendelenburg position but maintained in a neutral position on the table. The accessory ports are then placed. Entry into the peritoneum through a safe site can be ascertained by transilluminating the abdominal wall to avoid vessels and observing the entry of trocars under direct vision from within the abdomen.

FIGURE 12–3. The left lobe of the liver should be retracted using a liver retractor placed in the right midclavicular port. The left triangular ligament should *not* be incised. Doing so will make elevation of the left lobe significantly more difficult because the retractor will not be able to create a "tent" effect. The liver retractor should be maintained by the second assistant, who is positioned at the patient's right side. This is an important part of the procedure, and the second assistant must be alert not only to maintain adequate elevation of the lobe but also to guard against applying too much pressure to the liver, thus risking bleeding or subcapsular hematoma. Alternatively, an instrument holder may be used to elevate the left lobe and expose the hiatus.

FIGURE 12–3

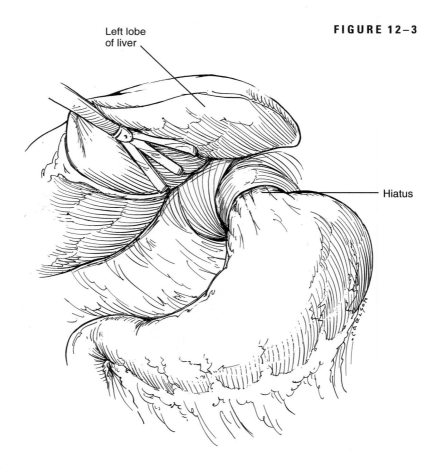

Left lobe of liver

Hiatus

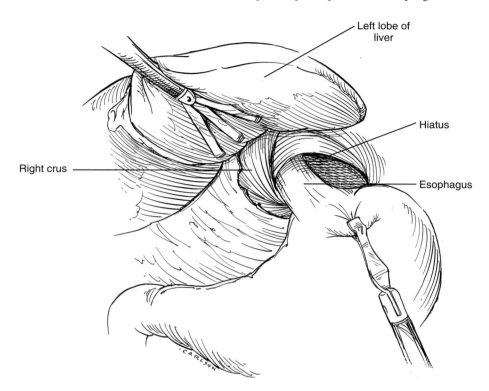

Left lobe of liver

Hiatus

Right crus

Esophagus

FIGURE 12–4

FIGURE 12–4. After positioning the first and second assistants, the surgeon begins dissection at the hiatus. In the typical patient a large defect is seen extending from the hiatus to the left at the level of the hiatus. Variable amounts of the gastric fundus are in the hernia, and portions of colon and small bowel may be present in the hernia as well. The first maneuver in the procedure is preliminary reduction of the contents of the hernial sac. The surgeon, positioned between the legs of the patient, uses a hand-over-hand technique to gently reduce the stomach into the abdomen using grasping instruments with broad surfaces that will not traumatize the gastric serosa. The positive pressure used to maintain the pneumoperitoneum is an adversary in this procedure. The surgeon must maintain constant caudal pressure on the stomach to prevent it from immediately returning to the chest. The surgeon is assisted in this endeavor by the first assistant who, using the left midabdominal port, maintains steady caudal retraction on the body of the stomach with an atraumatic bowel grasper such as a Babcock clamp, either a 10- or 5-mm instrument. As each new segment of stomach is reduced, a more proximal segment

is passed to the first assistant, who maintains traction on it while the surgeon reaches into the sac and reduces more. These maneuvers are repeated sequentially until the entire fundus has been reduced. Occasionally, when the stomach has been completely reduced, caudal retraction can be released, and the stomach may stay within the abdomen. This is not the typical situation, however, and in general traction must be maintained.

When the stomach has been completely reduced, the hernia ring can be easily identified, and the sac will become evident. The sac may be attached to the fundus of the stomach, but in my experience this is an infrequent finding. During open surgery for paraesophageal hernias, the sac is invariably taken during the repair. In my early experience excision was not always performed. As technique has evolved, however, it has become evident that reduction and excision of the sac, whenever possible, is important to minimize the chance of recurrence.

The sac should be grasped at the anterior margin of the hernia defect and excised circumferentially. This will eliminate a potential dead space in the mediastinum that will fill with fluid in the postoperative period and may contribute to postoperative symptoms. Additionally, excision of the sac at the margin of the hernia ring will create a raw surface that will facilitate healing of the defect when the margins have been sutured. Excision of the sac at the site of the normal hiatus and the gastroesophageal junction may be difficult, and the surgeon may decide to stay somewhat lateral at this point if a clear margin cannot be maintained.

When the stomach has been reduced and the sac excised, the surgeon must then determine whether or not a concomitant antireflux procedure will be performed. This decision will already have been suggested on the basis of the patient's symptoms and objective preoperative tests, such as manometric and pH studies.

Repair of Paraesophageal Hernia Without Antireflux Procedure

FIGURE 12-5. The diaphragmatic defect can be closed using one of two methods. In my early experience, the defect was closed by placing a suitably sized segment of polypropylene mesh over the defect and stapling it to the freshly cut edges of the hernia ring. The defect is sized by measuring the anteroposterior and lateral lengths and trimming a sufficient segment of mesh to cover the flaw with a 2-cm margin. The mesh is then introduced into the abdomen through a 12-mm cannula positioned over the defect and sutured or stapled circumferentially around the defect in two rows. The staples are typically started away from the gastroesophageal junction and brought toward the fundic portion of the stomach. The surgeon will find that placement of the final staples at the gastroesophageal junction is difficult because the margins are often obscured by the fundus and by a poorly identified margin at this location.

The mesh technique has several obvious advantages. It can be accomplished quickly and easily, and in elderly patients this may be a significant advantage. Also, it may be the most suitable repair for large hernias in which closure

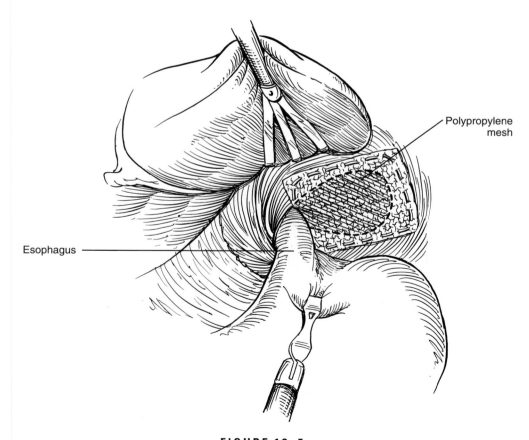

Polypropylene mesh

Esophagus

FIGURE 12-5

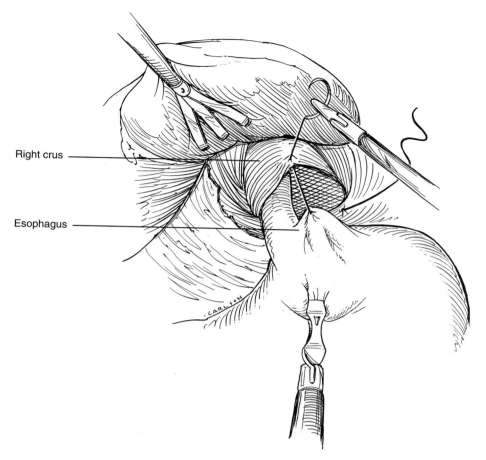

FIGURE 12-6

of the defect might significantly compromise respiratory function. There are several drawbacks, however. These include placement of prosthetic mesh in direct contact with the gastrointestinal tract and the possibility of subsequent erosion into the gut, and the difficulty of creating a tight closure at the left margin of the hiatus where the esophagus enters the abdomen. Additionally, the mesh allows accumulation of fluid in the posterior mediastinum in the early postoperative period, and this may compromise esophageal and respiratory function.

FIGURE 12-6. Primary suture closure of the defect obviates many of the objections to the use of mesh and can be performed quickly once the surgeon is comfortable with laparascopic suturing and knot-tying. Additionally, the recent introduction of suturing devices has greatly facilitated the ease with which this type of closure can be performed.

Closure is performed using heavy nonabsorbable sutures such as 0 or 2–0 Dacron or silk. The initial suture is placed in the most lateral extent of the defect. Intracorporeal or extracorporeal knots may be used, and either a running or interrupted closure is satisfactory. Running closure must be performed under a significant amount of tension to bring the defect together. Tension must be maintained by the surgeon using his nondominant hand, and this may be difficult as the first few sutures are being placed. Alternatively, the surgeon may use a lock stitch to facilitate this maneuver.

FIGURE 12-7

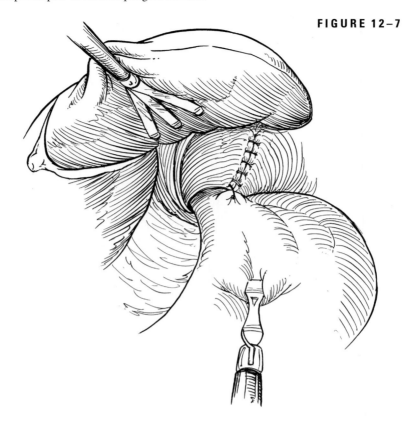

FIGURE 12-7. A snug closure at the hiatus completes this portion of the operation, and the surgeon finishes by securing the stitch with an intracorporeal knot. The closure must not be too tight, and if there is any concern that the newly reconstructed hiatus is too narrow, a bougie is placed to size the opening.

Repair of Paraesophageal Hernia With Antireflux Procedure

If an antireflux procedure is to be performed, dissection begins along the lesser curve to identify the right crus and create a retroesophageal window. This can be more difficult than it is during a typical antireflux procedure performed for a Type 1 hiatal hernia because the lesser omentum in a paraesophageal hernia tends to be thicker and more bulky. This situation apparently results from the chronic traction placed on the lesser curvature as it is drawn to the left.

Beginning at the midportion of the gastrohepatic ligament, the fatty tissue is incised and divided, taking care to avoid large vascular structures in this area. A frequent finding is a large accessory left hepatic artery in this area.

The dissection is continued cephalad and to the left, clearing the esophageal fat pad from the anterior surface of the gastroesophageal junction but sparing the anterior vagus nerve. The dissection continues posteriorly at the hiatus until the right crus has been identified and separated from the esophagus. The posterior vagus nerve is typically left posterior, and the retroesophageal window is established anterior to this nerve. In most cases of paraesophageal hernia, the fundus, because of its chronic traction into the posterior mediastinum, is sufficiently floppy to allow creation of a wrap without dividing the short gastric vessels. This must be ascertained by wrapping the fundus and determining the amount of tension on it. If the fundus reduces itself when traction is removed, the short gastric vessels must be divided.

The hiatus is then closed posteriorly with several 0 nonabsorbable sutures. Knot-tying may be performed either intracorporeally or extracorporeally, depending on the surgeon's preference. The wrap is then constructed over a large bougie (58 to 60 French) in the usual fashion.

After the wrap has been constructed, the surgeon must close the primary defect in the diaphragm. The preferred method for this is by suture, incorporating the wrap into the uppermost portions of the arch of the hiatus on both the right and left sides. This method brings the gastroesophageal junction as far anterior as possible. Angulating the gastroesophageal junction anteriorly is helpful in preventing postoperative reflux. Alternatively, the defect may be closed with mesh. Both techniques have been described previously.

X. Postoperative Medications

A. Analgesia
 1. Patient-controlled analgesia (PCA), or
 2. Intermittent injections of narcotics supplemented with ketorolac
B. Antiemetics (prochloperazine maleate [Compazine], droperidol, metoclopramide, or ondansetron)
C. H$_2$ blockers or proton blockers continued for at least 2 weeks if patient was taking them preoperatively

XI. Advancement of Diet

A. Clear liquids *ad libitum* are provided as soon as the nasogastric tube has been removed.
B. Patients are cautioned not to consume anything by mouth if they have a sense of nausea or are not thirsty.
C. After clear liquids are tolerated, the diet is advanced to full liquids and subsequently to pureed meals for 10 days.

XII. Determinants of Discharge

Patients may be discharged on the day after surgery if they are able to tolerate clear liquids and are having minimal incisional pain. The nasogastric tube is typically removed on morning rounds the morning after surgery, and clear liquids are encouraged. Assuming that no significant nausea and minimal pain are present, patients may be discharged. In certain situations, particularly in patients with significant coronary artery disease, a rule-out protocol may be necessary, which may delay discharge somewhat.

XIII. Return to Normal Activity

Patients may return to their normal activities within 10 to 12 days. Because most of these patients are elderly, the degree of heavy work they will be required to perform is limited. There is no limitation to their activities, however, with the exception of heavy lifting. Because of concern that a Valsalva maneuver might stress the repair, patients are requested to refrain from lifting more than 25 pounds for 6 weeks. Other activities such as driving, walking, climbing stairs, bicycle riding, and so on can be performed immediately. Patients are typically asked to return for office follow-up in 3 weeks. Postoperative radiographs are not ordinarily obtained.

Chapter 13

Laparoscopic Heller Myotomy

STEVE EUBANKS, M.D.

I. Indications

Achalasia

II. Contraindications

A. Inability to tolerate general anesthesia
B. A sigmoid esophagus is a relative contraindication since this condition compromises results

III. Factors Important in Patient Selection

A. History of dysphasia
B. Contrast study indicative of achalasia
C. Elevated lower esophageal pressures
D. Decreased esophageal body pressures

IV. Preoperative Preparation

A. Same-day admission or admission night before surgery
   1. Pureed diet for a week prior to surgery
   2. Gastric enteral feedings preoperatively if patient is malnourished or dehydrated
B. Preoperative medications including medication patches
   1. Preoperative antibiotics
   2. Aspiration precautions on intubation
C. Bowel preparation: none

V. Choice of Anesthesia

General endotracheal anesthesia

VI. Accessory Devices

A. Foley catheter (first choice)
B. Pneumatic compression stocking
C. Video gastroscope set-up

VII. Instruments and Telescopes

A. 30-degree, 10-mm telescope
B. Laparoscopic liver retractor
C. 5-mm laparoscopic scissors
D. Two 5-mm laparoscopic atraumatic graspers
E. Two 5-mm laparoscopic needle drivers

VIII. Position of Monitors and Placement and Size of Trocars

FIGURE 13–1. The camera trocar is placed by direct cutdown in the midline, approximately halfway between the umbilicus and the xiphoid process. A 30-degree angled telescope is employed. The abdomen is then briefly explored. A second 10-mm trocar is inserted in the midline just below the xiphoid to allow placement of a liver retractor. The next two trocars are the working ports of the primary surgeon. One is placed on the right costal margin just lateral to the midclavicular line, and the other splits the distance between it and the camera port. One of these can be a 5-mm port, depending on which hand the surgeon uses to perform sutures. Last, a 5-mm port is inserted lateral to the left clavicular line on the costal margin for the assistant.

Port placement can make or break the ability to complete this procedure. It is pivotal to plan port placement in relation to the individual patient's body habitus. The described port locations are estimates based on ideal anatomy. Special circumstances exist in all cases, and judgment is invariably required for optimal port positioning. One pitfall is placing the camera too far from the xiphoid. The dissection progresses above the diaphragm, requiring the camera to travel greater distances than is usual in other abdominal endoscopic procedures. Another important pearl relates to the relationship between the camera and the two ports of the primary surgeon. A distance of least 4 cm is desirable between each of these ports to minimize conflict between instrument and instrument or between instrument and camera. In addition, proper triangulation of these ports with the operative target provides the most working angles and image viewpoints from which to choose.

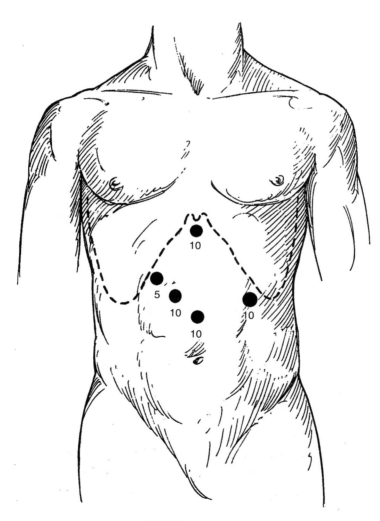

FIGURE 13-1

IX. Narrative of Surgical Technique

FIGURE 13-2. After placement of the trocars, the liver retractor is used to elevate the left lateral segment, and the gastrohepatic ligament is identified overlying the caudate lobe of the liver. This peritoneal reflection is divided using electrocautery as needed. The celiac branch of the vagus is in this plane and is preserved as the peritoneal incision is carried in the direction of the diaphragm. One hazard at this point is injury to a replaced left hepatic artery. If present, this structure courses within the gastrohepatic ligament. This anomaly can be anticipated and measures taken to preserve it. The peritoneal incision is carried from the gastrohepatic ligament in a cranial direction to a level about 4 to 6 cm proximal to the gastroesophageal junction.

The peritoneum of the gastrohepatic ligament is continuous with that overlying the esophagus. The line of incision is turned to the left, and the peritoneum over the esophagus is incised in a horizontal direction. This line of incision is carried to an area past the anticipated location of the left diaphragmatic crus. It is important to limit the initial incision to the peritoneum itself. This helps avoid blood staining of the tissues, injury to the celiac branch and replaced left hepatic artery, and injury to the vagus trunks when the dissection is carried over the esophagus. The peritoneum is elevated with one hand, and the underlying tissues are swept down with the other prior to cutting. The assistant has one hand on the liver retractor, leaving one hand free to assist in the dissection.

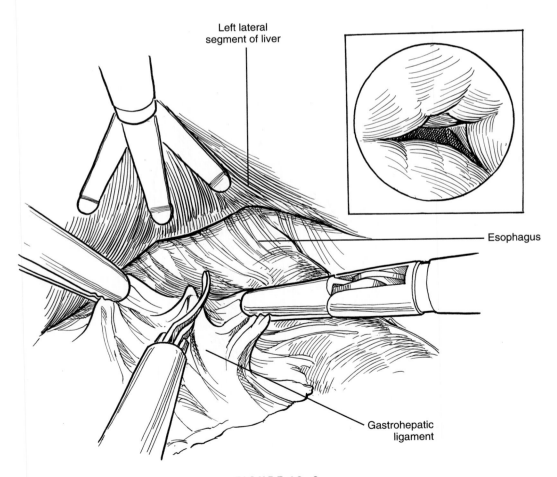

Left lateral
segment of liver

Esophagus

Gastrohepatic
ligament

FIGURE 13-2

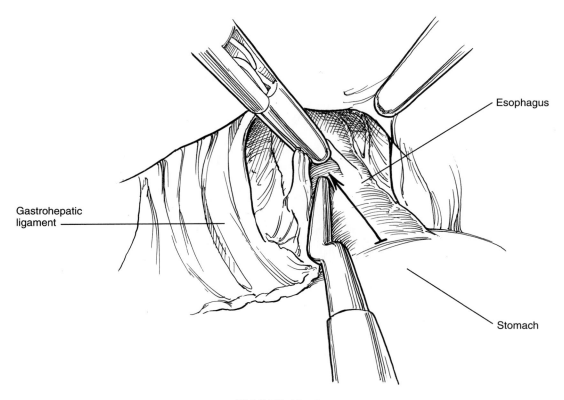

Gastrohepatic
ligament

Esophagus

Stomach

FIGURE 13–3

FIGURE 13-3. Next, the assistant applies gentle distal and posterior retraction to the anterior surface of the stomach approximately 3 to 4 cm below the gastroesophageal junction. This will increase the length of intra-abdominal esophagus. Retroesophageal dissection is avoided. The surgeon employs gentle blunt techniques to free the esophagus from its attachments at the diaphragmatic hiatus. These attachments are usually loose, and gentle blunt dissection is all that is required. Scarring and chronic paraesophageal hernia occasionally lead to more developed attachments from the esophagus and stomach to the diaphragmatic hiatus. In these cases, careful sharp dissection with proper tissue retraction is needed. The blunt dissection is taken into the mediastinum, freeing as much esophagus as will be required to complete the planned myotomy. The posterior and distal retraction of the stomach is the key element in acquiring accessible esophageal length.

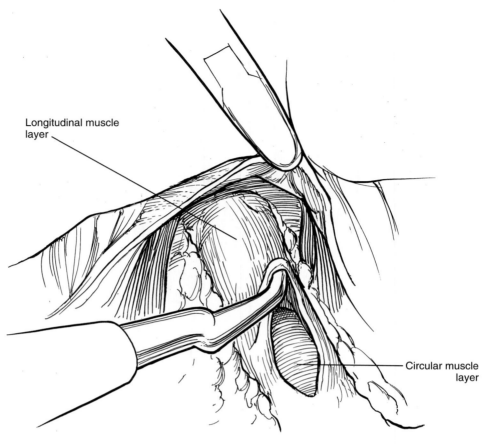

Longitudinal muscle
layer

Circular muscle
layer

FIGURE 13-4

FIGURE 13-4. Establishment of a defined muscular plane is necessary for safe completion of this procedure. Dissection in the area of the gastroesophageal junction is often made more difficult by scarring. This fibrosis is augmented by longstanding disease and multiple esophageal dilatations. For these reasons, the muscular dissection is initiated about 5 to 7 cm above the gastroesophageal junction. Here the muscular planes are more likely to be preserved. The anterior surface of the esophagus is cleared of the overlying areolar tissue underneath the peritoneal reflection. This exposes the longitudinal muscle fibers of the esophagus. The myotomy is established in the middle of the anterior surface of the esophagus because it will be extended bilaterally to encompass 180 degrees of the final external esophageal circumference. Usually this exteriormost muscular plane is easily split in its axis. Either scissors or hook cautery can be used for the muscular dissection. It is important to take small portions of muscle with each bite and elevate each off the underlying layers before applying heat or scissoring because there is a chance of fusion of the muscular planes, particularly in patients with advanced disease.

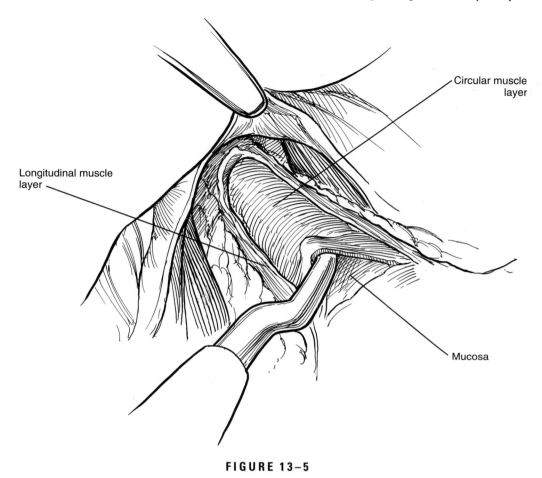

Circular muscle
layer

Longitudinal muscle
layer

Mucosa

FIGURE 13–5

FIGURE 13–5. After a window has been constructed in the longitudinal layer, the circular layer becomes apparent. Care is taken to expose a large enough space in the longitudinal muscle before dividing any circular muscle. Once a plane below the circular muscle and above the mucosa has been established, there is no reason to divide the two muscle layers individually, but they can be approached together if the mucosa is out of harm's way. Intraoperative endoscopy is helpful in this setting. Gentle insufflation and transillumination assist in defining the mucosal-muscular plane.

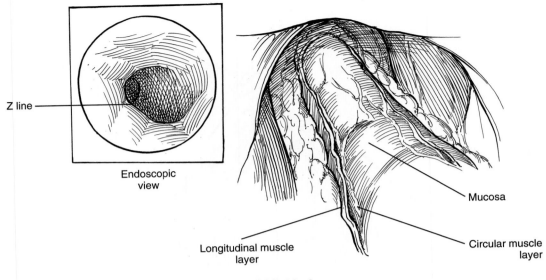

Z line

Endoscopic
view

Mucosa

Longitudinal muscle
layer

Circular muscle
layer

FIGURE 13–6

FIGURE 13-6. The proximal extent of the myotomy is established based on the extent of the disease. The distal extent of the myotomy is 1 cm past the gastroesophageal junction. Definition of the distal end point is also aided by intraoperative esophagogastroscopy. The internal (endoscopic) location of the gastroesophageal junction is defined by the Z line.

FIGURE 13-7. The external (laparoscopic) location of this internal transition zone can be correlated by pushing on the external surface at various external locations until the indentation is seen at the Z line on the endoscopic view.

FIGURE 13-8. Once the proximal and distal end points have been completed, the myotomy is checked for retained circular smooth muscle. When the esophagus is insufflated with the endoscope, constrictive bands are seen because they produce an hourglass or waistlike appearance in the myotomy bed. These bands are then individually taken down. Encroachment of the myotomy side walls likewise causes constriction of the myotomy. These tight areas are identified from the endoscopic view as focal narrow areas. The lateral side walls of the myotomy are extended to complete an 180-degree anterior myotomy. To extend the side walls, the cut edge of the myotomy edge is elevated, and the mucosa is exposed laterally by undermining the circular muscle.

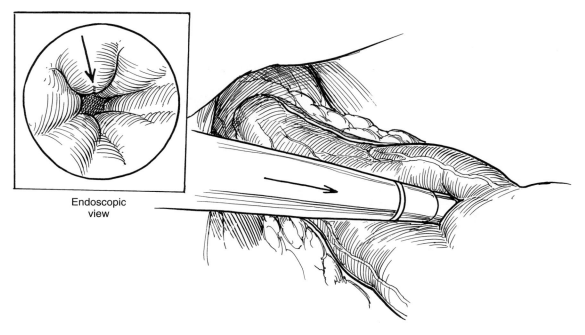

Endoscopic
view

FIGURE 13–7

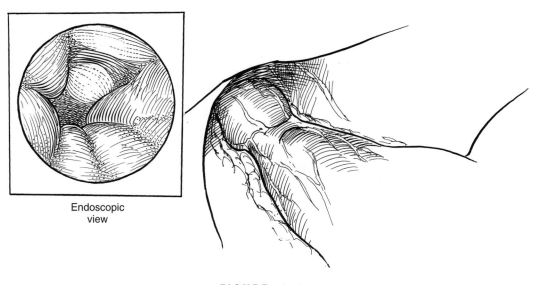

Endoscopic
view

FIGURE 13–8

FIGURE 13-9. Next, the myotomy bed is checked for perforations by submerging the esophagus in an irrigation fluid and insulating it with the endoscope. Care is taken to keep the endoscope centered in the esophagus because the new myotomy is susceptible to iatrogenic injury. The laparoscopic view can be used by the endoscopist to help avoid myotomy bed injury.

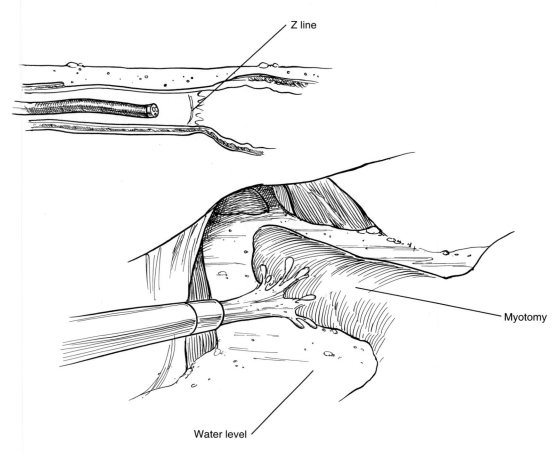

Z line

Myotomy

Water level

FIGURE 13-9

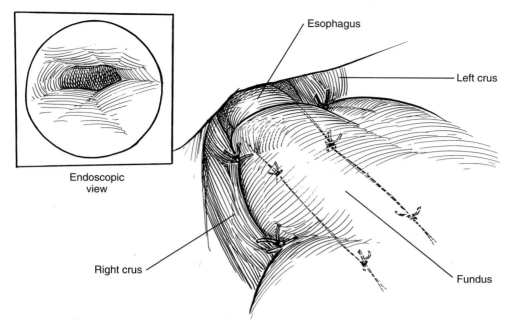

Endoscopic
view

Esophagus

Left crus

Right crus

Fundus

FIGURE 13–10

FIGURE 13–10. The last part of the procedure is the creation of an antireflux barrier. The wrap of choice is the Dor fundoplication. The retroesophageal space is left undissected. The fundus is grasped and brought from the left upper abdomen to cover the lower myotomy and gastroesophageal junction. If undue tension is created in performing this wrap, the short gastric vessels are taken down until a loose 180-degree wrap results. The wrap is secured to the left diaphragmatic crus first, and then to the left edge of the myotomy. The next sutures are placed from the posterior surface of the gastric wrap to the right myotomy edge. In the final wrap the myotomy is stented in the open position by stitching the myotomy edges in place to the underside of the Dor wrap. Finally, the anterior wrap is fixed to the right diaphragmatic crus. A fundoplication that is too tight will re-create dysphagia. A retroflexed view of the gastroesophageal junction can be used to visualize the fundoplication. Passing and withdrawing the scope through the gastroesophageal junction with insufflation provides information on the distensibility of the antireflux barrier.

X. Postoperative Medications

Antiemetic protocol

XI. Advancement of Diet

Clear liquids at breakfast of postoperative day 1

XII. Determinants of Discharge

A. Tolerating diet
B. Ambulating
C. Afebrile
D. Voiding
E. Moving bowels
F. Oral analgesia is controlling pain

XIII. Return to Normal Activity/Work

The patient can resume normal activities in 2 to 3 weeks.

Part IV

LAPAROSCOPIC SURGERY OF THE STOMACH

Chapter 14

Laparoscopic Highly Selective Vagotomy

GARTH H. BALLANTYNE, M.D.

I. Indications

A. Failure of medical therapy for peptic ulcer disease
1. Recurrence of an ulcer despite eradication of *Helicobacter pylori* and continuous treatment with a proton pump inhibitor
2. Recurrence of an ulcer in a noncompliant patient
B. Desire of the patient to avoid taking H_2 blockers or proton pump inhibitors for treatment of peptic ulcer disease for an indefinite period of time
C. Performance of a laparoscopic fundoplication for gastroesophageal reflux disease in a patient who is also afflicted with peptic ulcer disease
D. A highly selective vagotomy may be performed in conjunction with plication of a perforated duodenal ulcer.

II. Contraindications

A. Highly selective vagotomy is more effective in the treatment of duodenal ulcers than pyloric channel ulcers or gastric ulcers, and as a result these may be considered relative contraindications.
B. Patients with severe restrictive pulmonary disease who may not be able to tolerate the carbon dioxide of the pneumoperitoneum
C. Patients who have previously undergone fundoplications for gastroesophageal reflux

disease because the wrap makes the proximal gastric fibers from the vagal nerves inaccessible

III. Factors Important in Patient Selection

A. The magnified image telecast from the video telescope provides a vastly superior view for the surgeon than that obtained through conventional incisions. Consequently, once a surgeon gains experience in this technique, laparoscopy facilitates the performance of a highly selective vagotomy in most patients.
B. Several factors make a laparoscopy approach more difficult, although these factors tend to impede open operations as well. These include:
1. Previous upper abdominal operations
2. Obesity

IV. Preoperative Preparation

A. All patients should be fully evaluated for peptic ulcer disease prior to elective surgery. This generally includes:
1. Upper gastrointestinal endoscopy
2. Test for *H. pylori*
3. Serum gastrin level
B. Patients are admitted on the morning of surgery.

C. Patients are given Zofran 4 mg intravenously prior to the induction of anesthesia.
D. Patients are given one dose of antibiotic prophylaxis such as a cephalosporin 1 g intravenously (IV).

V. Choice of Anesthesia

All patients receive general anesthesia.

VI. Accessory Devices

A. A nasogastric tube is inserted after induction of anesthesia.
B. A urinary catheter is inserted after induction of anesthesia.
C. The patient's legs are wrapped with pneumatic compression stockings prior to the induction of anesthesia.

VII. Instruments and Telescopes

A. 10-mm, 30-degree telescope
B. Aesop 3000 robot (Computer Motion, Santa Barbara, CA)
C. Five 10/11-mm trocars

D. LCS Harmonic Scissors (Ethicon Endo-Surgery, Cincinnati, OH)
E. Laparoscopic curved dissector/grasper
F. Laparoscopic Babcock clamp
G. Roticulating Endo-Grasp (United States Surgical Corporation, Norwalk, CT)
H. Laparoscopic fan or paddle retractor
I. Laparoscopic suction/irrigation device
J. Small Penrose drain
K. Laparoscopic surgical clips

VIII. Position of Monitors and Placement of Trocars

FIGURE 14–1. The room is set up in a manner similar to that used by the surgeon for a laparoscopic cholecystectomy or laparoscopic fundoplication. The two monitors are positioned near the shoulders of the patient. If the primary monitor is suspended by a boom, it is best placed directly over the patient's head. The surgeon can operate between the patient's legs in the French position or from the right side with the patient in a supine position. The assistant stands on the patient's left side. If Aesop is used to hold the video camera, it can be positioned by the patient's left hip.

FIGURE 14–1

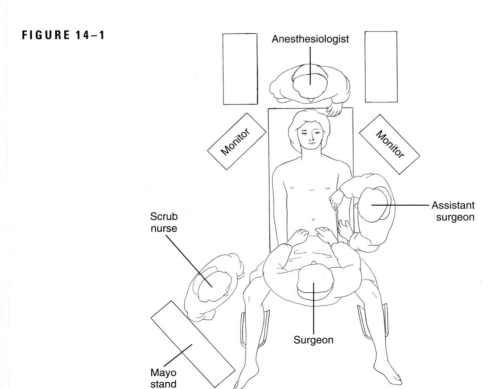

FIGURE 14-2. The 10/11-mm camera port is inserted through the midline about three finger breadths cephalad to the umbilicus. In tall men, this port is inserted even closer to the xyphoid. The surgeon uses two working ports for his or her left and right hands. These two 10/11-mm trocars are inserted on either side of the midline. The 10/11-mm or 12-mm trocar for the liver retractor is inserted on the right anterior axillary line below the costal margin. Traction will be placed on the stomach with a Babcock clamp inserted through a 10/11-mm trocar in-serted on the left anterior axillary line below the costal margin.

IX. Narrative of Surgical Technique

FIGURE 14-3. The typical appearance of the anterior vagus nerve and its many branches is shown here. The dotted line indicates the course of the planned anterior highly selective vagotomy commencing at the "crow's foot" and extending to the angle of His.

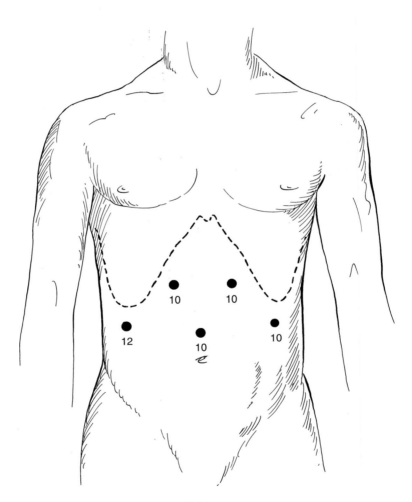

FIGURE 14-2

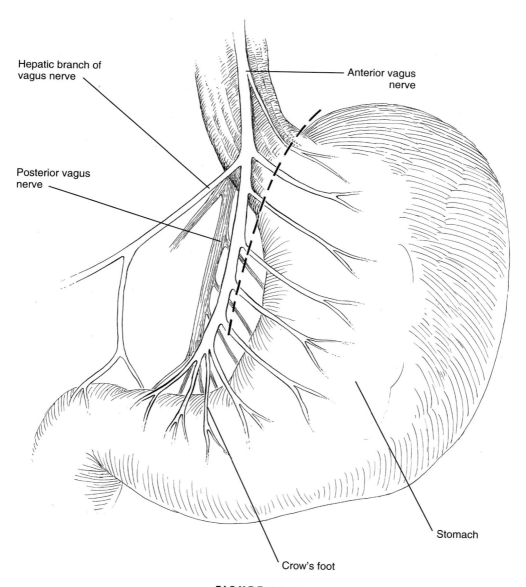

Hepatic branch of
vagus nerve

Anterior vagus
nerve

Posterior vagus
nerve

Stomach

Crow's foot

FIGURE 14–3

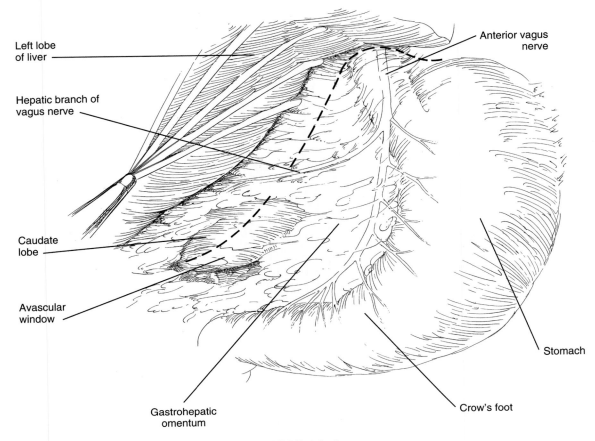

Left lobe
of liver

Anterior vagus
nerve

Hepatic branch of
vagus nerve

Caudate
lobe

Avascular
window

Gastrohepatic
omentum

Crow's foot

Stomach

FIGURE 14-4

FIGURE 14-4. The dissection begins in the same manner used for a fundoplication. This mobilizes the esophagus from the hiatus and delivers at least 6 cm of the esophagus from the mediastinum into the abdomen. Once the esophagus is mobilized in this manner, the anterior and posterior vagal nerves are easily identified. The planned course of dissection is indicated by the dashed line. The left lobe of the liver is elevated with a fan or paddle retractor.

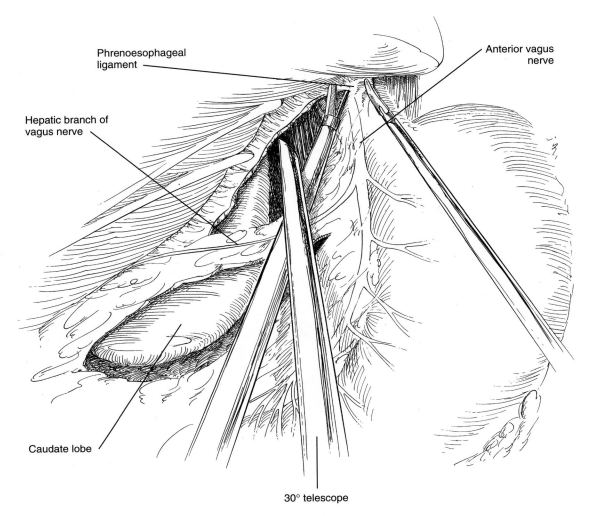

Phrenoesophageal ligament

Anterior vagus nerve

Hepatic branch of vagus nerve

Caudate lobe

30° telescope

FIGURE 14–5

FIGURE 14–5. The lesser sac is entered through the avascular window of the gastrohepatic omentum over the caudate lobe of the liver. The hepatic branches of the anterior vagus nerve are preserved. In about 7 per cent of individuals, an aberrant left hepatic artery traverses the gastrohepatic omentum in the same vicinity. This aberrant artery should be pre-served whenever possible. The incision of the gastrohepatic omentum skips over the hepatic vagal branches and then continues to the hiatus. The phrenoesophageal ligament is incised anteriorly over the esophagus. Rotation of the 30-degree telescope permits excellent visualization of this dissection from different perspectives.

FIGURE 14-6. The esophagus is mobilized from the hiatus. The incision of the phreno-esophageal ligament continues posteriorly along the left crus. Congenital adhesions between the greater curve of the stomach and the diaphragm are incised with the LCS harmonic scissors. The esophagus is bluntly pushed medially away from the left crus. Ideally, this dissection is continued posteriorly until the junction of the left and right crura is encountered. At this point, dissection starts again from the top of the hiatus. The right crus is followed posteriorly until its junction with the left crus is reached. The left crus is followed anteriorly. The esophagus is elevated with the blunt side of the curved dissector. A retroesophageal window is opened through the flimsy connective tissue directly over the posterior junction of the left and right crura. Using this technique, the posterior vagus is elevated with the esophagus and is easily identified. Flimsy adhesions between the esophagus and the hiatus are bluntly separated around the circumference of the esophagus.

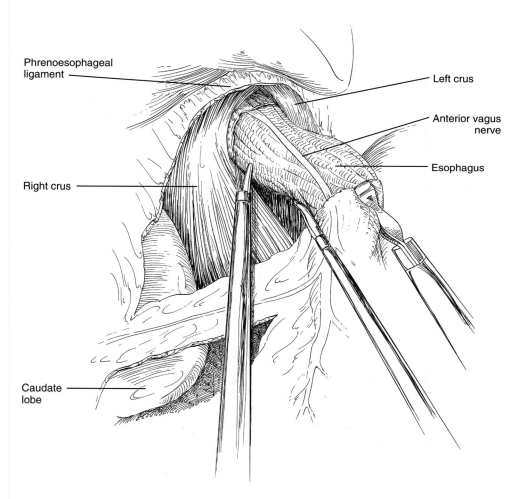

FIGURE 14-6

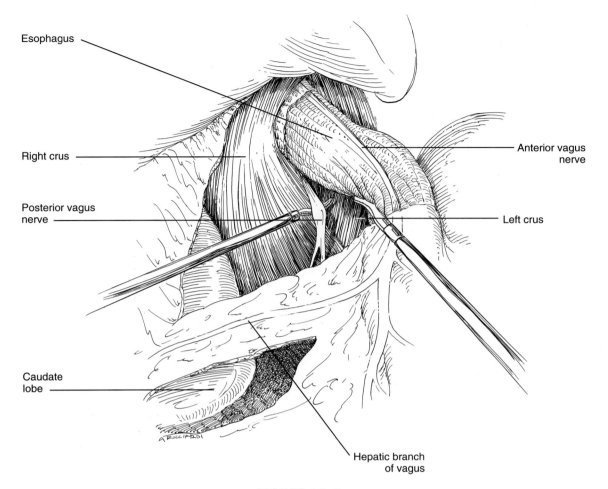

Esophagus

Right crus

Posterior vagus
nerve

Caudate
lobe

Anterior vagus
nerve

Left crus

Hepatic branch
of vagus

FIGURE 14–7

FIGURE 14–7. The anterior and posterior vagus nerves are identified. The posterior vagus nerve is freed from the back wall of the esophagus and allowed to drop back toward the crura. Similarly, the trunk of the anterior vagus nerve is freed from the vicinity of the gastroesophageal junction.

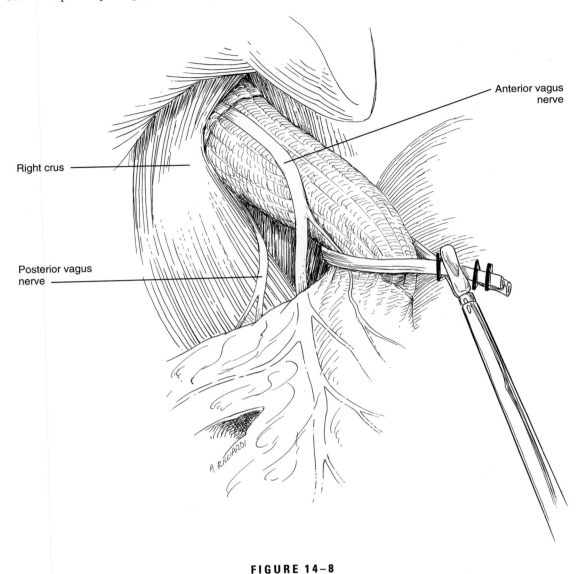

Right crus

Anterior vagus
nerve

Posterior vagus
nerve

A. RICCIARDI

FIGURE 14-8

FIGURE 14-8. A Roticulating Endo-Grasp
(United States Surgical Corporation, Norwalk,
CT) is passed around the esophagus. It is used
to pull a small Penrose drain around the esophagus. The trunks of the vagus nerves are left
outside the Penrose drain. The Penrose drain is
secured to itself with surgical clips or with a
pre-tied laparoscopic suture. A grasper then retracts the esophagus with the Penrose drain. At
least 6 to 8 cm of the esophagus is mobilized
from the mediastinum and delivered into the
abdomen.

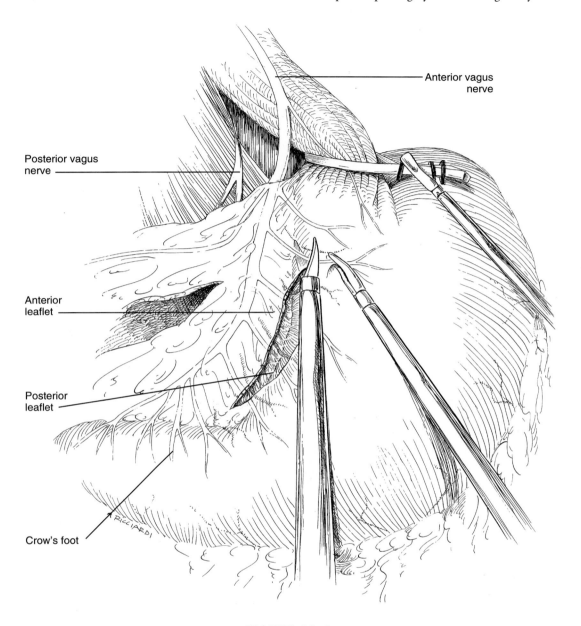

Anterior vagus nerve

Posterior vagus nerve

Anterior leaflet

Posterior leaflet

Crow's foot

RICCIARDI

FIGURE 14–9

FIGURE 14–9. The stomach and esophagus are now set up for the highly selective vagotomy. The dissection commences at the "crow's foot" made by the gastric vessels as they insert into the lesser curvature. The anterior leaflet of the gastrohepatic omentum is divided close to the lesser curve. Larger vessels can also be clipped with surgical clips to augment the sealing of the vessels by the LCS Harmonic Scissors (Ethicon Endo-Surgery, Cincinnati, OH). Dissection continues up to the Penrose drain.

FIGURE 14-10. The posterior leaflet is then divided up to the Penrose drains. Both the anterior and posterior leaflets are usually easily identified as discrete layers. The dissection of the anterior leaflet is continued across the anterior surface of the stomach. The entire lesser curve of the stomach is now freed from the crow's foot to the gastroesophageal junction. The lesser curve can be rotated anteriorly to allow confirmation of the complete division of the vagal fibers along the lesser curve.

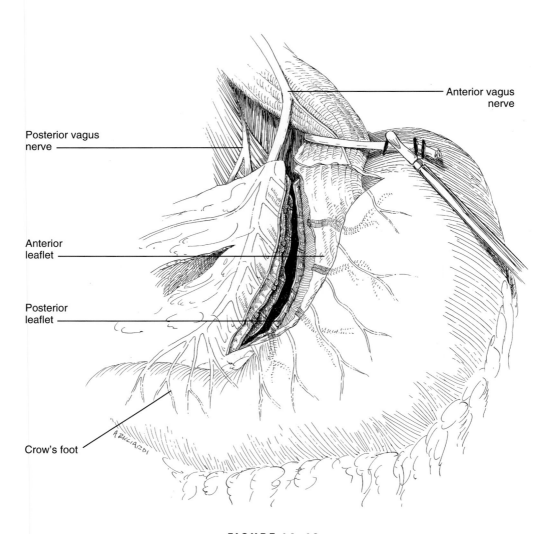

FIGURE 14-10

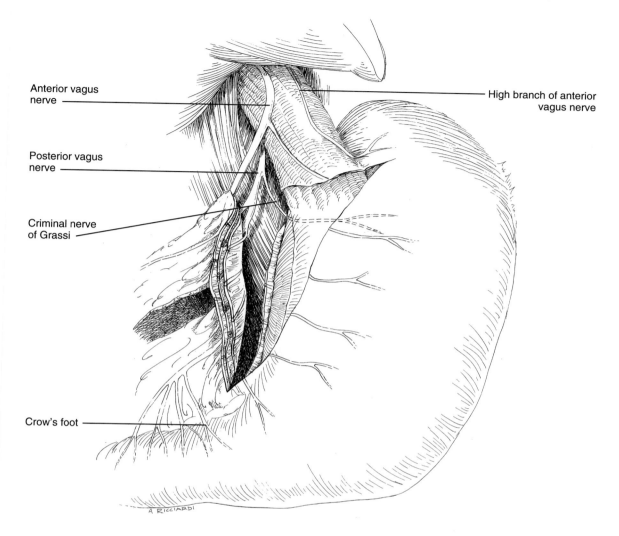

Anterior vagus nerve

Posterior vagus nerve

Criminal nerve of Grassi

Crow's foot

A RICCIARDI

High branch of anterior vagus nerve

FIGURE 14-11

FIGURE 14-11. The most common reason for failure of a highly selective vagotomy is failure to divide the vagal branches that separate from the main vagal trunks proximally to the gastroesophageal junction. These include the angle of His fibers that originate from the anterior vagus nerve and the "criminal" nerve of Grassi, which branches from the posterior vagus nerve. Extensive mobilization of the esophagus facilitates visualization of these branches. Dissection continues at least 4 cm along the esophagus proximally to the gastroesophageal junction. Any possible vagal branches are divided. Retraction anteriorly with the Penrose drain generally exposes the criminal nerve of Grassi.

If this is not seen from the right side of the esophagus, the Penrose is used to retract the esophagus to the left, allowing exposure of the hiatus from a different perspective. Again, any fibrous branches that may represent vagal branches are divided. This completes the highly selective vagotomy.

The abdomen is inspected for hemostasis, and the paddle retractor is removed. The pneumoperitoneum is deflated to a pressure of about 6 to 8 mm Hg. The abdomen and trocar sites are again examined for evidence of hemorrhage. The pneumoperitoneum is then completely deflated. The trocars are removed, and the fascial defects are closed with a 0 absorbable suture such as Vicryl on a UR-6 needle. The skin edges are approximated with subcuticular stitches, and the wounds are again infiltrated with marcaine. The patient is extubated in the operating room. The nasogastric tube, urinary catheter, intravenous catheter, and pneumatic compression stockings are left in place overnight and are removed the next morning.

X. Postoperative Medications

A. The patient receives Zofran 4 mg IV at the beginning of the operation, at the end of operation, and again about 4 hours after the operation.
B. The patient receives narcotics intramuscularly and then orally as needed.
C. The patient receives only one preoperative prophylactic dose of antibiotic.
D. The patient does not receive any antacids, H_2 blockers, proton pump inhibitors, or prokinetic agents after the operation.

XI. Advancement of Diet

A. The patient is allowed sips of clear liquids on the night of surgery.
B. The nasogastric tube is removed the morning after surgery.
C. The patient starts on a clear liquid diet after the nasogastric tube is removed.

D. The patient is advanced to a regular diet as tolerated.

XII. Determinants of Discharge

The patient is discharged to home when:
1. He or she can drink liquids without difficulty.
2. He or she can urinate without problems.
3. Pain is adequately controlled by oral agents.
4. The patient can ambulate without assistance.
5. The patient's social condition allows a safe home environment. For patients who live alone, hospitalization may be prolonged several days until they are better able to care for themselves.

Patients are typically discharged 24 to 48 hours after the operation.

XIII. Return to Normal Activity/Work

A. Patients are asked to avoid strenuous activity for at least 2 weeks because wounds require 10 to 14 days to reach 90 per cent of their ultimate strength.
B. Patients can sometimes return to work within a week if the job is primarily sedentary.
C. A sense of being tired often persists for 2 to 3 weeks.

Laparoscopic Management of Complications of Peptic Ulcer Disease

NAMIR KATKHOUDA, M.D., STEVE W. GRANT, M.D.,
MELANIE H. FRIEDLANDER, M.D., KRANTHI ACHANTA, M.D.,
and JEAN MOUIEL, M.D.

Laparoscopic treatment of intractable duodenal ulcers aims at treating patients who have not healed after a trial of intensive treatment such as H₂ blockers and/or therapy aimed at eradication of *Helicobacter pylori*. There is also a category of patients who are *H. pylori* negative who can be offered laparoscopic treatment of their ulcer by vagotomy. Patients who have earlier relapses on stopping medical treatment are also candidates for vagotomy. In patients with duodenal ulcer disease, complications of the disease such as bleeding or pyloric outlet obstruction represent valid indications to perform surgery. Since most of these complications are life-threatening and usually cannot be dealt with medically, the laparoscopic approach is a good option as long as common sense guides the surgeon performing the procedure. The laparoscopic approach is not recommended in patients with very severe disease such as diffuse peritonitis with septic shock, life-threatening hemorrhage, or patients who are at very high risk and need an operation that can be done as quickly and as simply as possible. Nevertheless, some plications, such as early perforated duodenal ulcers with chemical peritonitis, gastric outlet obstruction, recurrences, and moderate bleeding, can all be addressed laparoscopically.

I. Management of Gastric Outlet Obstruction

Two types of procedures are possible laparoscopically:

1. Laparoscopic total truncal vagotomy and gastrojejunostomy
2. Laparoscopic total truncal vagotomy and antrectomy with a Billroth II reconstruction.

The first operation is a simpler operation and is known to have a lower morbidity and mortality in open surgery. It is associated with a higher recurrence rate and is probably physiologically less satisfying when the stomach is chronically distended, because in such patients an element of gastric atony can contribute to poor gastric emptying.

Laparoscopic vagotomy and antrectomy, on the other hand, is a more radical approach; it not only denervates the stomach but also takes the gastrin-secreting part of the stomach as well as a nonfunctional antrum and probably speeds gastric emptying. It does have a higher mortality and morbidity, at least in inexperienced hands, and should be reserved for the more experienced surgeon. This latter procedure can be performed either intra-abdominally or in a laparoscopically assisted fashion, which we personally think is preferable.

Technique of Laparoscopic Total Truncal Vagotomy

FIGURE 15-1. The patient is placed in a supine position with the legs spread apart. The surgeon stands between the patient's legs in the so-called French position. Operating bimanually is comfortable if the monitor is placed in front of the surgeon.

FIGURE 15-2. Pneumoperitoneum is created by insufflation of carbon dioxide at a pressure of 14 mm Hg. Five trocars are then introduced into the upper part of the abdomen. The introduction of the trocars is very important because a misplaced trocar renders the procedure very difficult to perform. Trocar positioning is the same as for any laparoscopic foregut operation except that the video laparoscope is inserted at

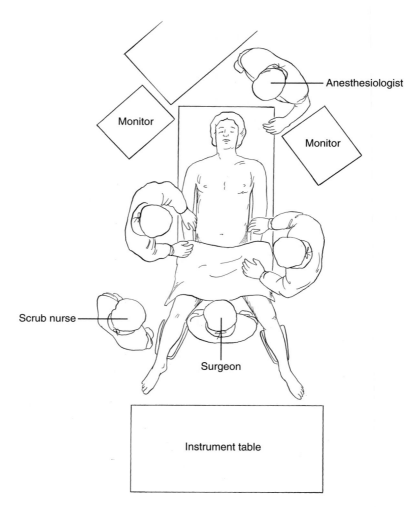

Anesthesiologist

Monitor

Monitor

Scrub nurse

Surgeon

Instrument table

FIGURE 15-1

the level of the umbilicus in order to gain good access not only to the hiatus but also to the different parts of the stomach. Mobilization of the greater curvature requires some juggling with the laparoscope, and it is best located in the umbilicus. Two trocars are inserted, one for the right hand of the surgeon for the operating instruments and the second for the left hand of the surgeon to hold the grasping forceps. These two trocars are triangulated with the umbilical video laparoscope. Finally, the next trocar is placed for the grasping forceps of the first assistant, and the last trocar is the xiphoid trocar, inserted at the left side of the falciform ligament for retraction of the left lobe. This retraction makes use of an irrigation suction device that can serve both purposes: irrigation of the hiatus and gentle retraction of the left lobe (American Hydrosurgical Instruments, Inc.).

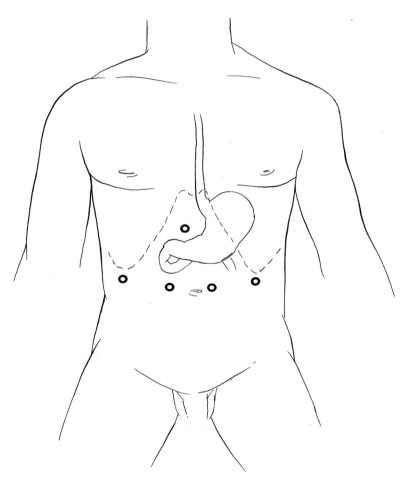

FIGURE 15–2

FIGURE 15-3. The abdomen is entered, and a thorough exploration of the peritoneal cavity is undertaken to exclude intra-abdominal lesions that might have been missed by the preoperative work-up. The liver is then retracted and the procedure is begun.

Access to the hiatus is straightforward with recognition of the following landmarks: The avascular aspect of the lesser sac, the caudate lobe, and the right crus of the diaphragm. The avascular aspect of the lesser sac is opened using electrical scissors to allow recognition of the caudate lobe and the right crus of the diaphragm. A gastric vein may be encountered in the upper part of the lesser omentum; if so, it should be divided between clips. The purpose of the meticulous dissection is to avoid any bleeding, minimizing trauma and blood loss. The right crus is then grasped with the left hand while the patient's head is tilted upward in a reverse Trendelenburg position. This allows the stomach and the greater omentum to fall down, providing access to the hiatus safely, even in obese patients.

The avascular plane between the esophagus and the right crus is entered, and care is taken not to dissect within the fibers of the esophagus.

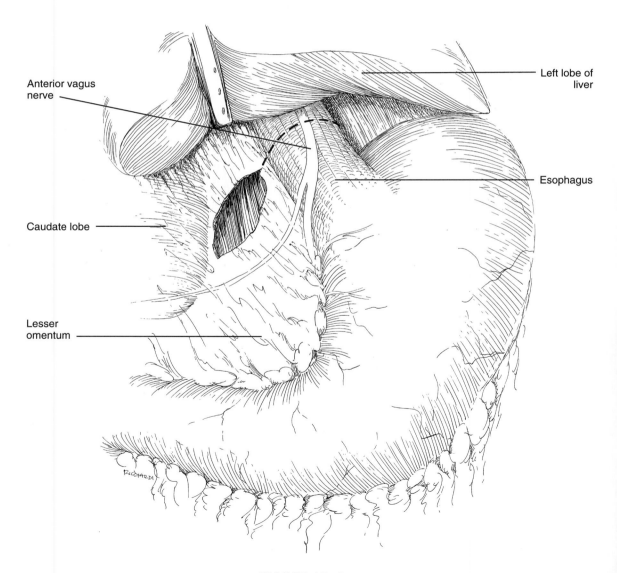

FIGURE 15-3

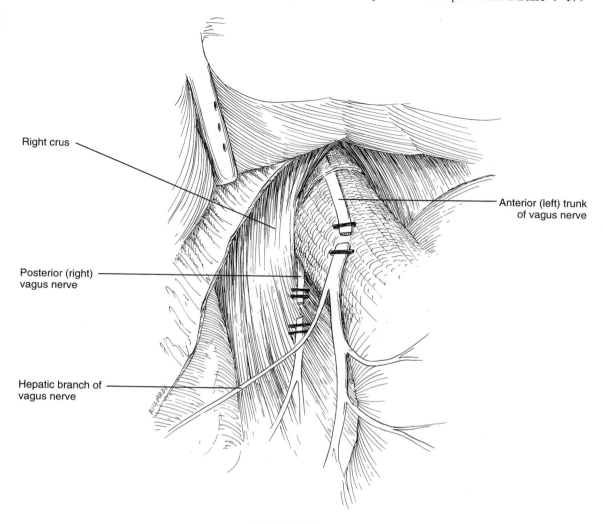

Right crus

Posterior (right)
vagus nerve

Hepatic branch of
vagus nerve

Anterior (left) trunk
of vagus nerve

FIGURE 15–4

The right vagal trunk is usually easily recognized because it lies on the left crus and is divided between clips. Care should be taken to look for a second right vagal trunk, which, however, was rarely encountered in our series. The phrenoesophageal membrane is then divided, allowing division of all small branches of the left vagal trunk.

FIGURE 15–4. The fat pad is removed, allowing identification of the inconstant left trunk of the vagus nerve. At this point, dissection behind the esophagus and under the left crus allows identification of other branches of the vagus nerve (e.g., criminal nerve of Grassi).

Division of these nerves and the nerve trunks completes the bilateral truncal vagotomy. At the end of this step, the esophagus is cleared of all the fatty tissues and nerve fibers using a hook dissector coagulator if necessary.

The Harmonic Scalpel and/or scissors is an interesting new instrument that allows safe hemostasis of this area with minimal trauma to the surrounding tissue. The principle of this instrument is an oscillating blade that moves at 55,000 cycles per second, producing heat and coagulation of small vessels, thereby reducing the number of clips required during this step of the procedure. This instrument can also serve as an atraumatic grasper.

Technique of Laparoscopic Gastrojejunostomy

FIGURE 15-5. This step is straightforward because only a minor dissection of the gastric pouch is required. The technique of performing an efficient gastrojejunostomy is to realize that it should be performed on the posterior aspect of the stomach about 8 cm proximal to the pylorus. Mobilization of the greater curvature of the stomach begins at the level of the entrance of the left gastric gastroepiploic artery in the gastrocolic ligament. It is not necessary to divide the gastroepiploic artery because dissection can be performed distal to the gastroepiploic arcade, thereby preserving it. The gastrocolic ligament is then opened using electrical scissors, and again the Harmonic Scissors may allow a safe and fast dissection of this plane. Superior retraction of the stomach allows exposure of the posterior aspect of the stomach. Division of any adhesions between the stomach and the anterior surface of the body of the pancreas allows better mobilization of the gastric pouch.

The jejunal loop is then chosen, and it is easier for the surgeon to move from the position between the legs to the right side of the patient to perform this step. Tilting the patient into a Trendelenburg position facilitates exposure of the small bowel. The best way to recognize the jejunal loop is to follow the jejunum toward the angle of Treitz, which can be recognized by its tension. It is mandatory at this point not to exert much traction on the angle of Treitz because a mesenteric tear could result, as happened in one of our cases. This tear must be repaired using intracorporeal suturing techniques and 3–0 Prolene threaded on a SH needle. When the second jejunal loop is identified it is mobilized and approximated to the stomach using two Babcock clamps. At this point in the procedure the left lateral trocar is removed and is replaced by an 18-mm trocar, which allows an endolinear cutter (ELC) 60 to be introduced with the tip of the cutter pointing toward the liver. It is also advantageous in our experience to use a 35 cutter, which is easier to handle because of its smaller size. A gastrotomy and enterotomy is then performed; the stapler is introduced, and two shots of the ELC 35 or one shot of the ELC 60 is then fired. The lumen of the anastomosis is then checked carefully for hemostasis, and one suture is placed at the end of the staple line as in open surgery. This stitch is placed using intracorporeal nylon. Finally, the two enterotomies are closed, using either two more triangulated firings of the ELC 35 or, even simpler, a running suture of Prolene 3–0 knotted intracorporeally. The operation is then completed by carefully introducing a nasogastric tube in the efferent loop of the jejunum, enabling decompression of the efferent loop in the immediate postoperative period. This nasogastric tube is removed the following day.

The postoperative course is usually very simple, but care is taken not to feed the patient immediately the next day because some stasis might be present from the previous distention due to the gastric outlet obstruction. The patient is usually fed on the third day after a Gastrografin swallow shows the integrity of the anastomosis.

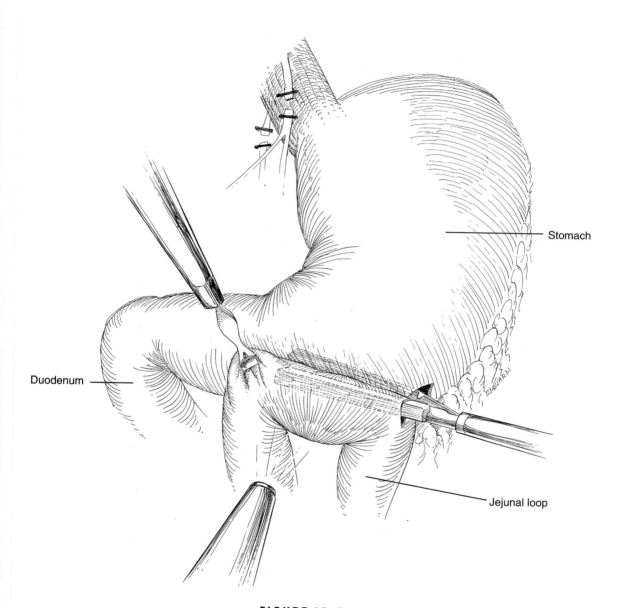

Stomach

Duodenum

Jejunal loop

FIGURE 15–5

Technique of Distal Gastrectomy or Antrectomy

FIGURE 15-6. The first step is the opening of the gastric colic ligament under the right gastroepiploic vessel as described earlier for the gastrojejunostomy. Careful use of the Harmonic Scissors may render this step very easy. Clips will secure all large vessels to prevent any hemorrhage, allowing anterior retraction of the stomach using Babcock clamps, which expose the duodenum in its posterior aspect. The area of the posterior aspect of the first part of the duodenum is carefully dissected as in open surgery using an atraumatic right-angle dissector.

At this point, it is usually necessary to ligate the right epiploic vessel after it has been divided from the gastroduodenal artery. The upper limit of the duodenum is dissected at the point where the right gastric artery is found, and it is ligated between two clips to secure the hemostasis. The next step is the transection and closure to the duodenum using an endolinear cutter 60 (Ethicon, Inc., Cincinnati, Ohio). Once the stapler has been fired, the line of sutures is inspected, and the hemostasis is meticulously completed. This maneuver allows the distal part of the antrum to be exposed with one grasper, and dissection along the lesser curve is then performed step by step using the Harmonic Scis-

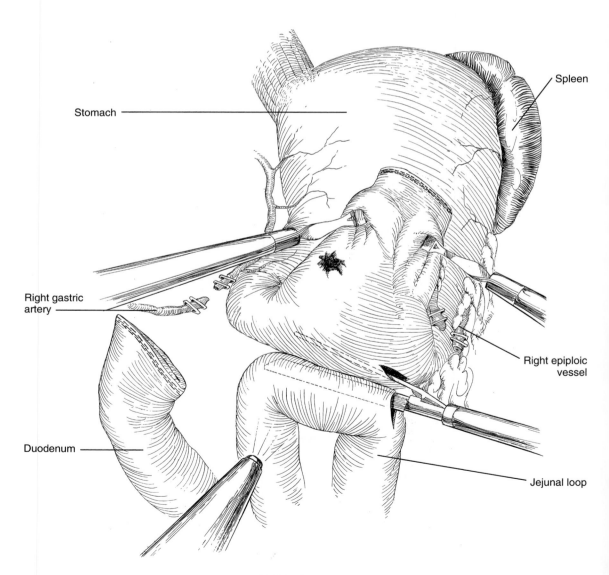

FIGURE 15-6

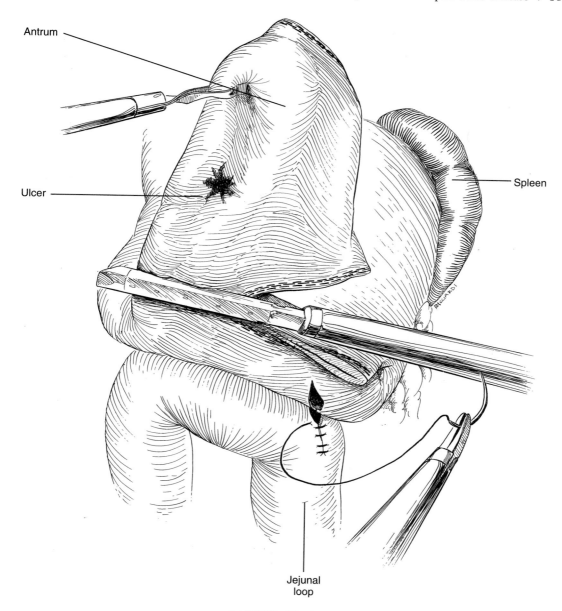

Antrum

Ulcer

Spleen

Jejunal
loop

FIGURE 15–7

sors or the clip applier as needed. It is important to be able to use the 30-degree telescope, which provides a good view of the posterior aspect of either the stomach or the lesser sac. Any large vessel encountered is dissected and cut between two clips. At this point one of two techniques is chosen: intra-abdominal or extra-abdominal anastomosis.

FIGURE 15–7. The intra-abdominal technique involves firing the ELC 60 between the stomach and the jejunum, which allows performance of a gastrojejunostomy in a Billroth II fashion, and the specimen can be resected with several shots of the ELC 60 with gastric green staples.

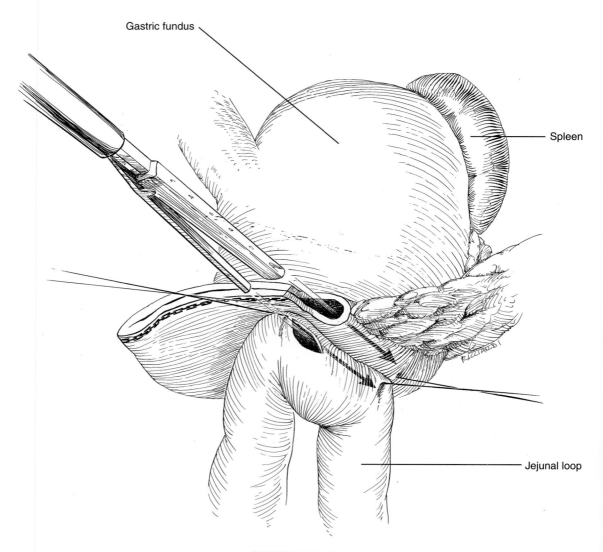

FIGURE 15–8

FIGURE 15-8. Another possibility is to re-move the specimen and use the staple line to introduce the cutter between the jejunum and the posterior aspect of the stomach. The enter-otomies and the gastrotomies are then closed with running sutures.

FIGURE 15-9. The extra-abdominal tech-nique involves a laparoscopically assisted antrec-tomy and a small abdominal incision (4 cm), which allows exteriorization of the stomach and jejunum, permitting completion of the resection and anastomosis outside the abdomen. This technique is probably quicker, easier, and safer and is probably amenable to most surgeons; it is our preferred technique because it cuts the time of the operation by 2 hours, leading to a mean of 2.5 hours for the total time of the procedures. No drains are needed after vigorous irrigation of the abdomen, but care is taken to close all trocar ports because small bowel her-nias are possible through the trocar holes.

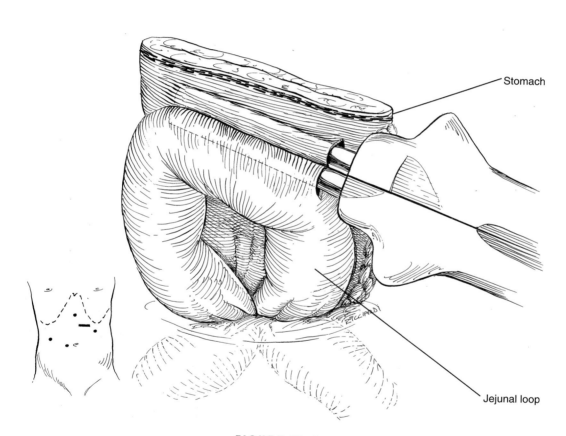

Stomach

Jejunal loop

FIGURE 15-9

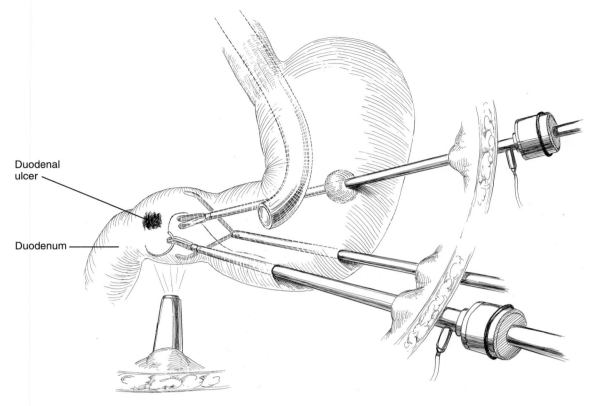

Duodenal ulcer

Duodenum

FIGURE 15–10

II. Treatment of Hemorrhagic Peptic Ulcers

FIGURE 15–10. This is a life-threatening situation owing to a visibly bleeding gastroduodenal artery, the treatment of which is controversial. Laser energy or electrocautery or even the application of clips except in the hands of a few experts is not ideal because there is a significant risk of recurrent bleeding. A definitive and reliable option is open surgical treatment using the Weinberg procedure. This consists of opening the duodenum, localizing the bleeding, suturing the bleeder, closing the duodenum, and then performing a truncal vagotomy if the patient's condition will tolerate the extra time needed for this procedure.

This procedure may be possible laparoscopically, but usually the patient is not hemodynamically stable enough for a longer laparoscopic procedure, and the open approach is preferable in most cases. If the patient is hemodynamically stable, the procedure can be attempted laparoscopically.

An interesting futuristic idea is the laparoscopic endo-organ concept. This could prove to be of great use in the future for the control of bleeding duodenal ulcers. It consists of the introduction of the laparoscope in the abdomen with simultaneous introduction of trocars into the gastric pouch. This allows the introduction of a grasper instrument into the stomach itself, with the possibility that, after pyloric dilation, one could localize precisely the bleeding area and achieve its hemostasis. This could be performed using a specially devised clip, an intragastric suture, or even an external suture tied on the external aspect of the duodenum. The concept of endo-organ surgery is still experimental but is probably going to develop into a very interesting alternative in the near future.

III. Management of Perforation of Duodenal Ulcers

Description of the various instruments can be found elsewhere in this book. The ability to place sutures and tie surgical knots is extremely important when performing emergency interventional laparoscopy. Laparoscopic closure of a perforated duodenal ulcer can only be accomplished with sutures because no stapling device can perform this closure safely at this point. A variety of laparoscopic needle holders are now available. Each one has advantages and disadvantages. The choice of suture material depends on the surgeon's preference. For most laparoscopic procedures we prefer a monofilament material such as Prolene 3–0. The laparoscopic suture of a perforated ulcer represents in our experience a straightforward operation that should be possible by most laparoscopic surgeons. This statement presupposes that the patient is stable and the perforation is seen early in the first 12 hours before massive bacterial contamination has ensued.

Operative Technique

Usually four trocars are needed for this procedure. One is placed in the umbilicus for the video laparoscope. A lateral trocar is placed on either side of the camera for each hand of the surgeon, and the final trocar is placed under the right costal margin for suction irrigation that will also serve as a retractor. After all four trocars have been inserted, intra-abdominal exploration is undertaken to locate the suspected duodenal lesion. Diagnosis of perforation is confirmed by the presence of free fluid overlying the distal stomach and duodenum and the presence of food fragments and fibrous membranes. In patients with a perforated duodenal ulcer there are often numerous false membranes over the intra-abdominal organs, and the ulcer perforation is usually completely covered by the gallbladder. These inflammatory adhesions must be gently removed usually beginning at the inferior edge of the liver. Once the left lobe and the right lobe of the liver are free, the liver and gallbladder are retracted superiorly. The dissection is then continued along the surface of the duodenum until the margin perforations are clearly visible. At that time, a small-caliber palpating probe can be safely introduced in the

perforation to determine the exact size of the opening and the extent of the inflammation of the surrounding tissues.

It is mandatory to perform a thorough peritoneal lavage using at least 8 liters of fluid to which antibiotics have been added. Each quadrant of the abdomen deserves individual attention, and we think that this is probably the single most important step of this procedure. This step will eliminate all contaminating fluids, and the procedure should only be continued after the lavage is finished. This process also helps to stabilize the patient's vital signs because fewer bacteria will be present in the abdomen and are therefore less likely to invade the bloodstream.

Closure of the Perforation

Before closure of the perforation is attempted, the duodenum should be gently and economically debrided from any necrotic material. Care should be taken in the debridement not to end up with a larger hole than can be sutured. Several different methods of closure have been employed; however, all require the use of intracorporeal knot-tying techniques. If it has been the surgeon's practice to perform Graham patches in open surgery he should perform the same operation laparoscopically and patch the perforation using an omental patch. Two or three sutures will then catch the edges of the ulcer, the omental patch, and the other edge of the ulcer. Another technique is to suture the edges of the ulcer, tie the knots, and then apply an omental patch. Both techniques are acceptable, and the decision depends on the surgeon's own preference. Care is taken not to damage the duodenum. The delicate and fragile nature of the duodenum in such patients mandates that sutures be performed intracorporeally. Extracorporeal tying results in excessive tension on the suture, which results in tearing of the inflamed tissues. Prolene, 2–0 or 3–0 threaded on an SH needle, is usually our suturing material of choice, and it is usually cut short at 15 cm. Small perforations can be managed with a direct suture closure. If the patient has no history of peptic ulcer disease, our recommendation is to stop the operation at this point and treat the patient medically with eradication of *H. pylori* if tests for this are positive in the postoperative period.

FIGURE 15-11. If the patient has a long history of chronic duodenal ulcer with repetitive and intractable disease or with relapse while under thorough medical treatment, a vagotomy should be added to the procedure. Two choices are possible. One is highly selective vagotomy, which is probably a more tedious and longer operation in the emergency setting. Another alternative is posterior truncal vagotomy and anterior seromyotomy as we described them in 1989. This is an easy and straightforward operation that carries minimal mortality and morbidity. It consists of a laparoscopic right truncal vagotomy that spares the left anterior trunk and an anterior lesser curve seromyotomy that extends from the posterior aspect of the angle

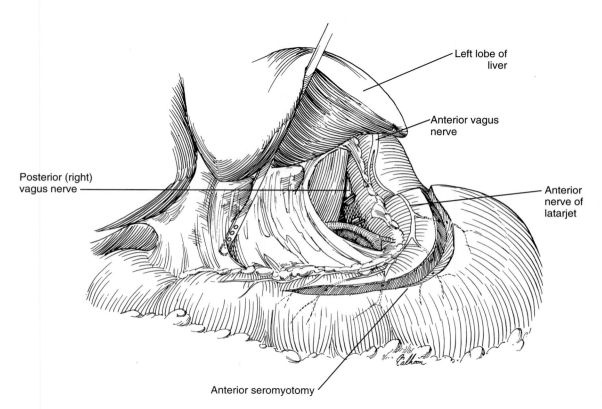

FIGURE 15-11

of His to the first branch of the crow's foot, terminal branches of the anterior gastric nerve of Latarjet. The remaining branches of the nerve of Latarjet are sufficient to ensure adequate antral motility and emptying.

FIGURE 15–12. The divided seromuscular layer is then closed in an overlapping fashion to prevent nerve regeneration and control postoperative hemorrhage from the seromuscular incision.

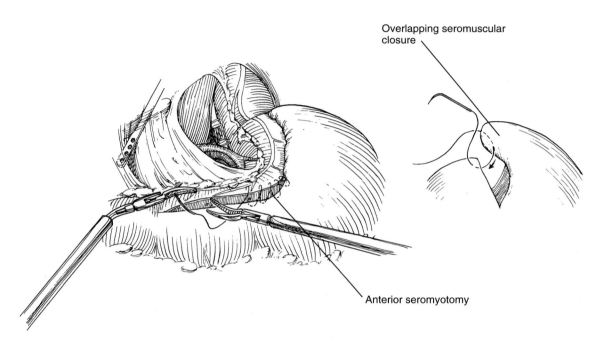

Overlapping seromuscular closure

Anterior seromyotomy

FIGURE 15–12

Chapter 16

Laparoscopic Gastrectomy

DENNIS L. FOWLER, M.D.

I. Indications

A. Benign conditions of the stomach requiring resection
 1. Nonhealing gastric ulcer
 2. Arteriovenous malformation
 3. Benign neoplasms of the stomach that are not locally or endoscopically resectable
  a. Mucosal lesions such as adenomas
  b. Submucosal lesions such as leiomyomas
B. Malignant conditions of the stomach
 1. For palliation when lesions are not resectable for cure
 2. For cure when performed within the confines of a prospective study

II. Contraindications

A. Any contraindication to laparoscopy
B. Active bleeding

III. Factors Important In Patient Selection

A. Location of disease in the stomach
 1. Disease in the antrum allows distal gastrectomy (less difficult)
 2. Proximal disease requires proximal gastrectomy (more difficult)
B. Average or lean body habitus

IV. Preoperative Preparation

A. Evaluation with EGD
B. CT scan if lesion is malignant
C. Same day admission unless coexisting conditions dictate prior admission
D. Patient kept nil per os (NPO) 8 hours before procedure
E. Continue medications until time of NPO

V. Anesthesia

General anesthesia

VI. Accessory Devices

A. Nasogastric tube
 1. Insert initially to decompress the stomach.
 2. Pull back into esophagus after stomach has been decompressed to avoid including tube in resection line of stomach.
 3. After anastomosis, reposition in gastric remnant.
B. Foley catheter
C. Pneumatic compression boots

VII. Instruments and Telescopes

A. Laparoscopes
 1. 0-degree, 10-mm scope for routine use

2. 30-degree, 10-mm scope for better visualization of gastroesophageal junction if needed

B. Video camera with two monitors

C. High flow insufflator

D. Energy sources
   1. Electrocautery
   2. Ultrasonic generator for ultrasonically activated shears or scalpel (Harmonic Scalpel, Ethicon Endo-Surgery, Cincinnati, OH)

E. Trocars and accessories
   1. 10-mm and 15-mm trocars with flap valves
   2. Nonslip devices for trocars
   3. Veress needle
   4. 33-mm port for using circular stapler or for specimen removal (Ethicon Endopath 33-mm trocar, Ethicon Endo-Surgery, Cincinnati, OH)

F. Hand instruments
   1. Atraumatic graspers
      a. Babcock clamps
      b. Allis clamps
      c. Bowel graspers with atraumatic jaws
   2. Curved or angled dissectors
   3. Clip applier
   4. Scissors
   5. Ultrasonically activated shears (Laparo-Sonic Coagulating Shears, Ethicon Endo-Surgery, Cincinnati, OH)
   6. Needle holders
   7. Suction/irrigation device
   8. Fan retractor for liver (not always needed for distal gastrectomy)

G. Endoscopic staplers
   1. Linear cutting stapler (Endo GIA 30 and Endo GIA 60, United States Surgical Corporation, Norwalk, CT)
   2. Linear noncutting stapler (Endo TA, United States Surgical Corporation, Norwalk, CT)
   3. Circular stapler for Billroth I or esophagogastrostomy (Endopath ILS Endoscopic Curved Intraluminal Stapler, Stealth Circular Stapler, Ethicon Endo-Surgery, Cincinnati, OH)

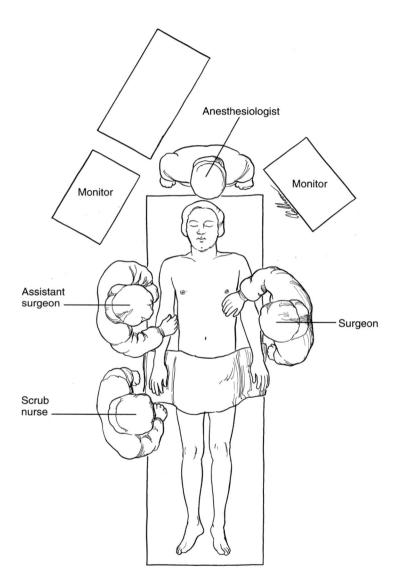

FIGURE 16–1

VIII. Position of Monitors and Trocar Placement

FIGURE 16-1. The equipment in the operating room is arranged so that the surgeon and assistant can stand on each side of the patient and comfortably look across the table and toward the head and see a monitor (see Fig. 16–2). The surgeon works from the patient's left side, and the assistant from the opposite side. The scrub nurse stands beside the assistant.

FIGURE 16-2. Four ports are usually sufficient to complete a distal gastrectomy, and this arrangement has the advantage of requiring only one assistant. If the liver is large or particularly difficult to dissect, or if the operation is a proximal gastrectomy, a fifth port site is necessary for a fan retractor to hold the liver anteriorly and cephalad. The scope is placed through a 10-mm port in or just caudal to the umbilicus, and another 10-mm port is placed in the upper midline to hold the stomach as necessary. Two 15-mm ports are used to facilitate the use of the 60-mm linear cutting stapler. The 60-mm stapler is preferable to the 30-mm stapler for dividing the stomach. Each of the two 15-mm ports is placed at the level of the umbilicus, just lateral to the rectus abdominis on each side. The port on the left is placed at an appropriate angle to divide the stomach with the linear stapler, and the port on the right is at an appropriate angle to divide the duodenum. A 33-mm port can be used to replace one of the 15-mm ports if the circular stapler is to be used for a Billroth I or esophagogastric anastomosis.

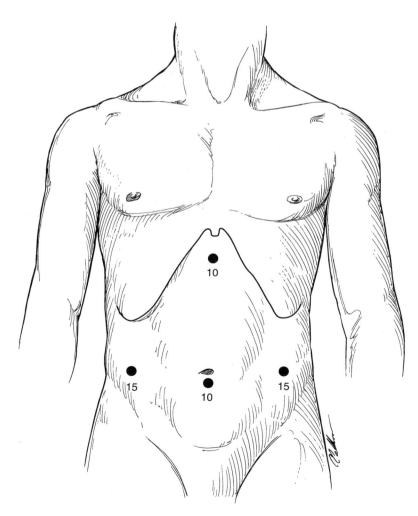

FIGURE 16-2

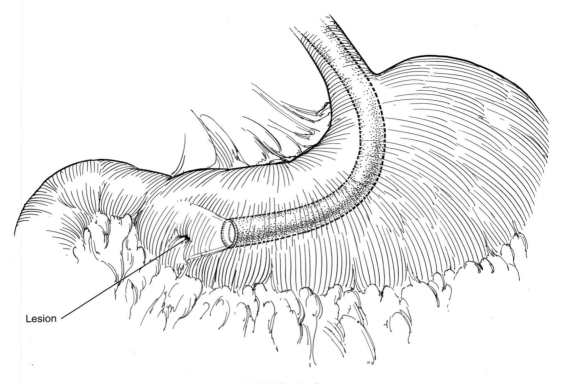

Lesion

FIGURE 16-3

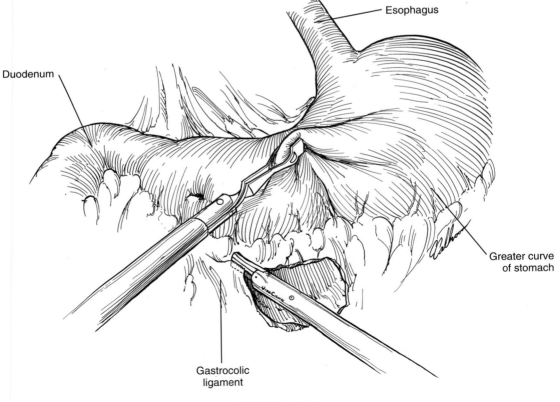

Esophagus

Duodenum

Greater curve
of stomach

Gastrocolic
ligament

FIGURE 16-4

IX. Narrative of Surgical Technique

FIGURE 16–3. Once all the ports are in place and the abdomen has been explored, the surgeon should localize the lesion. Intraoperative endoscopy with transillumination of the endoscope light through the stomach not only localizes the pathology but also conclusively identifies the location of the pylorus. Clips or a marking suture should be placed in the area of the pathology and also at the pylorus.

Distal Gastrectomy

FIGURE 16–4. The dissection is begun by dividing the gastrocolic ligament. A window is made bluntly through the gastrocolic ligament into the lesser sac. Although scissors, electro-

cautery, or even the linear stapler can be used for this dissection, the ultrasonically activated shears function most effectively for this. The dissection may be continued distally past the pylorus as previously described. Mobilization along the greater curvature of the stomach may be performed inside or outside the gastroepiploic arcade depending on the pathology and the individual need in each operation. The gastroepiploic vessels along the greater curvature and the gastric vessels along the lesser curvature may be divided with the shears or between clips.

FIGURE 16–5. The proximal line of resection in the stomach is then divided using the 60-mm linear stapler inserted through the left midabdominal port.

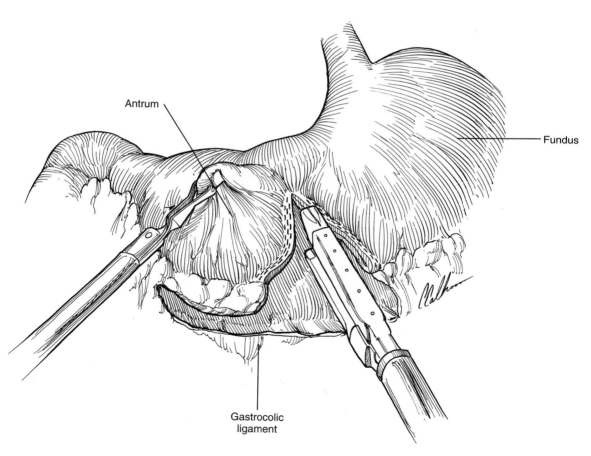

Antrum

Fundus

Gastrocolic
ligament

FIGURE 16–5

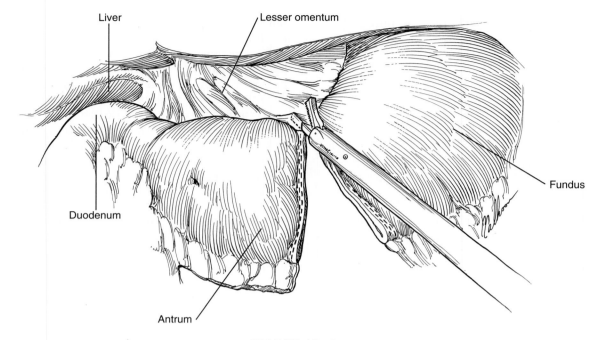

Liver

Lesser omentum

Fundus

Duodenum

Antrum

FIGURE 16–6

FIGURE 16–7

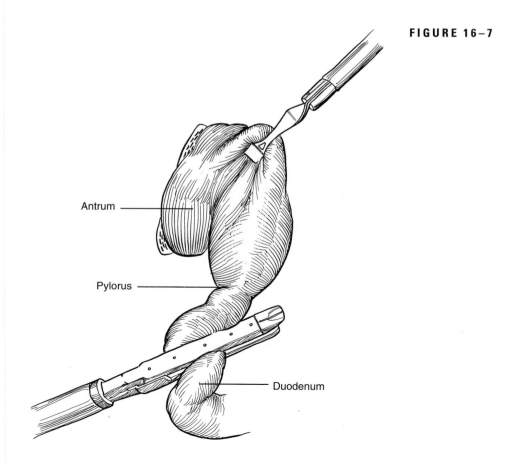

Antrum

Pylorus

Duodenum

FIGURE 16-6. The lesser omentum and gastric vessels along the lesser curvature can then be divided with the shears. Any posterior attachments of the antrum to the pancreas and retroperitoneum can also be divided with the shears. This leaves the duodenum as the only remaining structure attached to the specimen. Once the duodenum has been freed distally as far as necessary, the duodenum is divided. If a Billroth I anastomosis is planned, the duodenum should usually be kocherized at this time before the duodenum is divided.

FIGURE 16-7. Depending on the type of reconstruction anticipated, the duodenum may be divided with the linear stapler for a Billroth II or with scissors or shears for a Billroth I procedure.

The technique described can be used for any size distal gastrectomy. If a distal subtotal resection is necessary, the short gastric vessels along the proximal greater curvature may be divided with the shears or between clips, and the proximal line of resection is divided with the stapler at a more proximal location. For a radical subtotal gastrectomy, an en bloc splenectomy may be included in the dissection. Additionally, the left gastric or gastroduodenal vessels may be followed as high as necessary to perform appropriate lymph node dissection.

FIGURE 16-8. Although either a Billroth I or a Billroth II anastomosis can be completed with laparoscopic suturing techniques, it is faster to use staplers. A Billroth II can be completed relatively easily using the linear cutting stapler by constructing a side-to-side antecolic gastrojejunostomy.

FIGURE 16-8

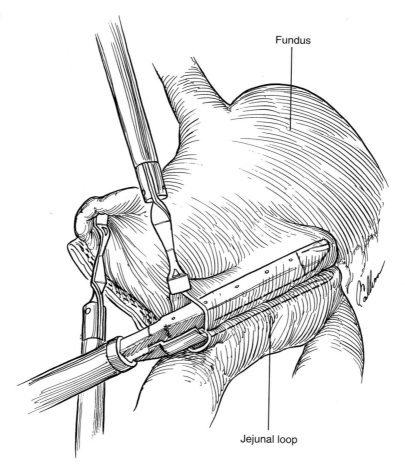

Fundus

Jejunal loop

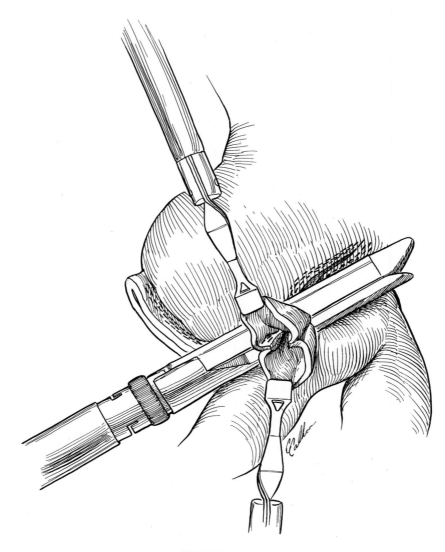

FIGURE 16–9

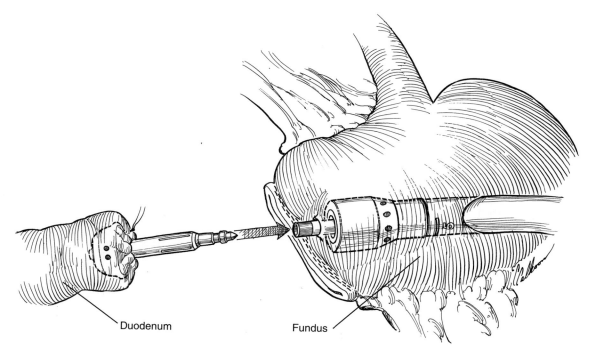

Duodenum   Fundus

FIGURE 16–10

FIGURE 16–9. The remaining defect can be sutured or closed with the linear noncutting stapler.

FIGURE 16–10. A Billroth I anastomosis can also be sutured, but the circular stapler can be passed through a 33-mm port to create a stapled gastroduodenoscopy. The circular stapler is introduced through the 33-mm port placed in the left midabdomen and then is inserted into the stomach through an anterior gastrotomy. The anvil is positioned in the open end of the duodenum. A purse-string suture must be placed in the end of the duodenum with laparoscopic suturing techniques to hold the anvil in place. With the circular stapler in the stomach, the stapler is "opened," and the spike in the stapler is passed through the anterior wall of the stomach. The anvil, which is in the duodenum, is connected to the spike, and the stapler is closed and fired. After the stapler is removed, the anterior gastrotomy is closed with sutures or the linear noncutting stapler.

The specimen can be placed in a bag and brought out through a short extension of the umbilical incision. If spleen is attached, it can be finger fractured in the bag before the bag is removed. Usually the incision needs to be only 2 to 3 cm in length. If the 33-mm port is used for the circular stapler, the specimen can be removed through that port or through that incision after the port is removed.

Proximal Gastrectomy

FIGURE 16–11. The dissection is begun by bluntly making a window in the gastrocolic ligament near the greater curvature at the anticipated distal line of resection. The greater omentum is then divided in a proximal direction parallel to the greater curvature. This dissection is best done with the ultrasonically activated shears. The dissection can be done either inside or outside the gastroepiploic arcade.

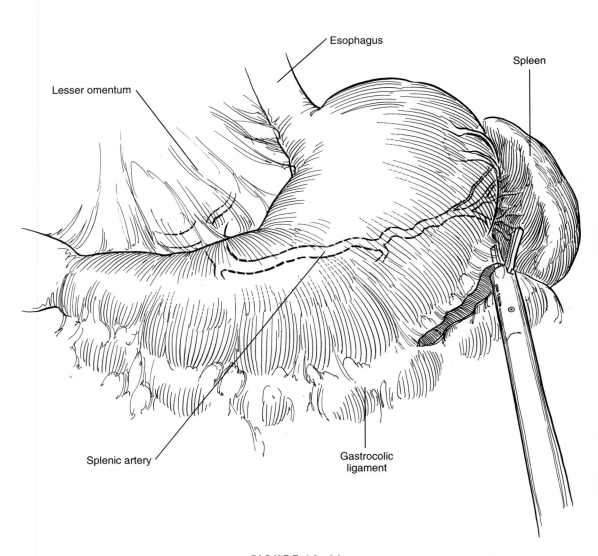

FIGURE 16–11

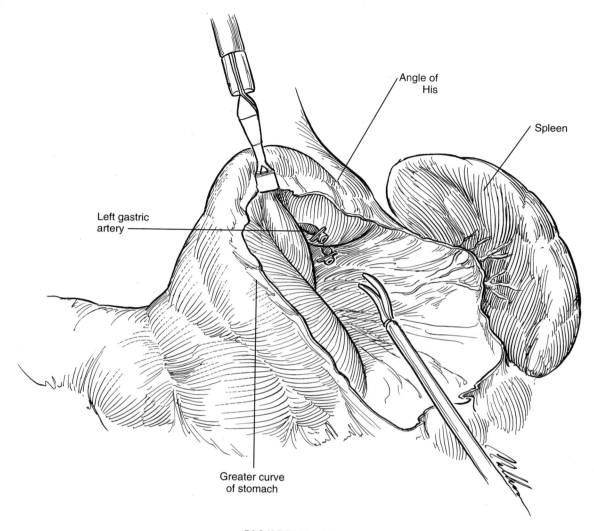

Angle of
His

Spleen

Left gastric
artery

Greater curve
of stomach

FIGURE 16–12

FIGURE 16–12. More proximally, the dissection is carried through the short gastric vessels all the way to the top of the fundus. The fundus is mobilized away from the diaphragm to the angle of His, and the left gastric artery is identified. It can be divided between clips or ligatures at a level appropriate for the type of resection.

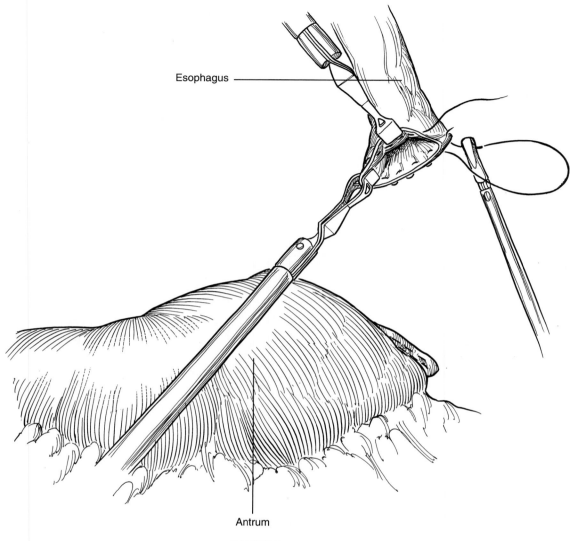

Esophagus

Antrum

FIGURE 16–13

FIGURE 16–13. The distal line of resection in the midportion of the stomach can be divided using the 60-mm linear cutting stapler. Next, the gastric vessels along the lesser curvature should be divided at the distal line of resection. The lesser omentum can then be divided all the way up to the diaphragmatic hiatus. This dissection is done with scissors, electrocautery, or even the linear stapler, but the shears are the preferred instrument. The only remaining structure attached to the proximal stomach should then be the esophagus. The esophagus can be divided with scissors or shears.

The anastomosis between the stomach and the esophagus can be completed with laparoscopic suturing techniques or with the circular stapler. If the stapler is used, a purse-string suture must be placed in the end of the esophagus using laparoscopic suturing techniques.

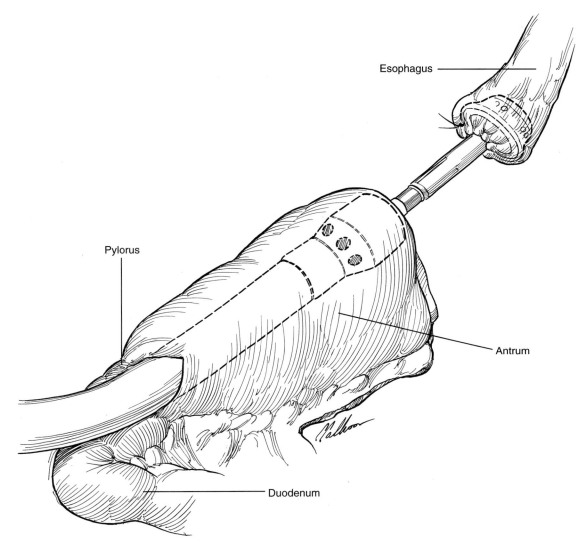

Esophagus

Pylorus

Antrum

Duodenum

FIGURE 16-14

FIGURE 16-14. The circular stapler is introduced into the abdominal cavity through the 33-mm port, which is placed in the right midabdomen. A transverse incision is made across the pylorus, and the stapler is inserted into the stomach through the pyloric incision. The stapler is "opened," and the spike of the stapler is pushed through the anterior wall of the gastric remnant. The anvil, which is held in the end of the esophagus with the tied purse string, is attached to the spike of the stapler. The stapler is then closed and fired to create the anastomosis. The pyloric incision is closed transversely to create a Heineke-Mikulicz pyloroplasty. This can be done using either sutures or the linear noncutting stapler. The specimen is placed in a bag and then is removed through the 33-mm port or that incision. If there is attached spleen, it can be finger fractured in the bag prior to removal.

X. Postoperative Medications

A. Patient-controlled analgesia (PCA) using morphine or Demerol for pain control
B. H$_2$ blocker for 2 weeks
C. Although it is not always necessary, a prokinetic agent such as metoclopramide or cisapride may help reestablish gastric motility
D. A nasogastric tube may be helpful overnight but can be removed on the first postoperative morning

XI. Advancement of Diet

A. A clear liquid diet is given on the morning after surgery when the nasogastric tube is removed.
B. The diet is advanced to a regular diet when it can be tolerated, usually on the second morning after surgery.
C. Depending on the size of the resection, the patient may need more frequent, smaller feedings (i.e., a postgastrectomy six-feeding diet).

XII. Determinants of Discharge

A. Adequate oral intake
B. Ambulatory
C. Adequate pain control

XIII. Return to Normal Activity/Work

A. Gradual resumption of normal activities
B. Return to work in 2 to 3 weeks

Chapter 17

Laparoscopic Partial Gastrectomy and Billroth II Gastrojejunostomy

JOSEPH F. UDDO, JR., M.D.

I. Indications

A. Gastric lipomas
B. Gastric leiomyomas
C. Gastric polyps
D. Gastric angiodysplasia

II. Contraindications

A. Gastric cancer may be considered a relative contraindication at this time
B. Patients who cannot tolerate general anesthesia

III. Factors Important in Patient Selection

A. The lesion should be in the gastric antrum and away from the gastroesophageal junction.
B. Previous upper abdominal surgery or obesity make the operation more difficult.

IV. Preoperative Preparation

A. The lesion should be evaluated by endoscopy and biopsy prior to surgery.
B. A preoperative upper gastrointestinal series is helpful in establishing the location of the lesion in the stomach and planning the operation.
C. The patient is admitted on the morning of surgery.

D. Preoperative antibiotic prophylaxis is administered.
E. Deep venous thrombosis prophylaxis is used.

V. Choice of Anesthesia

General anesthesia is required.

VI. Accessory Devices

A. A nasogastric tube is inserted after general endotracheal anesthesia is induced.
B. A urinary catheter is inserted.

VII. Instruments and Telescopes

A. Laparoscopes: 10-mm, 0-degree laparoscopes are used. A 10-mm, 30-degree laparoscope and a 5-mm laparoscope should be available.
B. Video equipment: Two full camera systems with individual light sources and two monitors are used.
C. Insufflation device: A rapid insufflation device with a smoke evacuator is preferred.
D. Electrocautery: A monopolar electrocautery device with an assortment of wands is needed.
E. Four noncrushing bowel graspers
F. Laparoscopic probes and retractors
G. Laparoscopic clip applier (large)
H. Laparoscopic loop ties

I. Laparoscopic needle holder, knot pusher, and suture material
J. Curved laparoscopic scissors capable of conducting electrocautery
K. An assortment of laparoscopic dissectors capable of conducting electrocautery
L. Laparoscopic stapling devices:
   1. Endo GIA 60 and Endo GIA 30
   2. Endo TA 60

VIII. Position of Monitors and Placement of Trocars

The patient is placed supine on the operating table with both arms secured at the patient's side. Use of an electric table facilitates positioning of the patient and bowel retraction. Two monitors are used. One is placed on either side of the head of the patient. Care should be taken not to place the instruments in such a way that movement around the operating table is impeded.

FIGURE 17–1. Laparoscopic gastric surgery is similar to laparoscopic cholecystectomy in that the operative site is relatively fixed. The exact placement of laparoscopic trocars for this procedure is still evolving; however, it has been most useful to place a 10-mm port through the umbilicus for the laparoscope. Two additional ports are placed in the right upper quadrant and two in the left upper quadrant. A lower midline 15-mm port has been used for the introduction of the laparoscopic 60-mm stapling device. This lower midline placement allows adequate maneuverability of the 60-mm device. Ports that are closer hinder proper positioning of the stapler.

FIGURE 17–1

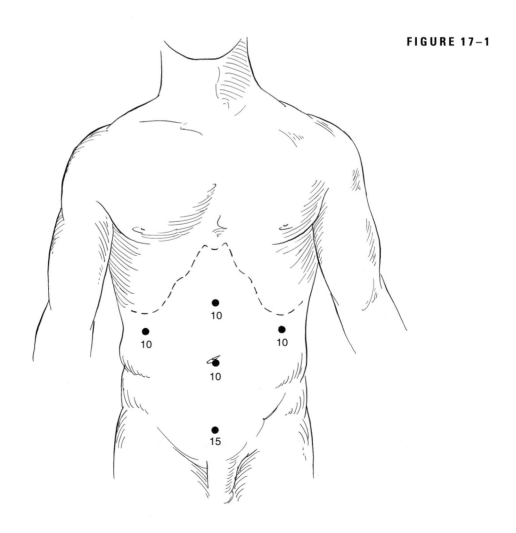

IX. Narrative of Surgical Techniques

FIGURE 17-2. After the abdomen has been thoroughly explored laparoscopically, the stomach is grasped and held cephalad while the colon is retracted caudally. The gastrocolic ligament is then taken down, and the lesser sac is entered. The vessels in the gastrocolic ligament are clipped proximally and distally and divided. Alternatively, this structure can be divided using a laparoscopic stapling device. The lesser omentum is then taken down; this can be accomplished for the most part with electrocautery. The stomach and duodenum are transilluminated using an intraoperatively placed gastroscope to be certain that the pylorus is included in the distal extent of resection and that the lesion is clearly identified. These points are marked with laparoscopic clips. The duodenum is then mobilized distally. A laparoscopic 60-mm stapling device is used to divide the duodenum just distal to the pylorus. One application of this instrument is adequate to completely divide the duodenum. The proximal line of transection is then identified. A 60-mm stapling device is used to transect the stomach. Two applications of this device may be required; however, one application of the 60-mm device followed by application of a 30-mm device to complete the transection may be adequate. At this point, all attachments to the specimen have been divided. The specimen is then placed in the right upper quadrant to be retrieved after the anastomosis has been completed.

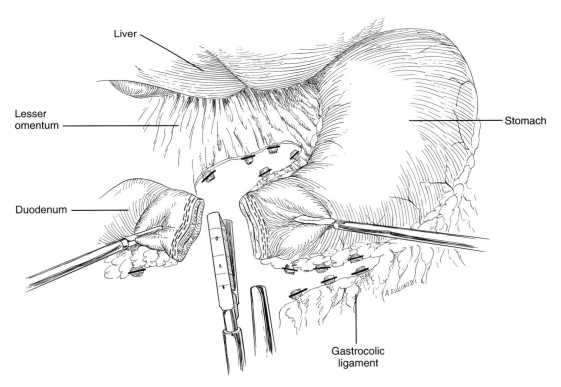

Liver

Lesser omentum

Stomach

Duodenum

Gastrocolic ligament

FIGURE 17-2

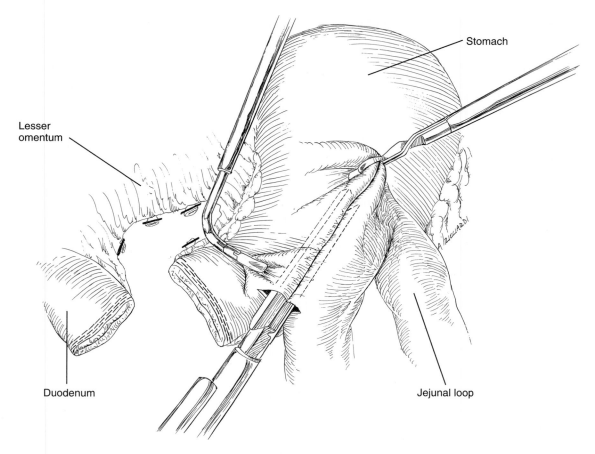

Stomach

Lesser
omentum

Duodenum

Jejunal loop

FIGURE 17–3

FIGURE 17-3. The ligament of Treitz is identified, and a loop of small bowel is brought into approximation with the gastric remnant in an anticolic fashion. The two limbs to be anastomosed can be kept in secure approximation using a laparoscopic atraumatic Babcock clamp. A gastrotomy is fashioned in the stomach and an enterotomy in the small bowel. The 60-mm stapling device is introduced through the lower midline incision. The forks of the device are placed through the previously fashioned openings and, once proper positioning of the device has been confirmed, the instrument is closed and then fired. The anastomosis can be easily inspected with the laparoscope.

FIGURE 17-4. The remaining enterotomy is closed using an Endo TA stapling device introduced through the lower midline 15-mm port. Care should be taken to identify the full extent of the enterotomy to be certain that it is fully and securely closed.

The specimen is then removed through the lower midline port site. Minimal extension of the excision may be required. Choosing the lower midline port site for extraction of the specimen yields better cosmesis as well as less postoperative pain.

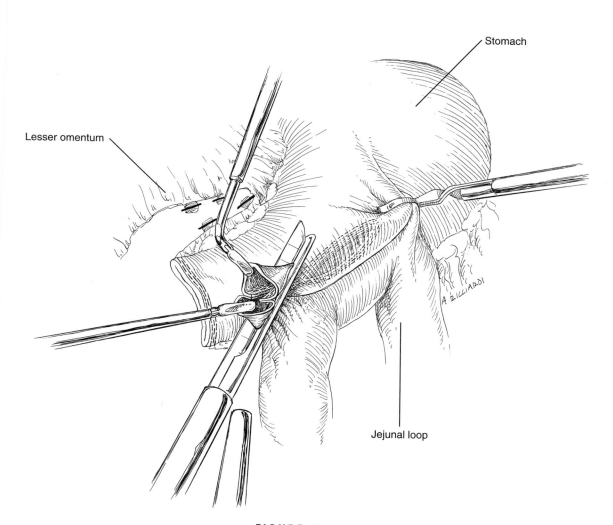

FIGURE 17-4

Closure

All fascial incisions for ports 10 mm or greater are closed with interrupted absorbable sutures. Skin incisions are closed with staples or subcutaneous stitches. The Foley catheter is removed in the recovery room.

X. Postoperative Medications

Minimal postoperative pain control is required.

XI. Advancement of Diet

A. The nasogastric tube is left in place until the first signs of recovery of bowel function appear.

B. Liquids are started shortly after the nasogastric tube is removed (48 to 72 hours).

C. Clear liquids continue until the patient has a strong desire to advance to a solid diet.

XII. Determinants of Discharge

A. Discharge takes place in 3 to 5 days.

B. Patients must be ambulatory, tolerating a liquid diet, and using oral analgesics.

XIII. Return to Normal Activity/Work

The patient can return to unrestricted activity shortly after discharge.

Chapter 18

Laparoscopic Resection of Benign Gastric Tumors

W. PETER GEIS, M.D., and CONSTANTINO STRATOULIAS, M.D.

I. Indications

A. Polyps that cannot be completely excised by endoscopic techniques—more than 2 cm in diameter, sessile, difficult location (e.g., gastroesophageal junction, pyloric area)
   1. Asymptomatic adenomatous polyps
   2. Symptomatic polyps
B. Leiomyomas and other intramural mesenchymal tumors
C. Pancreatic rests (causing pain or obstruction)
D. Brunner's gland adenomas (causing pain or obstruction)
E. Symptomatic duplication cysts

II. Contraindications

A. Benign polyps that can be completely excised by endoscopic techniques
B. Asymptomatic biopsy-proven hamartomatous, inflammatory, or hyperplastic polyps
C. Patients who cannot undergo pneumoperitoneum
D. Patients who cannot tolerate general anesthesia

III. Factors Important in Patient Selection

It is mandatory that the patient can tolerate general anesthesia and muscle-paralyzing agents. It is also preferable if the patient has had no prior surgery. There should be a normal coagulation profile, and hemoglobin should be replaced if gastric bleeding has occurred.

The surgeon should have reasonable assurance that the lesion is benign, although this is often impossible to know for certain preoperatively. Table 18–1 delineates the classification of benign gastric tumors. The surgeon should recognize that only 7 per cent of gastric tumors are benign. Upper gastrointestinal endoscopy and contrast radiographs are the major diagnostic tools used for these lesions. Symptomatic

Table 18–1. Classification of Benign Gastric Tumors

Polyps
Hyperplastic
Adenomatous
Mixed
Inflammatory
Peutz-Jeghers (hamartomatous)
Intramural
Leiomyoma
Lipoma
Neurogenic tumors
Fibroma
Vascular tumors
Heterotopic pancreas
Brunner's gland adenoma
Adenomyoma
Cysts
Mucocele (intramucosal cyst)
Gastritis cystica profunda (submucosal cyst)
Duplication cyst

polyps causing pain, bleeding, or obstruction, as well as asymptomatic adenomatous polyps should be completely removed for histologic diagnosis. Four per cent of adenomatous polyps less than 2 cm in diameter are associated with adenocarcinoma, whereas 25 per cent are malignant if the lesion is greater than 2 cm. Leiomyomas should be excised to provide symptom relief and for histologic diagnosis; the benign nature of these lesions cannot be established by segmental biopsy alone. Pancreatic rests and Brunner's gland adenomas should be excised if they cause pain or obstruction (usually in the prepyloric antrum) or if the biopsy is indeterminant. Symptomatic duplication cysts should also be surgically removed.

IV. Preoperative Preparation

A. Same day admission unless patient has:
  1. Chronic obstructive pulmonary disease (COPD) or coronary artery disease (CAD); admit patient 1 day preoperatively to optimize cardiopulmonary systems.
  2. Overt hemorrhage; control blood loss and proceed urgently.
  3. Gastric outlet obstruction; admit patient for gastric decompression and fluid and electrolyte replacement.
B. Preoperative medications
  1. Intravenous antibiotics
  2. Hyperalimentation if nutrition is impaired
C. Bowel preparation
  1. Gastric decompression
  2. Mechanical bowel preparation to diminish size of colon during laparoscopy

V. Choice of Anesthesia

A. General anesthesia
B. Muscle paralyzing agents
C. Avoid nitrous oxide
D. Associated issues:
  1. Reverse Trendelenburg position
  2. Invasive monitoring for high risk patients

VI. Accessory Devices

A. 50 to 52 French bougie (for lesions in the vicinity of the gastroesophageal junction)

B. Urinary catheters
C. Pneumatic compression stockings
D. Two carbon dioxide insufflators for
  1. Peritoneal cavity
  2. Stomach

VII. Instruments and Telescopes

A. 10-mm and 5-mm laparoscopes (0 and 30 degrees, respectively)
B. Flexible endoscope
C. Endoscopic Babcock clamps
D. Endoscopic linear stapler/cutter with thick tissue staples
E. Radial expanding dilator transgastric ports
F. Ultrasonic scalpel
G. Liver retractor
H. Laparoscopic needle holders
I. Laparoscopic bowel clamp
J. Endo-loops

VIII. Position of Monitors and Placement and Size of Trocars

FIGURE 18–1A. The patient is placed in a modified lithotomy position. Two primary monitors are placed above the right and left shoulders of the patient. The monitors are suspended on overhead ceiling columns, if possible, for more versatility. In most cases, four 10/12-mm ports are used, one for the liver retractor, one for the laparoscope, and two working ports. The patient is placed in the reverse Trendelenburg position, and the left lateral segment of the liver is retracted cephalad. If the exact location of the lesion is in question, most commonly when the lesion is adjacent to the pylorus or adjacent to the gastroesophageal junction, intraorgan assessment is performed using radial expanding dilator RED ports. Two or three 5-mm ports are placed in the epigastrium to accomplish this step. The radial dilating port is placed through the anterior gastric wall, and a second carbon dioxide insufflator is used to insufflate the stomach to a pressure of approximately 15 mm Hg. The size of the stomach is increased (distended) by diminishing the pressure of carbon dioxide insufflation into the abdominal cavity, thus increasing the pressure gradient across the gastric wall. The exact location of the lesion is determined. Lesions within the pylorus require gastric resection, while lesions proximal to the pylorus may be excised locally. Lesions at the gastroesophageal junction must be excised very carefully to avoid destruction of the gastroesophageal junction. These patients may require associated Nissen fundoplication. A 5-mm laparoscope and a second camera system are used to perform gastroscopy/gastroduodenoscopy to assess the antrum of the stomach, pylorus, and first portion of the duodenum.

For lesions near the gastroesophageal junction and body of the stomach, one port is placed in the right upper quadrant a few centimeters above the umbilicus in the midline, and two are placed in the left upper quadrant. Laparoscopic port positions for the resection of benign gastric tumors located in the area of the gastroesophageal junction and the body or fundus of the stomach are:

1. Right midclavicular line
2. Supraumbilical midline
3. Left midclavicular line
4. Left anterior axillary line

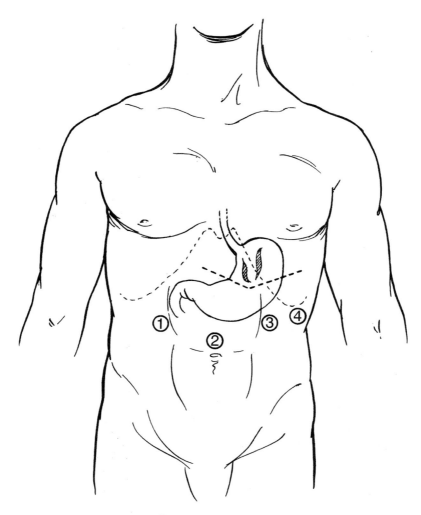

FIGURE 18–1A

FIGURE 18-1B. For lesions in the pyloric area and antrum, the ports are placed lower: one in the right lower quadrant, one in the midline a few centimeters below the umbilicus, one in the left lower quadrant, and one in the left upper quadrant or almost at the level of the umbilicus. The transgastric ports are 5-mm ports and are placed after the location of the stomach and the preoperative information about the location of the lesion have been evaluated intraoperatively.

IX. Narrative of Surgical Technique

FIGURE 18-2A. Excision of a benign gastric tumor with an endoscopic linear stapler inserted through an anterior gastrotomy. The tumor is retracted using an atraumatic endoscopic clamp.

FIGURE 18-2B. Staple line on posterior gastric wall after excision of benign gastric tumor through an anterior gastrotomy.

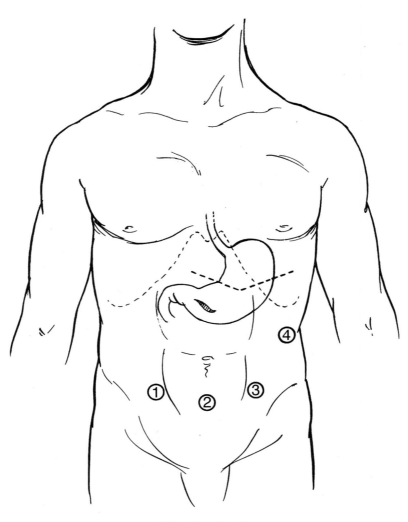

FIGURE 18-1B

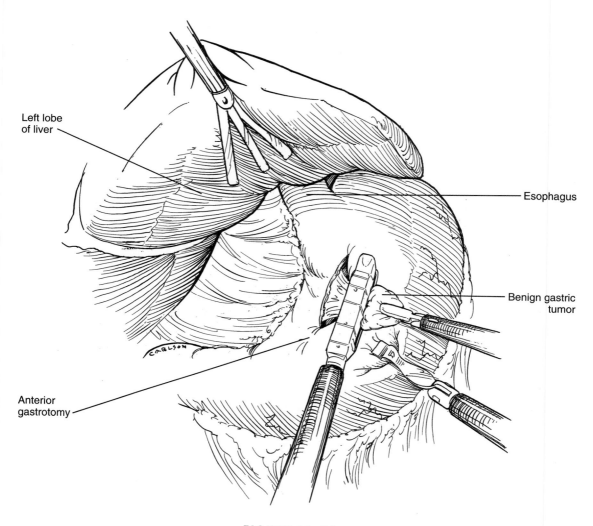

Left lobe
of liver

Esophagus

Benign gastric
tumor

Anterior
gastrotomy

FIGURE 18–2A

FIGURE 18–2B

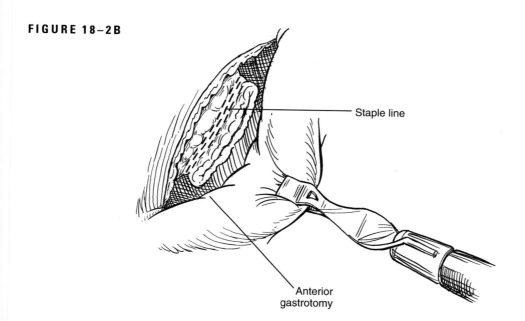

Staple line

Anterior
gastrotomy

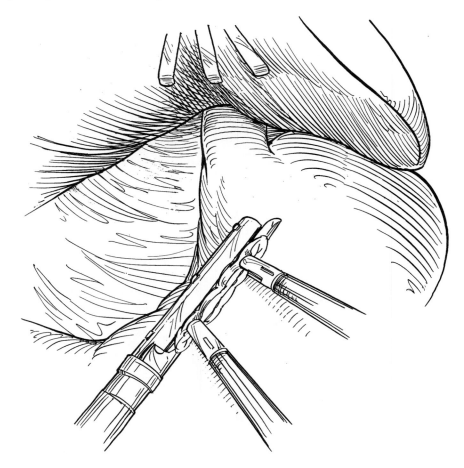

FIGURE 18–2C

FIGURE 18–2C. Closure of the anterior gastrotomy with an endoscopic linear stapler after excision of a gastric tumor. The edges of the gastrotomy are approximated with atraumatic endoscopic clamps. The staple line is later reinforced with interrupted sutures.

FIGURE 18–3. Excision of a benign gastric tumor by intraorgan excision using radial expanding dilator ports. One intragastric port is used for the laparoscope, and there are two working ports. The proximal jejunum is clamped with an atraumatic endoscopic clamp to avoid distention of the small bowel by the insufflated gas.

FIGURE 18–4A. Transection of the first portion of the duodenum with a linear endoscopic stapler for excision of a tumor in the pyloric area.

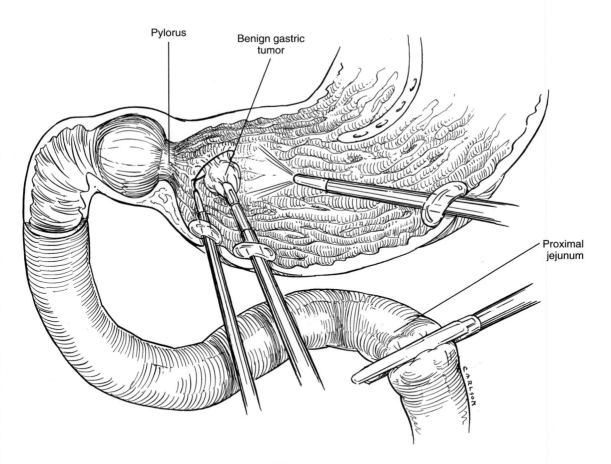

Pylorus

Benign gastric tumor

Proximal jejunum

FIGURE 18–3

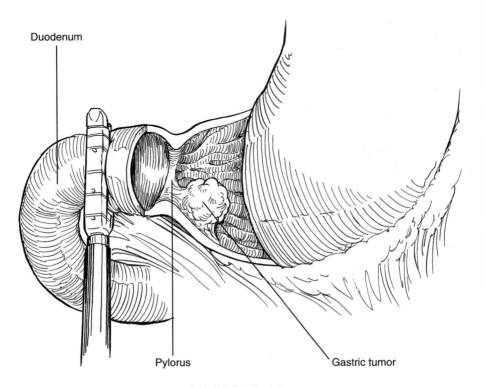

Duodenum

Pylorus

Gastric tumor

FIGURE 18–4A

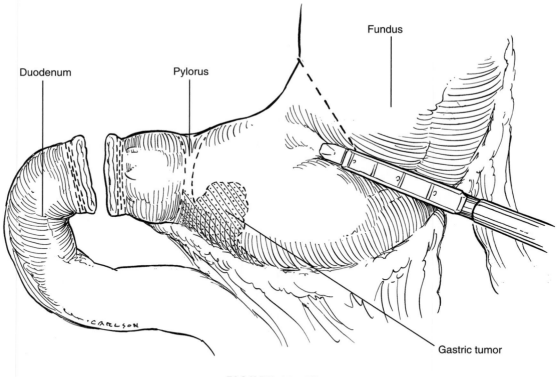

Duodenum

Pylorus

Fundus

Gastric tumor

·CARLSON·

FIGURE 18–4B

FIGURE 18–4B. Transection of the proximal stomach with a linear endoscopic stapler during laparoscopic distal gastrectomy.

FIGURE 18–4C. Completion of transection of the proximal stomach with sequential firing of the endoscopic linear stapler during laparoscopic distal gastrectomy.

FIGURE 18–4C

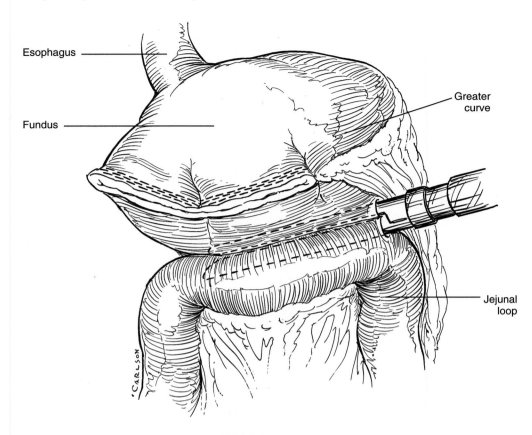

Esophagus

Fundus

Greater
curve

Jejunal
loop

CARLSON

FIGURE 18–4D

FIGURE 18–4D. Performance of gastrojejunal Billroth II anastomosis using an endoscopic linear stapler. This step can also be performed at the skin level through a mini-incision if a larger anastomosis is desired.

FIGURE 18–4E. Closure of the final opening after performance of a stapled Billroth II gastrojejunostomy at the skin level. A linear stapler or hand suture technique can be used for this step of the procedure.

X. Postoperative Medications

A. Intravenous or intramuscular pain medication as needed

B. Oral pain medication when oral diet is instituted

C. Associated issues:
   1. Nasogastric decompression
   2. Gastrografin swallow is performed on the second postoperative day.
   3. Liquid diet after gastrografin swallow

D. H_2 blockers are given intravenously and then orally.

XI. Advancement of Diet

A. Liquid diet is instituted following satisfactory results on Gastrografin swallow/UGI

B. Progress to mechanically soft diet in 24 hours

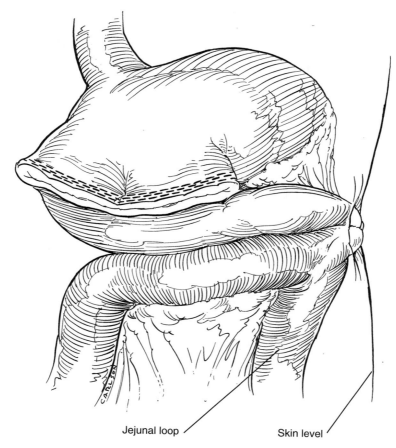

Jejunal loop   Skin level

FIGURE 18–4E

XII. Determinants of Discharge

The patient is discharged on the third or fourth postoperative day if he or she is tolerating the mechanically soft diet and has normal bowel function and if there are no other medical contraindications to discharge owing to concomitant illnesses.

XIII. Return to Normal Activity/Work

Normal daily activities are allowed on discharge except for heavy lifting and strenuous exercise during the first 2 weeks after the operation. Most patients are able to return to work on postoperative day 5 if the work does not involve strenuous activity. Minimal amounts of narcotic analgesics are required after the patient is discharged from the hospital.

Chapter 19

Laparoscopic Vertical Banded Gastroplasty

JOSEPH F. AMARAL, M.D.

I. Indications

A. Patients must meet all of the following criteria:
  1. Current body weight more than 100 pounds over ideal
  2. Failed attempts at medically supervised diets
  3. No endocrine disease
B. No peptic ulcer disease
C. Concomitant obesity-related disease:
  1. Hypertension
  2. Diabetes
  3. Sleep apnea
  4. Severe arthritis

II. Contraindications

A. Intolerance of general anesthesia
B. Severe coagulopathy
C. Alcoholism
D. Drug abuse

III. Factors Important in Patient Selection

Because of the technical difficulty of operating on obese patients, laparoscopic vertical banded gastroplasty is limited to patients who are 100 to 250 pounds over their ideal body weight. Before attempting this procedure the surgeon should have had extensive experience in laparoscopic surgery (more than 100 laparoscopic cases) and should be familiar with open bariatric surgery.

IV. Preoperative Preparation

A. Same day admission
B. Preoperative medications: metoclopramide hydrochloride intravenously (IV), 2 g cefazolin IV, 5000 units heparin subcutaneously
C. Bowel preparation: none

V. Choice of Anesthesia

General endotracheal anesthesia

VI. Accessory Devices

A. Nasogastric tube
B. Urinary catheter
C. Pneumatic compression stockings

VII. Instruments and Telescopes

A. 10-mm, 0-degree laparoscope
B. One curved dissector
C. Two tissue graspers
D. Two Babcock forceps
E. One curved grasper or dissector (Roticulating Grasper, United States Surgical Corporation, Norwalk, CT)
F. Ultrasonically activated scalpel and/or laparosonic coagulating shears (LCS) (Har-

222

monic Scalpel, Ethicon Endo-Surgery, Cin-cinnati, OH)
G. Polypropylene mesh
H. Endo GIA 30 (United States Surgical Cor-poration) or EZ 35 (Ethicon Endo-Surgery, Cincinnati, OH)
I. Endo TAO 60 (United States Surgical Cor-poration) or ECL 60 (Ethicon Endo-Sur-gery, Cincinnati, OH)
J. CEEA 28 mm (United States Surgical Cor-poration) or CDH 29 (Ethicon Endo-Sur-gery, Cincinnati, OH)
K. Suction irrigation device
L. Pressurized irrigation system (EndoFlow, Davol, Inc)

VIII. Operating Room Set Up and Trocar Positions

FIGURE 19–1A. The patient is placed in the supine position on the operating table. Al-though the lithotomy position is desirable, the large size of these patients usually makes it im-possible. Two monitors are used, located at the patient's right and left sides at about the level of the shoulders. The surgeon stands on the patient's right side, and the camera operator stands on the patient's left side. A second assis-tant stands on the right. The surgeon uses a two-handed technique. The procedure is per-formed with the patient in the supine position.

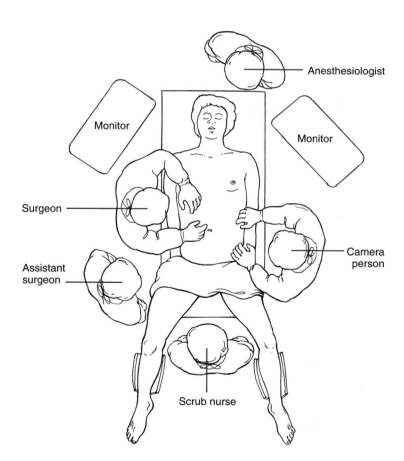

FIGURE 19–1A

FIGURE 19–1B. Laparoscopy is initiated with an open (Hasson) technique. The procedure is performed by making a 10- to 12-mm vertical incision approximately midway between the xiphoid and the umbilicus and spreading the subcutaneous tissue to the fascia with a hemostat. The fascia is then grasped on either side of the midline with Kocher clamps, and the midline fascia is divided with a scalpel. Heavy sutures, such as 0 silk or polyglycolic acid, are placed on either side of the midline incision for traction and for later closure of the defect. Under direct vision, the preperitoneal fat and posterior sheath are identified and divided, and the peritoneum is identified and incised. Confirmation of entrance into the abdominal cavity is achieved either by visualization of the bowel or omentum or by the ability to pass a blunt instrument freely into the abdominal cavity. A blunt, trocar-cannula system designed for open laparoscopy is then placed in the abdomen. Prior to insufflation, the cavity is visually explored with the laparoscope to ensure its appropriate location and the absence of visceral or vessel injury.

Five cannulas are used for the procedure: four 10-mm cannulas and one 5 mm cannula. Their locations are shown in Figure 19–1A. They comprise a 5-mm subxiphoid cannula that enters the abdomen to the left of the patient's falciform ligament, a 10-mm right midclavicular cannula adjacent to the costal margin, a 10-mm left midclavicular cannula adjacent to the costal margin, and a 10-mm cannula midway between the xiphoid and the 10-mm cannula used for open laparoscopy in the midline. During the procedure the midclavicular left cannula will be changed to a 33-mm cannula, and the supraumbilical cannula will be changed to a 15-mm cannula.

FIGURE 19–1B

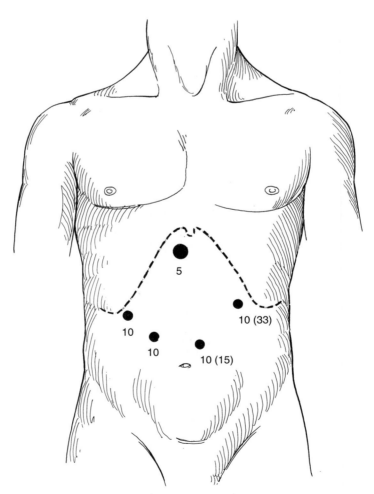

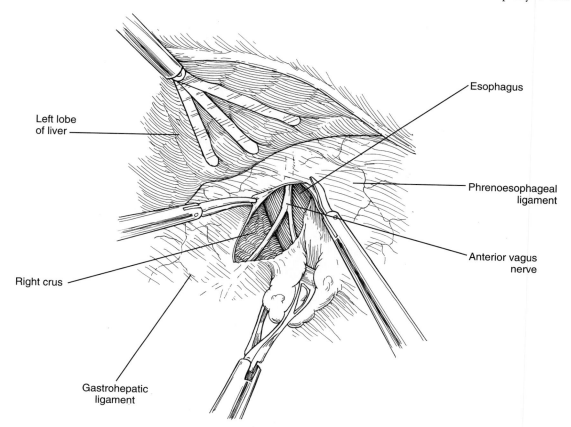

FIGURE 19–2

IX. Narrative of Surgical Technique

FIGURE 19–2. Once the cannulas are inserted the liver is elevated with a retractor through the right midclavicular cannula. We prefer not to use an open fan-type retractor because the limbs tend to cut into the liver. Instead, a 10-mm flat retractor or a closed fan-type retractor is used. The fatty liver of these obese patients is very easy to penetrate. Care must be taken to avoid doing this because it results in bleeding that will interfere with crural dissection. The stomach is then grasped with a 10-mm Babcock-type forceps inserted through the lower 10-mm cannula, and traction is exerted on the stomach toward the pelvis. This forceps should not be twisted during traction because it can tear the stomach. Additionally, the instrument itself should not be traumatic. Surgical dissection is started with the surgeon using a two-handed technique through the 5-mm subxiphoid and the 10-mm left midclavicular cannulas. The phrenoesophageal ligament is grasped with a dissector and divided using the sharp side of the LCS if the area is avascular. Vascular areas are transected with the blunt side of the LCS. Bleeding is stopped using the blunt side of the LCS by grasping the bleeding site and activating the LCS for 3 to 5 seconds. This dissection opens not only the phrenoesophageal ligament across the crura and esophagus but also a window in the gastrohepatic ligament. Blunt dissection using an endo-peanut or the suction irrigation device is used to identify the right crura and the esophagus. Care must be taken to avoid injury to the esophagus. If there is no hiatal hernia, the crura may be closely applied to the esophagus and may be mistaken for the esophagus itself. If there is difficulty in identifying the esophagus a lighted bougie may help.

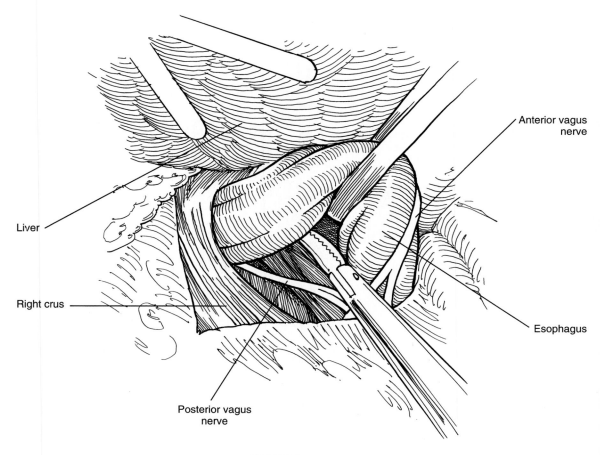

Liver

Right crus

Posterior vagus
nerve

Anterior vagus
nerve

Esophagus

FIGURE 19–3

FIGURE 19-3. No energized dissection is used in the hiatus until the esophagus and right crus are clearly visualized. To facilitate this dissection, we stay between the posterior vagus nerve and the esophagus because there is less fatty tissue here than below the vagus nerve. The LCS on the blunt side is used to divide small periesophageal blood vessels. The gastroesophageal fat pad is also removed using the LCS. The sharp edge of the LCS is used to remove the fat pad until the one or two vessels feeding it are found. These are coagulated with the dull side of the blade. Complete dissection of the crural area requires identification and clearing of the left crus as well as the right. This is necessary to identify the external cardioesophageal junction and create a large infraesophageal window that allows the esophagus to be encircled with a Penrose drain. A roticulating or curved instrument is helpful in getting around the esophagus. Working around the esophagus is a critical step during which the esophagus may be perforated or the left pleural cavity entered. To avoid these complications this dissection must be performed under direct vision and not by blind puncture. A space is created between the left crus and the stomach.

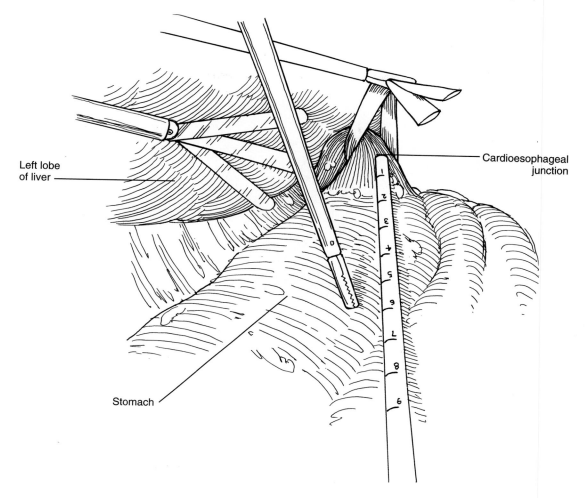

FIGURE 19–4

FIGURE 19–4. An endo-ruler is used to measure a point 6 cm caudad from the cardioesophageal junction; it is marked with methylene blue. This denotes the site where the gastric window will be created. In general, this point corresponds to the location of the first visible crossing vessel on the lesser curve.

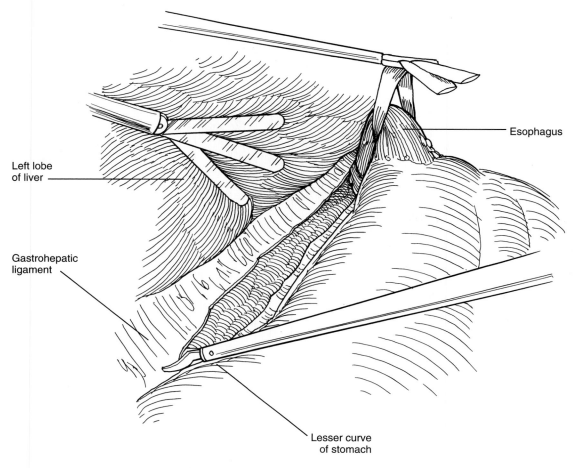

Esophagus

Left lobe
of liver

Gastrohepatic
ligament

Lesser curve
of stomach

FIGURE 19-5

FIGURE 19-5. Attention is next directed to the lesser curve of the stomach at the level of the methylene blue dot. Dissection aimed at clearing a 3-cm window on the lesser curve is begun by isolating vessels and dividing them with the blunt side of the LCS. It is important to refrain from using clips in this step so that the circular stapler can later be used without misfiring. Clear entrance into the lesser sac denotes the presence of an adequate window. Once this window has been created, a 32 French bougie is placed to determine where the circular staple and gastrotomy should be located.

FIGURE 19-6. The left midclavicular 10-mm cannula is changed to a 33-mm cannula. A 28-mm anvil is dropped into the abdomen through this 33-mm cannula.

FIGURE 19-7. The 28-mm anvil is grasped with a Babcock clamp placed through the right 10-mm midclavicular port and pushed through the stomach from posterior to anterior using two Babcocks. This maneuver is facilitated by making an incision on the anterior gastric wall using scissors at the point where the Babcock clamp is pushing against the anterior abdominal wall.

FIGURE 19-6

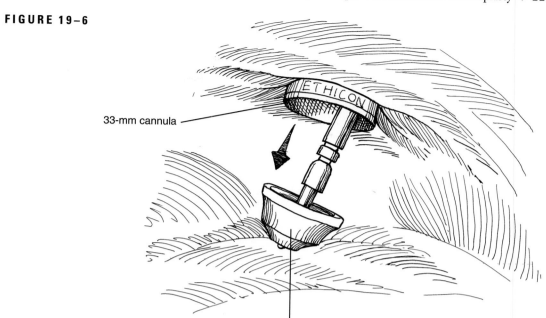

33-mm cannula

Anvil of circular
stapling device

FIGURE 19-7

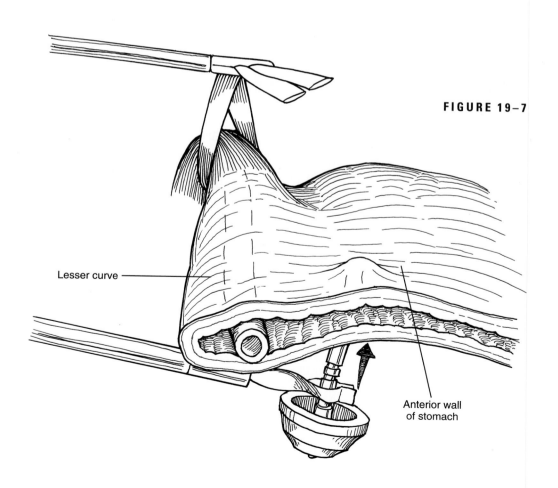

Lesser curve

Anterior wall
of stomach

FIGURE 19-8. Once the anvil is through the stomach, it is linked to the handle of the circular staple and fired, resulting in a stapled hole in the stomach. This staple line is inspected for any leaks, and the retrogastric space is examined to be sure subsequent staplers can be passed through this space to the cardioesophageal junction. A 32 French bougie is then passed down the esophagus into the stomach and guided through the narrow passage between the lesser curve and the gastrotomy.

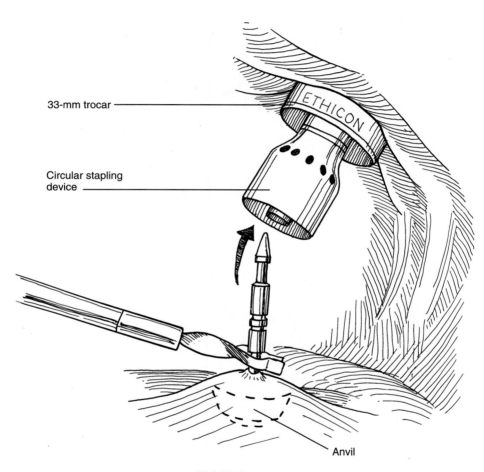

FIGURE 19-8

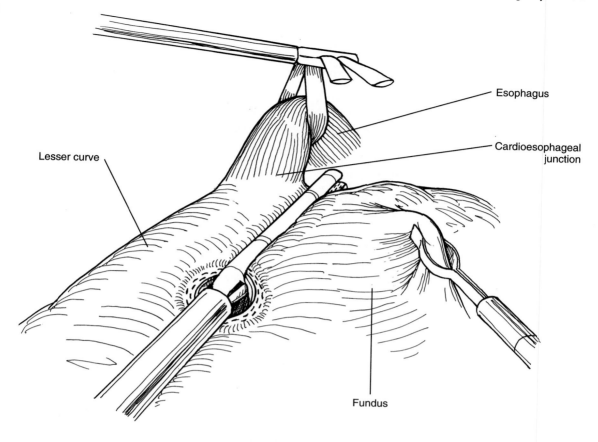

FIGURE 19–9

FIGURE 19–9. Although it is tempting to apply a TA 60 stapler through the gastric window along the bougie to the cardioesophageal junction at this time, it will not reach. Therefore, a 30-mm linear cutter (Endo GIA 30) is passed cephalad through the gastric window and fired alongside the 32 French bougie. A TA 60 device is then placed across the remainder of the stomach adjacent to the bougie, making sure that the stapler extends past the cardioesophageal junction. This is critical to ensuring a complete staple line.

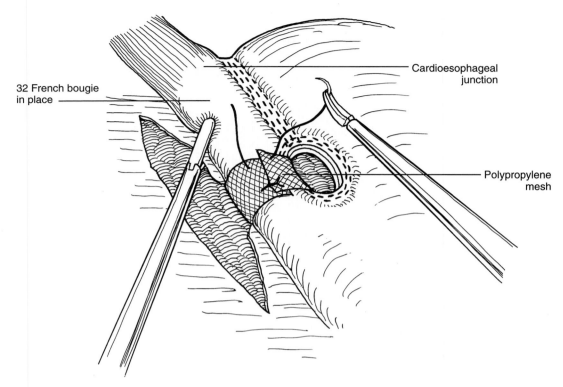

32 French bougie in place

Cardioesophageal junction

Polypropylene mesh

FIGURE 19–10

FIGURE 19–10. A 1.5- × 6-cm strip of polypropylene mesh is then inserted into the abdomen through an available empty port and passed around the stomach and the 32 French bougie at the circular stapler window. This is sutured with three interrupted sutures using an intracorporeal or extracorporeal knot-tying technique. This completes the vertical banded gastroplasty. The bougie is then removed and replaced by an 18 French nasogastric tube. The integrity of the pouch and the staple lines is tested with methylene blue and by insufflating the stomach under water. The trocars are removed under vision, the incisions are closed at the fascia with 0 Vicryl (10-mm sites only), the skin is closed with 4–0 nonabsorbable suture, and the incisions are infiltrated with bupivacaine.

X. Postoperative Medications

Patients are given intramuscular meperidine according to body weight in the recovery room. They then receive oral acetaminophen-codeine or oxycodone as needed. They also receive an additional 1-g dose of cefazolin in the recovery room.

XI. Advancement of Diet

The nasogastric tube is removed on the day following surgery if there is no tachycardia. The patient is given 30 ml per hour of water and advanced to clear liquids ad lib over the next 24 hours. He or she is advised by the dietitians about a soft diet and discharged on the third day.

XII. Determinants of Discharge

Patients are discharged when they can manage their pain with oral analgesics, are ambulatory, have no fever or tachycardia, and can eat soft food. This typically is the third postoperative day.

XIII. Return to Normal Activity/Work

Patients are allowed to return to activities as tolerated immediately after surgery. The only restriction is that they should not drive for 3 to 4 days and while taking analgesics.

Part V

OTHER LAPAROSCOPIC OPERATIONS OF THE UPPER GASTROINTESTINAL TRACT

Chapter 20

Laparoscopic Plication of a Perforated Duodenal Ulcer

J. COSGROVE, M.D.

I. Indications

The same indications that exist for open laparotomy and plication of a perforated duodenal ulcer hold for the laparoscopic approach to the perforated duodenal ulcer. In fact, the laparoscopic approach to the perforated duodenal ulcer is advantageous in that it allows for cleansing the peritoneal cavity with the suction irrigator and addressing the perforation with the placement of an omental patch. Additionally, when indicated, a definitive procedure can be performed (posterior truncal vagotomy and anterior seromyotomy).

II. Contraindications

The only contraindications to laparoscopic plication of a perforated duodenal ulcer are technical inability to perform the procedure (e.g., inability to attain a pneumoperitoneum), coagulopathy, or an unstable patient who is not able to tolerate pneumoperitoneum.

III. Factors Important in Patient Selection

Generally, all stable patients are candidates for the laparoscopic approach.

IV. Preoperative Preparation

A. The patient should have had fluid resuscitation with normal saline or lactated Ringer's solution.
B. A large-bore intravenous catheter should be used as well as a Foley catheter.
C. A broad-spectrum antibiotic should be administered preoperatively.
D. A nasogastric tube should be used for gastric decompression in all cases.

V. Choice of Anesthesia

The patient should undergo endotracheal intubation with general anesthesia.

VI. Accessory Devices

A. Trendelenburg table with foot rest
B. Nasogastric tube
C. Foley catheter
D. Pneumatic compression stockings

VII. Instruments and Telescopes

A. One video monitor
B. One high flow carbon dioxide insufflator
C. One 30-degree telescope

D. One 10-degree telescope
E. Camera and high intensity light source
F. Three trocars, including a Hasson port (for open technique) with reducer
G. One endoscopic Babcock clamp
H. One needle holder (K. Storz, Germany)
 I. One curved dissector
 J. One suction irrigator
K. One right-angle dissector
 L. 2–0 silk suture

VIII. Position of Monitors and Placement and Size of Trocars

FIGURE 20–1. The surgeon stands between the legs of the patient in the French position. The assistant surgeon stands to the left of the surgeon. A camera holder is optional; this task can be performed by the assistant surgeon. The primary monitor is placed near the patient's right shoulder so that the surgeon has a visual orientation at 90 degrees to the monitors. The scrub nurse stands to the right of the surgeon.

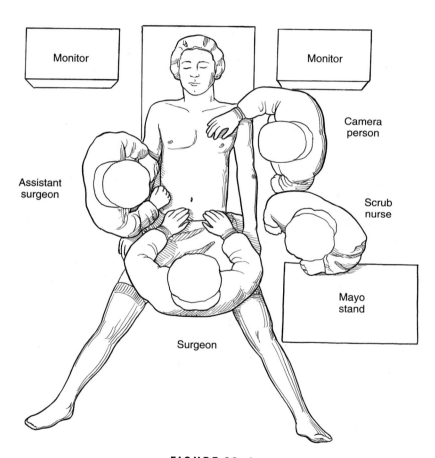

FIGURE 20–1

FIGURE 20-2. The initial 10/11-mm trocar is inserted through an infraumbilical incision using a Hasson technique. A 5-mm trocar is placed in the left upper quadrant on the mid- clavicular line. A third 12-mm trocar is placed in the right lower quadrant just medial to the midclavicular line.

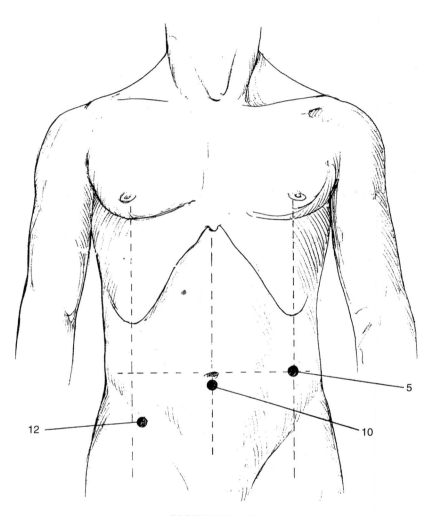

FIGURE 20-2

IX. Narrative of Surgical Procedure

FIGURE 20-3. The procedure is performed with the patient under general anesthesia. The surgeon is oriented perpendicular to the video monitor between the patient's legs. Three trocars are used: one 5-mm, one 12-mm, and one Hasson port for the camera. The right lateral port (12-mm) is used to insert the endoscopic Babcock clamp used to retract the omentum. The left midclavicular port (5-mm) is used for the endoscopic needle holder (K. Storz). The omentum is freed up, and the abdominal cavity is irrigated with 4 to 5 liters of saline. The endoscopic needle holder is then used to pass the silk sutures. Three 2–0 silk sutures are used as stay sutures placed through the seromuscular coats of the duodenum. The omentum is placed between the stay sutures, which are then tied intracorporeally. If there is a paucity of omentum, a tongue of greater omentum may be mobilized using sharp dissection with endoscopic scissors placed through the left midclavicular port.

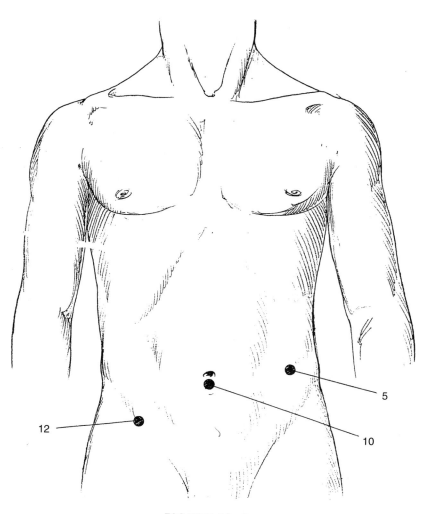

FIGURE 20-3

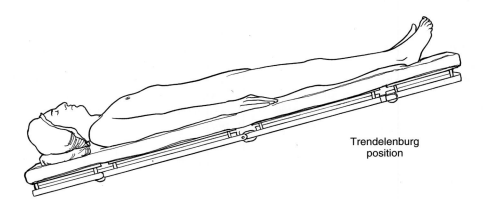

Trendelenburg
position

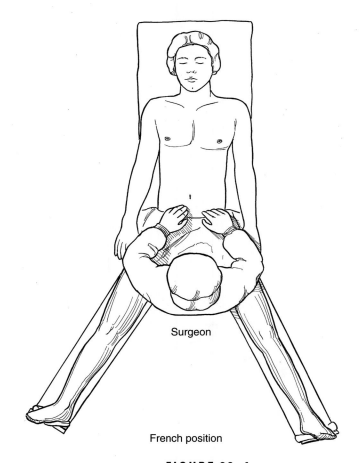

Surgeon

French position

FIGURE 20–4

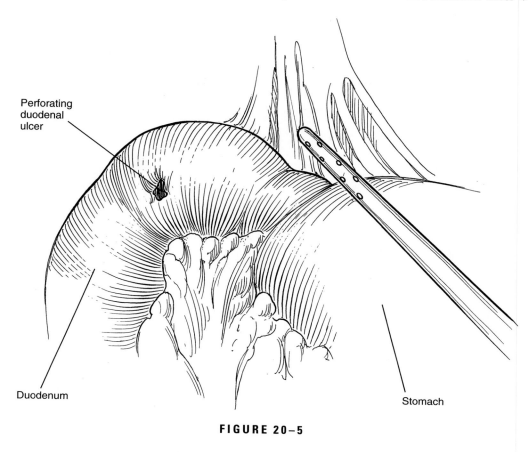

FIGURE 20–5

FIGURE 20–4. The Trendelenburg position facilitates intra-abdominal irrigation. Orientation is important in suturing.

FIGURE 20–5. The video laparoscope generally projects an excellent magnified image of the perforated duodenum.

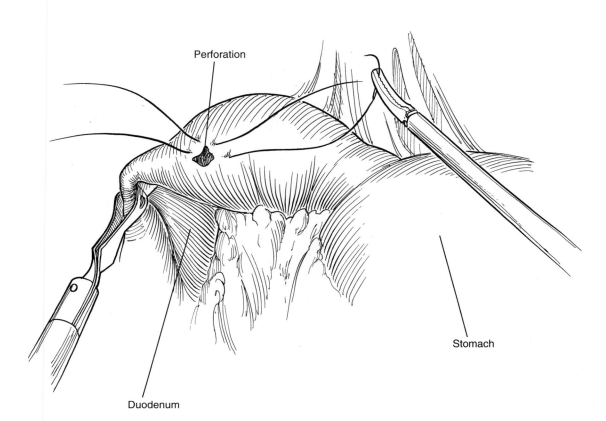

FIGURE 20–6

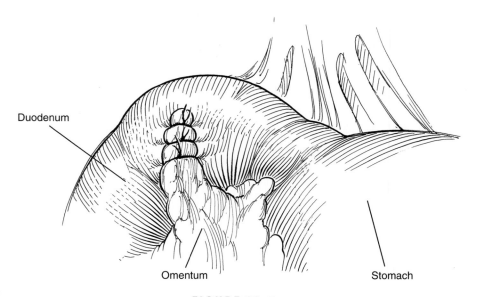

FIGURE 20–7

FIGURE 20–6. The duodenum is grasped with a laparoscopic Babcock distal to the perforation. Silk stay sutures are placed around the border of the perforation.

FIGURE 20–7. A tongue of omentum is pulled up to the duodenum and placed under the stay sutures. These sutures are used to secure the omentum in place over the perforation, completing the Graham patch.

X. Postoperative Medications

A. Patient-controlled analgesia (PCA) (morphine) administration
B. Patient is ambulating on the first postoperative day.

XI. Advancement of Diet

A. The nasogastric tube is removed when gastrointestinal function returns.
B. A clear liquid diet is begun when the patient passes flatus.

XII. Determinants of Discharge

Patients are discharged when they are tolerating a full liquid diet and are ambulating.

XIII. Return to Normal Activity

Patients return to normal physical activity upon discharge. Heavy physical activity can be performed after the staples have been removed one week postoperatively.

Techniques of Laparoscopic Enteral Access

JEFFREY H. PETERS, M.D., and THOMAS J. WATSON, M.D.

Laparoscopic Gastrostomy

I. Indications

A. Patients who require enteral alimentation in whom percutaneous endoscopic gastrostomy (PEG) is not feasible. These include:
   1. Patients with anatomic barriers such as obstructing pharyngeal or esophageal neoplasms.
   2. Patients with esophageal strictures.
   3. Patients who have previously undergone esophagectomy or gastrectomy so that the stomach is not available for access.
   4. Patients with wired mandibles due to fractures.
   5. Patients with intra-abdominal adhesions secondary to previous operations.
   6. Patients in whom the colon or liver overlies the stomach.
   7. Obese patients in whom endoscopic transillumination of the abdominal wall cannot be observed.

B. Patients who are undergoing laparoscopy for another reason and need a gastrostomy placed concomitantly.

II. Contraindications

Patients who require enteral alimentation in whom a percutaneous endoscopic gastrostomy can be safely accomplished and used without excessive danger of aspiration.

III. Factors Important in Patient Selection

Previous upper abdominal operations may make the procedure more difficult but are not a contraindication.

IV. Preoperative Preparation

A. Patients are admitted the same day as surgery if they are outpatients but are often already inpatients.

Jeffrey H. Peters, M.D., holds the copyright for the illustrations in this chapter.

B. All patients receive broad-spectrum intravenous antibiotics preoperatively.
C. No bowel preparation is required.

V. Choice of Anesthesia

A. General anesthesia
B. Local anesthesia with intravenous sedation

VI. Accessory Devices

A. A nasogastric tube is passed if this is feasible.
B. The bladder is decompressed with a Foley catheter.

VII. Instruments and Telescopes

A. 5-mm, 0-degree telescope
B. J-wire
C. 14 French Silastic balloon catheter
D. 12 French and 14 French dilators
E. Ross Flexiflo R 18F Introducer gastrostomy kit with Brown/Mueller T-fastener (Ross Industries, Columbus, OH)
F. Spinal needle

VIII. Position of Monitors and Placement and Size of Trocars

After a sterile preparation and drape is performed, pneumoperitoneum is established to a pressure of approximately 15 mm Hg with the use of a Veress needle. A 5- or 10-mm trocar is introduced, depending on the size of the laparoscope available. Alternatively, an open technique may be used in which a Hasson trocar is introduced into the peritoneal cavity through a curvilinear, infraumbilical incision. The laparoscope is inserted through this umbilical port, and a 5-mm trocar is introduced into the right abdomen under direct vision.

IX. Narrative of Surgical Technique

The patient is placed in the reverse Trendelenburg position. A grasping forceps is introduced through the second trocar and used to elevate the body of the stomach toward the anterior abdominal wall. If additional distention of the stomach is required, air may be introduced through the nasogastric tube. We use the technique described by Edelman and Unger, in which a 7-cm 18-gauge needle is used to pierce the skin in the left subcostal region and enters the stomach under direct vision. Under laparoscopic visualization a J-wire is inserted through the needle and into the stomach. The tract is dilated with 12 French and 14 French dilators before a 16 French peel-away sheath is introduced. A 14 French Silastic balloon catheter is advanced into the stomach, the balloon is inflated with 5 to 10 ml of water, and the peel-away sheath is removed. The catheter is affixed to the skin after the stomach has been pulled up to the anterior abdominal wall. The abdomen is thoroughly examined for hemostasis and leakage about the gastrostomy. The trocars are removed, and the fascia at the umbilical site is closed with interrupted absorbable sutures. The skin edges are reapproximated using a running, subcuticular absorbable stitch.

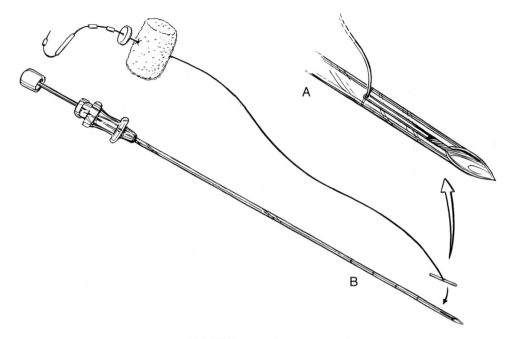

FIGURE 21–1A and B

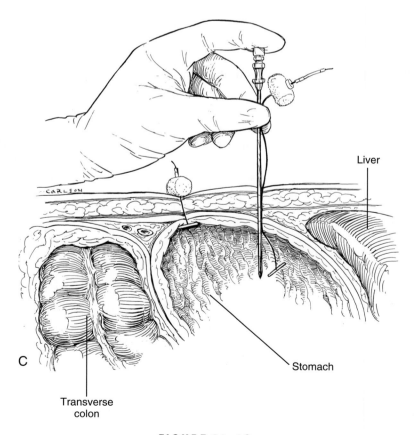

Liver

Stomach

Transverse
colon

FIGURE 21–1C

FIGURE 21-1A-C. Alternatively, T-fasteners may be used to provide four-point fixation of the stomach to the anterior abdominal wall, as described by Duh et al. Using a commercially available percutaneous gastrostomy kit (Ross Flexiflo R 18F Introducer gastrostomy kit with Brown/Mueller T-fastener), a T-fastener needle is introduced percutaneously in the left upper quadrant and advanced through the anterior wall of the stomach under direct vision (C). The stylet is inserted, and the T-fastener is released.

FIGURE 21-2. Three further T-fasteners are inserted 1 cm from the first to provide four-point fixation.

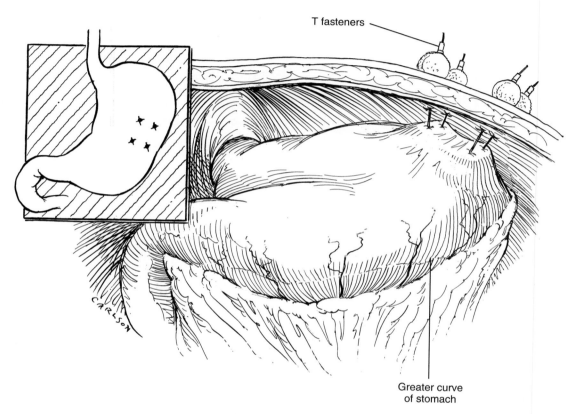

T fasteners

Greater curve
of stomach

FIGURE 21-2

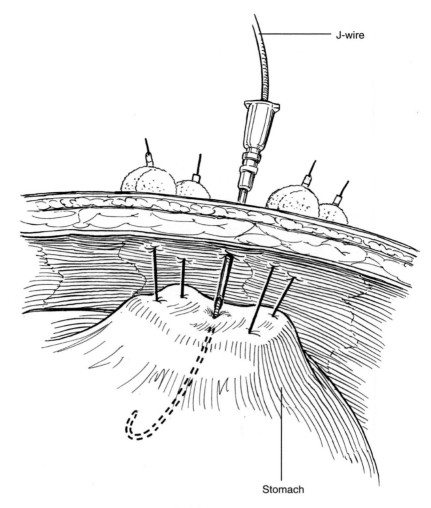

FIGURE 21-3

FIGURE 21-3. Using a spinal needle, a J-wire is then introduced into the stomach between and somewhat inferior to these two T-fasteners. The gastrostomy tract is gradually enlarged over the J-wire, using the dilators provided in the kit, up to 18F. Countertraction on the stomach is provided by the T-fasteners while the tract is dilated.

FIGURE 21-4. The gastrostomy tube is inserted over the J-wire into the stomach (A).

The anterior gastric wall is approximated to the anterior abdominal wall by exerting traction on the tube and the T-fasteners. The tube is sutured to the skin, and the T-fasteners are secured by crimping the metal washer with a blunt-tipped needle holder (B). The abdomen is examined, the trocars are removed, and the wounds are closed as previously discussed. The T-fasteners provide additional security if the gastrostomy balloon ruptures or the tube dislodges.

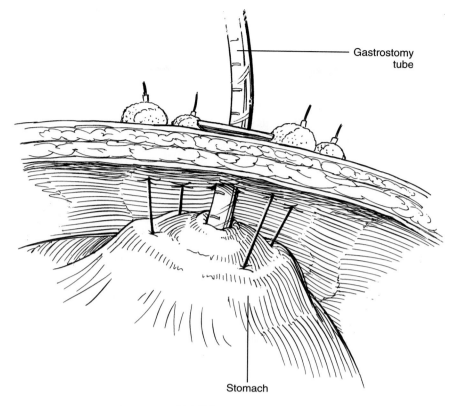

Gastrostomy
tube

Stomach

FIGURE 21–4A

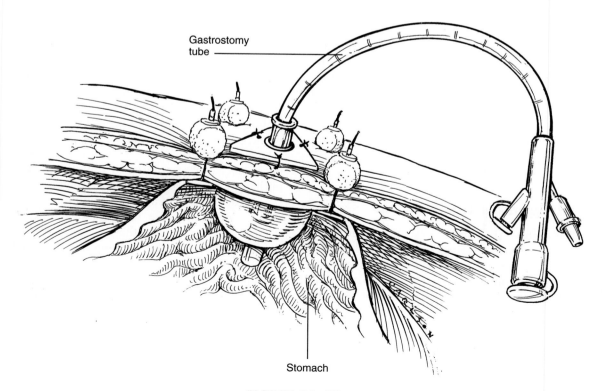

Gastrostomy
tube

Stomach

FIGURE 21–4B

X. Postoperative Medications

Analgesics are given as required.

XI. Advancement of Diet

Feedings are typically started 24 hours after surgery. We begin with full-strength formula at a rate of 15 ml per hour and gradually advance it, using a continuous drip infusion technique, by 15 ml/hour per day until the goal rate is attained. While a complete discussion of nutritional assessment and requirements is beyond the scope of this chapter, we typically administer 25 to 40 kcal/kg per day and 1.0 to 2.0 g/kg per day of protein, depending on the nature and severity of the patient's underlying illness. Serum albumin and transferrin levels, nitrogen balance, patient weight, and the overall clinical course are followed to assess the adequacy of nutritional support. Once an oral diet is resumed, the level of supplementation is gradually tapered off.

Patients who require continued enteral alimentation after discharge from the hospital are issued a portable pump (Ross Industries, Columbus, OH) that can be carried on a shoulder strap while the patient goes about daily activities. These pumps are reliable and easily maintained.

The stomach has the advantage of allowing bolus feedings, if this is desired. Once a continuous infusion of formula is tolerated, the patient can be slowly accustomed to receive the same total daily volume given in several discrete boluses. This method frees the patient from the burden of transporting and maintaining the feeding pump throughout the day and appears to be generally well tolerated.

XII. Determinants of Discharge

Ambulatory patients can be discharged home on the same day as surgery, although these procedures are more typically performed on inpatients. Patients are given instructions for the maintenance of the catheters and the advancement of tube feedings.

XIII. Return to Normal Activity

Patients may resume their normal activities as tolerated.

Laparoscopic Jejunostomy

I. Indications

A. Patients who require enteral alimentation and are scheduled for esophagectomy because a percutaneous endoscopic gastrostomy may interfere with later use of the stomach as an esophageal substitute.
B. Patients who require enteral alimentation but are at high risk for aspiration.
   These include:
   1. Patients with a mechanically incompetent lower esophageal sphincter.
   2. Patients with gastroparesis.
   3. Patients with gastric outlet obstruction.
   4. Patients with mental obtundation.

II. Contraindications

Patients who require enteral alimentation in whom a percutaneous endoscopic gastrostomy can be safely accomplished and used without excessive danger of aspiration.

III. Factors Important in Patient Selection

A surgical jejunostomy is considered when the stomach is either unavailable or unsuitable as a site for enteral access. The traditional open Witzel jejunostomy, which employs a 12-mm tube placed through a serosal tunnel, has not gained popularity owing to the frequent and potentially serious complications associated with it, such as intraperitoneal leakage, kinking of the tube or bowel, intestinal obstruction, and tube dislodgement. The incidence of these complications has been reduced by the introduction of the intramural needle–catheter technique described by Delaney et al. Their method involves the use of a 14-gauge needle and a catheter from a central venous catheterization set. The main problem with this technique is the small diameter of the tube, which frequently leads to clogging and a sluggish flow. We use a commercially available needle-catheter jejunostomy kit that provides a tube with a larger lumen, allowing the use of more viscous formulas at a faster rate and less frequent clogging. The tube is also somewhat stiffer and therefore kinks less often. It may be easily replaced through an established tract should it become dislodged.

The following technique of laparoscopic jejunostomy is a direct modification of our open procedure, as initially described by Roy and DeMeester.

IV. Preoperative Preparation

A. Patients are admitted the same day as surgery if they are outpatients but are often already inpatients.
B. All patients receive broad-spectrum intravenous antibiotics preoperatively.
C. No bowel preparation is required.

V. Choice of Anesthesia

A. General anesthesia
B. Local anesthesia with intravenous sedation

VI. Accessory Devices

A. A nasogastric tube is passed if this is feasible.
B. The bladder is decompressed with a Foley catheter.

VII. Instruments and Telescopes

A. 5-mm, 0-degree telescope
B. J-wire
C. 14 French Silastic balloon catheter
D. 12 French and 14 French dilators
E. Ross Flexiflo R 18F Introducer gastrostomy kit with Brown/Mueller T-fastener
F. Spinal needle

VIII. Position of Monitors and Placement and Size of Trocars

Same as for laparoscopic gastrostomy

IX. Narrative of Surgical Technique

Several techniques exist for placement of laparoscopic feeding tubes, including percutaneous T-fastener techniques similar to that described earlier for gastrostomy placement and percutaneous insertion under direct vision using suture fixation. We have used most of these approaches and have come to use the following technique most commonly. As with laparoscopic gastrostomy, all patients are given broad-spectrum in-travenous antibiotics perioperatively. Laparoscopic jejunostomy, however, usually requires general anesthesia. A Foley catheter and nasogastric tube are passed for urinary and gastric decompression. After sterile preparation and drape have been completed, a 10-mm Hasson trocar is introduced into the peritoneal cavity through a curvilinear infraumbilical incision using an open technique. The incision is made larger than usual to allow evisceration of the small bowel. The use of a Veress needle is not appropriate in this procedure because it is necessary to manipulate the bowel extracorporeally at the umbilical trocar site. Pneumoperitoneum is established to a pressure of approximately 15 mm Hg, and the laparoscope is inserted through this port. An additional 10-mm trocar is introduced in the left lower quadrant under direct vision, and a third is placed in the right lower quadrant.

FIGURE 21–5. As stated previously, we prefer to use a commercially available needle–catheter jejunostomy kit (Intestofix, Braun Melsungen AG, Germany). The kit contains two breakaway needles and a flexible 12 French catheter. The shorter needle is used to pass the catheter through the skin and the longer one to create an intramural tunnel within the jejunal serosa.

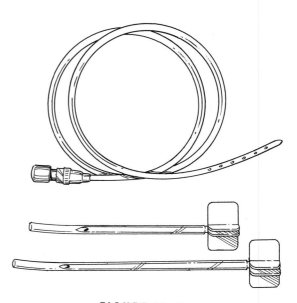

FIGURE 21–5

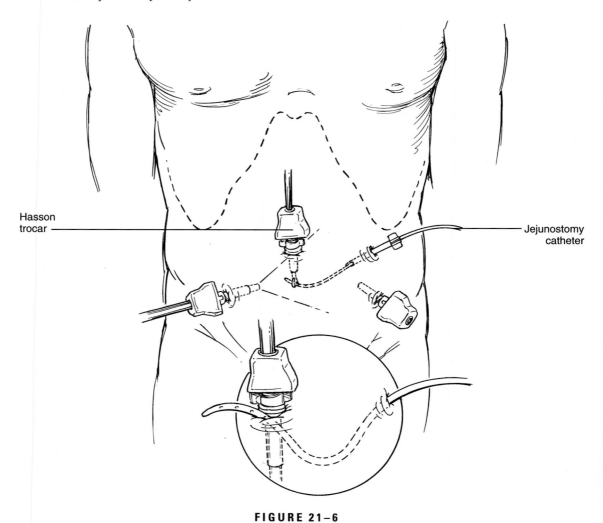

Hasson trocar

Jejunostomy catheter

FIGURE 21–6

FIGURE 21–6. The catheter is inserted into the peritoneal cavity in the left lower quadrant, tunneling it through the abdominal wall in a lateral to medial direction, and the breakaway needle is removed. The Hasson trocar and laparoscope are removed, and the tip of the catheter is brought out through the umbilical incision. This trocar and the laparoscope are then reinserted, and pneumoperitoneum is reestablished.

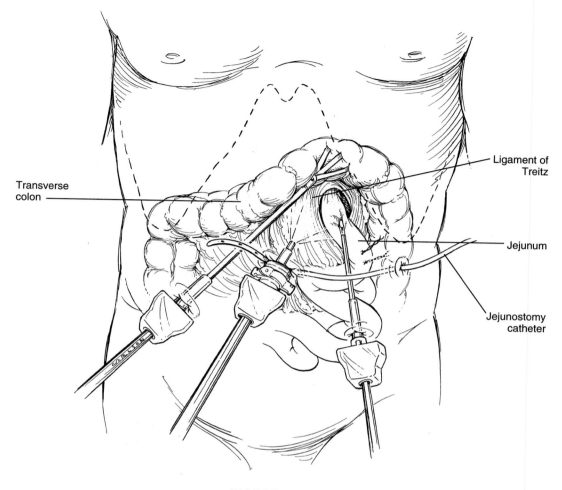

Transverse colon

Ligament of Treitz

Jejunum

Jejunostomy catheter

FIGURE 21-7

FIGURE 21-7. The patient is placed in a reverse Trendelenburg position to allow the small bowel to fall toward the pelvis. The ligament of Treitz is located after the transverse colon is lifted anteriorly. Sutures are placed to mark the proximal and distal bowel segments for later reference.

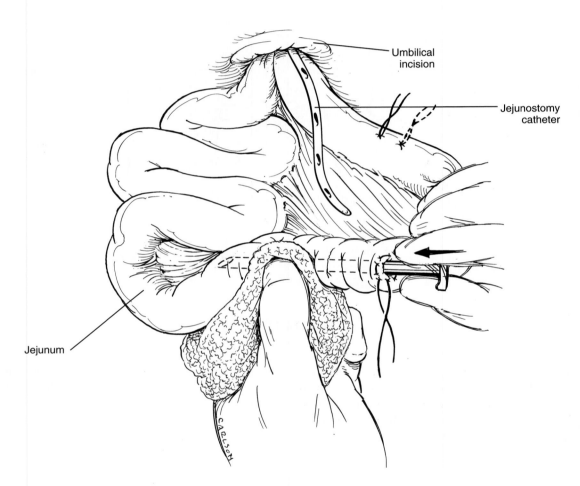

Umbilical
incision

Jejunostomy
catheter

Jejunum

FIGURE 21–8A

FIGURE 21–8. (A) A portion of the proximal jejunum approximately 25 cm distally is grasped, and 2 to 3 feet of small bowel at this site are brought out through the umbilical incision. A purse-string suture of 3–0 chromic is placed on the antimesenteric border of the bowel. To create the intramural tunnel, the serosa is pierced, the needle is held steady, and the wall of the bowel is advanced over it. The tip of the needle should be visualized through the translucent serosa as the wall of the gut is pulled over the shaft. (B) The length of the tunnel should be 12 to 15 cm, at which point the needle is angled in to pierce the mucosa. The catheter is threaded through the needle into the lumen for a distance of 25 to 30 cm. The needle is then split and removed, and the purse string is tied down. We make it a point to verify the intraluminal position of the catheter by occluding the bowel proximally and distally and irrigating the catheter with saline.

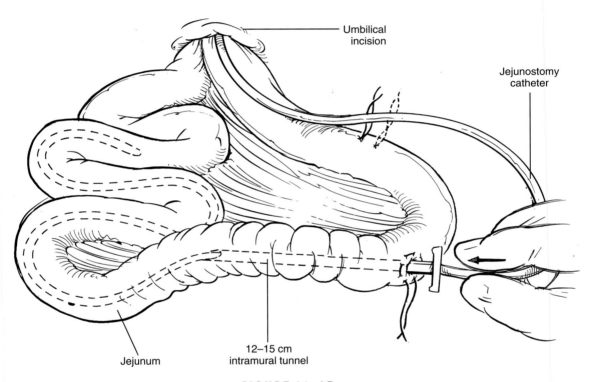

Umbilical incision

Jejunostomy catheter

Jejunum

12–15 cm intramural tunnel

FIGURE 21–8B

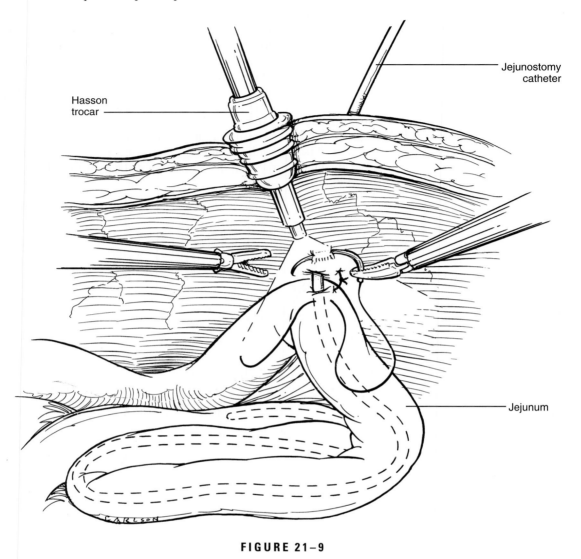

FIGURE 21–9

FIGURE 21–9. The loop of jejunum is returned to the peritoneal cavity, and the Hasson trocar is replaced. Under direct vision, the jejunum is affixed to the parietal peritoneum and the transversalis fascia with four silk sutures placed circumferentially around the catheter. To aid visualization, it is helpful to place the suture farthest from the laparoscope first. Care must be taken to ensure the proper orientation of the bowel with regard to proximal and distal to prevent iatrogenic volvulus and subsequent bowel obstruction. The trocars are removed, and the fascia of the infraumbilical incision is reapproximated with interrupted absorbable su-tures. The skin edges are closed with running subcuticular absorbable sutures. The catheter is sewn to the skin surface with 2–0 polypropylene sutures using a 14 French red Robinson catheter slit along one end as a bolster. We have found it useful to affix the external portion of the catheter in a U configuration oriented transversely to prevent kinking when the patient bends forward.

If the commercial kit is not available, we use a small gallbladder trocar to create the intramural tunnel. A 10 French infant feeding tube can be passed easily through the lumen of the trocar.

We have found this an entirely satisfactory, if less elegant, alternative. The only caveat is that the feeding tube must be passed once through the trocar before the latter is inserted because the proximal flared end may require trimming to allow removal of the trocar after the tube is in place.

Several other techniques of laparoscopic feeding jejunostomy tube placement have been reported in the literature. The technical elements are similar to those described here and include: (1) laparoscopic visualization of the ligament of Treitz and proximal jejunum, (2) fixation of the jejunum to the anterior abdominal wall using intracorporeal, extracorporeal, or percutaneous suturing techniques or T-fasteners, and (3) advancement of an appropriate feeding tube into the jejunal lumen. The number of cases reported is small, and few data are available on complications and long-term function. These procedures resemble the open Witzel technique in certain key respects and consequently may suffer from the same pitfalls. None of the techniques appear to offer any distinct advantages over the method we have described herein.

X. Postoperative Medications

Analgesics as required

XI. Advancement of Diet

Feeding is typically begun on the third postoperative day. We start with full-strength formula at a rate of 15 ml per hour and gradually advance it, using a continuous drip infusion technique, by 15 ml/hour per day until the goal rate is attained, as described in the earlier part of this chapter. As oral consumption is resumed, the amount of supplementation is gradually tapered off. Patients who require nutritional support after discharge from the hospital are issued a portable pump, as for the gastrostomy technique.

Any medications administered through the tube ideally should be in liquid form or at least pulverized thoroughly. Clogging of the catheters can be prevented by routine irrigation with 15 ml of Coca-Cola, cranberry juice, or vinegar. We have found a 1-ml tuberculin syringe useful for applying forceful pressure to the needle–catheter jejunostomy tube should a clog occur. Diarrhea is common, especially soon after placement of the tube. This may be controlled by adding Kaopectate or paregoric to the formula, by slowing the rate temporarily, or by switching to an isotonic formula. We have also found that intermittent administration of narcotic-based constipating agents, such as diphenoxylate with atropine (Lomotil) or tincture of opium, is useful in difficult cases. Of course, antibiotic-induced diarrhea and pseudomembranous colitis are always important considerations and must be ruled out when appropriate. Rarely should diarrhea lead to interruption of feedings. Should a catheter become dislodged or kinked after the first few days, a new one can easily be threaded in place under fluoroscopic guidance. Intraluminal positioning of the tube should be verified by injecting a small amount of water-soluble contrast agent and obtaining an abdominal radiograph. The semirigid character of these tubes allows them to be readily reinserted.

XII. Return to Normal Activity

Patients may resume their normal activities as tolerated.

References

Delany HM, Carnevale NJ, Garvey JW. Jejunostomy by needle catheter technique. Surgery 1973; 73:786–790.

Duh QY, Way LW. Laparoscopic jejunostomy using t-fasteners as retractors and anchors. Arch Surg 1993; 128:105–108.

Edelman DS, Unger SW. Laparoscopic gastrostomy and jejunostomy. Review of 22 cases. Surg Laparosc Endosc 1994; 4:297–300.

Roy A, DeMeester TR: Perioperative management of carcinoma of the esophagus: The reduction of operative mortality. *In* Delarue NC, Wilkins EW Jr, Wong J (eds): International Trends in General Thoracic Surgery Volume IV: Esophageal Cancer. St. Louis, C.V. Mosby, 1988, pp. 101–113.

Chapter 22

Laparoscopic Distal Pancreatectomy

BARRY A. SALKY, M.D.

I. Indications

A. Benign tumors of the tail of the pancreas
   1. Cystadenoma
   2. Neuroendocrine tumors

II. Contraindications

A. Acute pancreatitis
B. Suspicion of malignant disease
C. Previous left upper quadrant surgery (relative)

III. Factors Important in Patient Selection

A. Clear diagnosis based on preoperative evaluation
B. Nonoperated left upper quadrant best but not always possible
C. Thin patient rather than obese
D. No contraindication to general anesthesia

IV. Preoperative Preparation

A. Same day admission unless general medical condition of patient requires preoperative admission.
B. If the tumor is secreting hormonally active substances, preoperative control with medication may be needed.

C. Mechanical bowel preparation of the colon is recommended.

V. Choice of Anesthesia

General anesthesia is required.

VI. Accessory Devices

A. Foley catheter
B. Pneumatic compression stockings
C. Orogastric tube (removed at the end of the procedure)
D. Cardiac monitoring (Swan-Ganz catheter, arterial line) if clinically warranted

VII. Instruments and Telescopes

A. 45-degree laparoscope
B. High flow insufflator (at least 6 liters per minute)
C. Electrocautery scissors (5-mm)
D. 5- and 10-mm atraumatic grasping forceps
E. 30-mm vascular GIA-type stapler
F. Chromic or Vicryl pre-tied ligatures
G. Titanium clips
H. Laparosonic coagulating shears (UltraCision)
I. Specimen retrieval bag (Cook)
J. Needle holder (Ethicon)

VIII. Position of Monitor and Placement and Size of Trocars

FIGURE 22–1.

1. Modified lithotomy position with the thighs parallel to the trunk. A sandbag is placed beneath the left thoracic area to elevate it about 25 degrees.
2. Monitor located over head of patient.
3. Surgeon stands between the patient's legs, first assistant (camera holder) to the patient's left, and second assistant to the patient's right.
4. Nurse stands behind and to the left of the surgeon with a full view of the monitor.
5. Cannula A, 5 mm (atraumatic ratcheted forceps)
6. Cannula B, 5 mm (forceps, left hand operating port)
7. Cannula C, 10 mm (laparoscope)
8. Cannula D, 12 mm (right hand operating port, GIA stapler)
9. Cannula E, 10 mm (atraumatic grasper, assistant's port)

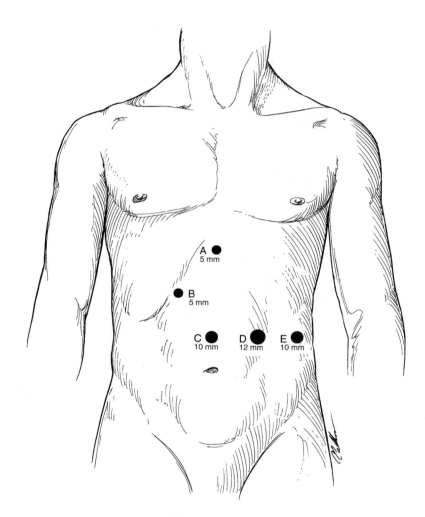

FIGURE 22–1

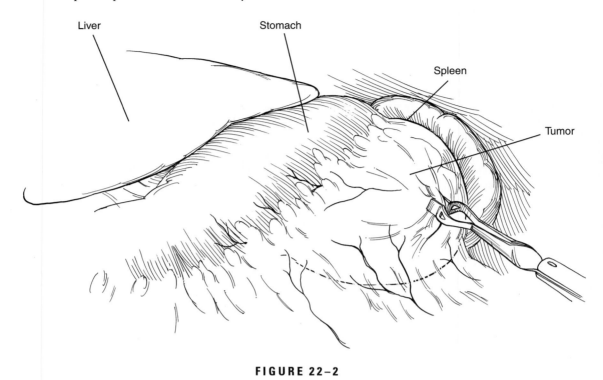

Liver Stomach Spleen Tumor

FIGURE 22–2

IX. Narrative of Surgical Technique

FIGURE 22–2. Once the five trocars and sleeves have been placed in the abdominal cavity, the 45-degree laparoscope is directed toward the left upper quadrant. The relationships of the stomach, spleen, and mass are demonstrated here.

FIGURE 22–3. The lesser sac is opened through the gastrocolic ligament at an avascular area. The blood vessels are clipped with titanium clips and divided. The laparosonic coagulating shears (LCS) can be used here as well. The greater omentum must be fully mobilized away from the mass to appreciate the retroperitoneal pancreas and its relationship to the splenic flexure of the colon and the posterior wall of the stomach. In this figure the lesser sac has been entered through the gastrocolic ligament. The stomach is to the left, and the mass is to the right.

FIGURE 22–4. The posterior inferior attachments of the pancreas to the retroperitoneum are divided with electrocautery scissors.

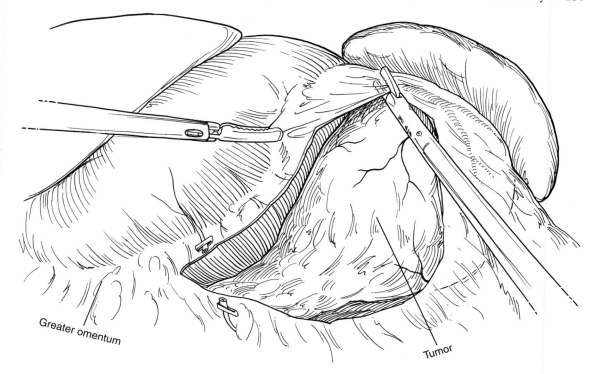

Greater omentum

Tumor

FIGURE 22–3

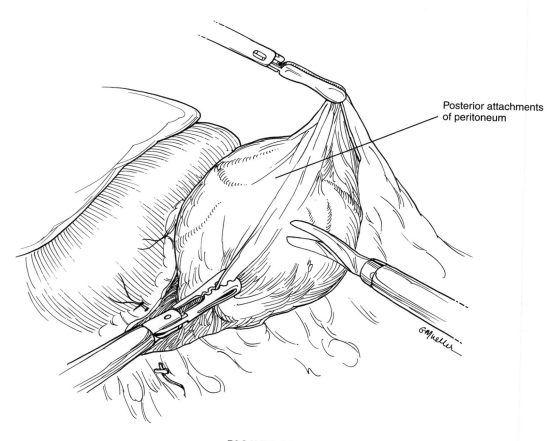

Posterior attachments
of peritoneum

FIGURE 22–4

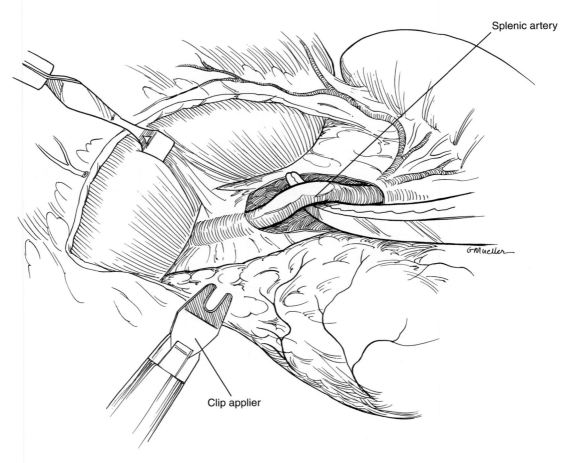

Splenic artery

Clip applier

FIGURE 22–5A

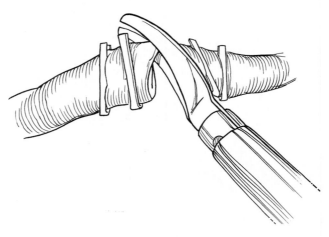

FIGURE 22–5B

FIGURE 22–5A. The relationship of the splenic vein to the pancreatic mass is ascertained by incising the peritoneum over the vein. If the vein is free, a spleen-saving distal pancreatectomy can be performed. However, if the splenic vein is adherent to the mass, distal pancreatectomy with splenectomy is required. The peritoneum over the splenic artery at the superior border of the pancreas is opened, and the splenic artery is dissected free. Its tortuous nature can be appreciated once the dissection is complete.

FIGURE 22–5B. The artery is doubly clipped and divided. The proximal artery is further secured with a pre-tied ligature of either chromic or Vicryl.

FIGURE 22–6. The stomach is retracted toward the midline (cannula A) and the spleen laterally (cannula E). This places the splenogastric tissues on stretch, exposing the proper dissection plane. The splenogastric ligament is divided using a vascular GIA stapling device. The LCS device can also be used here.

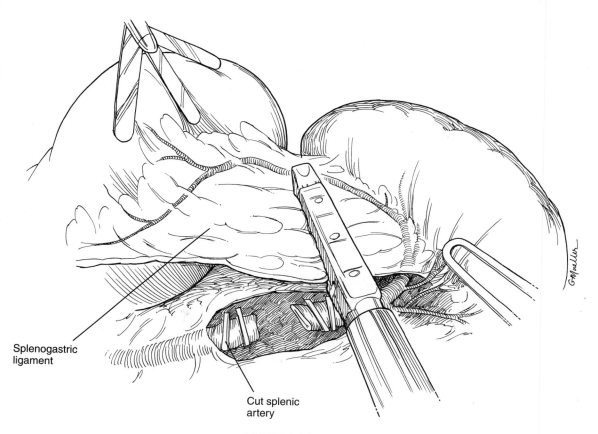

Splenogastric
ligament

Cut splenic
artery

FIGURE 22–6

FIGURE 22-7. The dissection is continued toward the short gastric vessels, which can be divided between clips or with the LCS.

FIGURE 22-8. After the spleen has been detached from the stomach, the posterior avascular attachments of the pancreas are bluntly dissected from the posterior abdominal wall. The dissection should be directly opposite the previously divided splenic artery. The inferior aspect of the pancreas is elevated by placing a 10-mm grasper beneath the pancreas. The pancreas is then divided using the vascular GIA stapler.

Two applications of the stapler are required to divide the whole pancreas. Suture ligatures of 3–0 silk should be available in case bleeding occurs from the cut end of the pancreas. Once the pancreas is divided, the remaining posterior attachments to Gerota's fascia are severed using either electrocautery and clips or the LCS.

FIGURE 22-9. After the spleen and distal pancreas are free, a sturdy, nonporous retrieval bag is placed in the abdomen in the left upper quadrant. It is held open with three-point traction (cannulas A, B, and E).

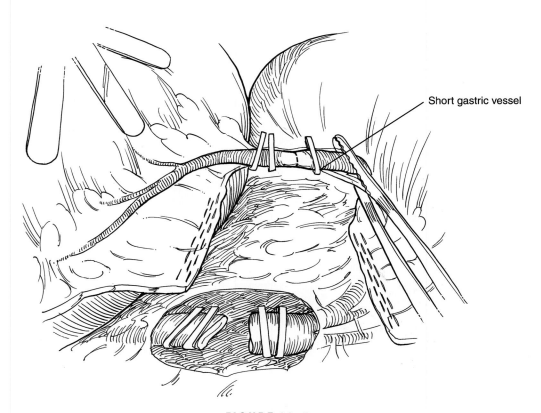

Short gastric vessel

FIGURE 22-7

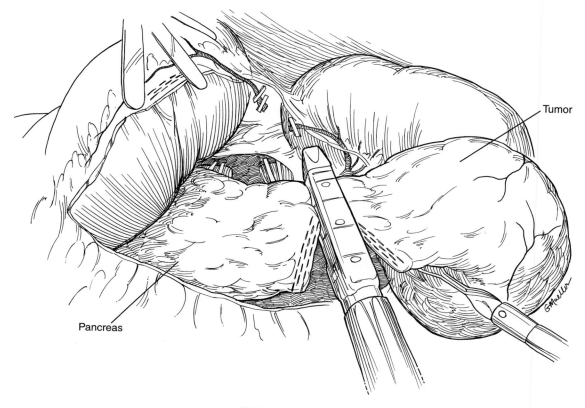

Tumor

Pancreas

FIGURE 22–8

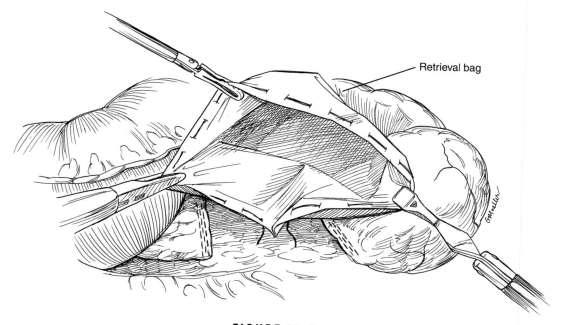

Retrieval bag

FIGURE 22–9

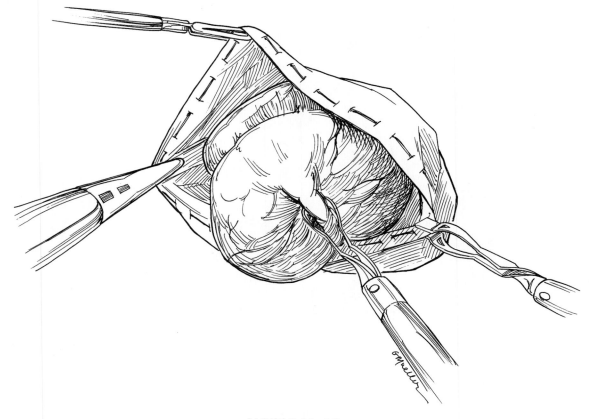

FIGURE 22-10

FIGURE 22-10. The specimen is captured, the drawstrings are closed, and the bag is extracted from the cannula D site.

FIGURE 22-11. The left upper quadrant is inspected, and a closed suction drain is left in place. The fascia is closed at all 10-mm and larger ports. All incisions are injected with ½ per cent bupivacaine, and they are closed with subcuticular sutures of 4–0 Vicryl.

X. Postoperative Medications

A. Injectable pain medication (meperidine) is given on the first postoperative evening, and oxycodone by mouth is prescribed thereafter.

B. No other specific medications are given.

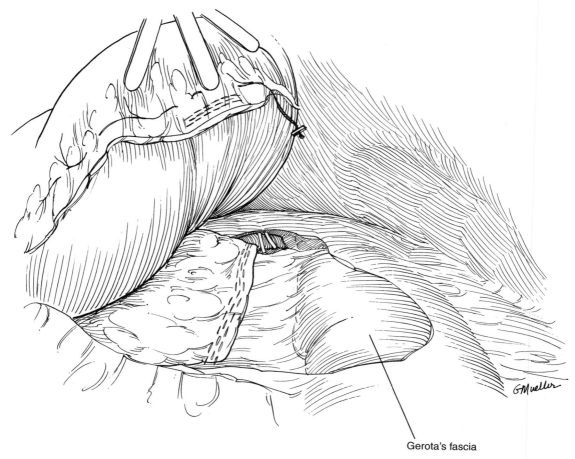

Gerota's fascia

FIGURE 22-11

XI. Advancement of Diet

The patient begins with clear fluids on postoperative day 1. A regular diet is started when flatus is passed (usually on postoperative day 3).

XII. Determinants of Discharge

The closed suction drain is removed by postoperative day 2 assuming that the drainage is serious in nature and the amylase content is within the normal range. The patient must be afebrile, ambulating, and able to tolerate a normal diet. Pain relief is achieved by either acetaminophen or oxycodone.

XIII. Return to Normal Activity/Work

Because of the small abdominal incisions, normal activity can usually be resumed around the tenth to fourteenth day postoperatively. I allow patients to do anything they feel their incisions will allow them to do.

Chapter 23

Anterior Approach to Laparoscopic Splenectomy

JOHN L. FLOWERS, M.D., and MICHAEL J. MASTRANGELO, JR., M.D.

I. Indications

A. Underlying splenic disease
  1. Splenic hamartoma/benign splenic tumors
  2. Splenic hydatid cyst
  3. Splenic cyst
  4. Infarct (symptomatic)
  5. Abscess
  6. Trauma
  7. Hereditary elliptocytosis
  8. Hereditary spherocytosis (splenomegaly/cholelithiasis)
  9. Autoimmune thrombocytopenia
  10. Idiopathic or immune thrombocytopenic purpura (ITP)
  11. Human immunodeficiency virus-associated thrombocytopenia
  12. Thrombotic thrombocytopenic purpura
B. Symptomatic hypersplenism
  1. Splenomegaly secondary to hemodialysis
  2. Enlarged spleen with filling defects
  3. Symptomatic hypersplenism
  4. Splenic vein thrombosis (sinistral portal hypertension)
  5. Sarcoid
  6. Felty's syndrome
  7. Chronic myelocytic leukemia
  8. Chronic leukocytic leukemia
  9. Agnogenic myeloid metaplasia
  10. Sickle cell disease
  11. Beta-thalassemia (major)
  12. Hemolytic anemia
  13. Gaucher's disease
  14. Leukemic infiltrative disease (hairy cell leukemia)
  15. Evans syndrome (acquired hemolytic anemia and thrombocytopenia)
C. Staging of Hodgkin's lymphoma
D. Diagnostic splenectomy in patients with a mass of unknown etiology

II. Contraindications

A. Absolute contraindications
  1. Inability to tolerate general anesthesia
  2. Intractable coagulopathy
B. Relative contraindications
  1. Portal hypertension
  2. Severe thrombocytopenia (platelet count less than 20,000 mm^3)
  3. Obesity
  4. Spleen long axis length 20 to 30 cm
  5. Pregnancy
  6. Previous upper abdominal surgery

III. Factors Important in Patient Selection

A. Age or body habitus: Anterior approach is more difficult in children and small adults because operating ports are encumbered by the left hip and thigh.

B. Obesity: In general, dissection and extraction are more difficult in obese patients.

C. Spleen size: Advantages of laparoscopic approach are less clear when the long axis length is more than 20 cm. The laparoscopic approach is not feasible in most patients with a spleen length of over 30 cm. Some authors prefer to perform preoperative splenic artery embolization for spleens longer than 20 cm. We have not used this approach.

D. Underlying thrombocytopenia or coagulopathy: In patients with severe ITP or hypersplenism, the platelet count can usually be corrected with aggressive administration of gamma globulin or platelet transfusion. An elevated prothrombin time can be corrected with vitamin K or fresh frozen plasma infusion. Increased intraoperative blood loss may be expected in patients with platelet counts of less than 50,000 mm³.

E. Underlying or coexisting medical problems: Patients with significant cardiopulmonary disease may not tolerate pneumoperitoneum or excessive hemorrhage. Patients on corticosteroid therapy or other immunosuppressive drugs may have an increased incidence of infectious or wound complications.

F. Prior upper abdominal surgery

IV. Preoperative Preparation

A. Preadmission
  1. Pneumococcal and *Haemophilus influenzae* type B vaccines are given at least 2 weeks preoperatively.
  2. IgG infusion is given 2 to 3 days preoperatively for refractory ITP with severe thrombocytopenia.
  3. Technetium-99-labeled heat-damaged red blood cell scan and computed tomographic scan for refractory thrombocytopenia are scheduled after splenectomy to search for accessory spleens.

B. Same day admission or night before surgery
  1. Consider angiographic embolization of splenic artery in patients with massive splenomegaly.
  2. Continue IgG or corticosteroid infusion in patients receiving those medications preoperatively.

C. Preoperative medications

  1. "Stress dose" corticosteroids
  2. Surgical antibiotic prophylaxis (single dose of first-generation cephalosporin)
  3. Platelet or fresh frozen plasma infusion in appropriate patients; platelets are usually administered after hilar ligation

D. Bowel preparation: not used routinely, though may be considered in patients with massive splenomegaly.

V. Choice of Anesthesia

A. General anesthesia
B. Multiple large-bore intravenous access catheters
C. Invasive hemodynamic monitoring is used in appropriate cases.

VI. Accessory Devices

A. Orogastric tube is placed after induction of anesthesia and removed prior to extubation; it is not used routinely postoperatively.
B. Urinary catheter is removed on the first postoperative day after adequate urine output has been documented.
C. Pneumatic compression devices are used on calves until the patient is ambulatory.

VII. Instruments and Telescopes

A. Angled (30- or 45-degree) laparoscope; a 10-mm scope gives better light delivery, but an experienced operator may wish to use a 5-mm scope.
B. 5- or 12-mm operating ports
C. Linear laparoscopic stapling device—length 30 mm, staple height 2.0 to 2.5 mm ("vascular" staple load)
D. Ultrasonic dissecting shears
E. Large (over 750 ml) specimen extraction sac
F. 5- or 10-mm laparoscopic clip applier
G. Suitable 5-mm graspers and dissecting instruments
H. 5- and 10-mm suction/irrigation cannulas; a 10-mm suction catheter is better for clot evacuation if hemorrhage occurs
I. Laparoscopic needle holders and knot pusher (optional)
J. Fan retractor (optional)

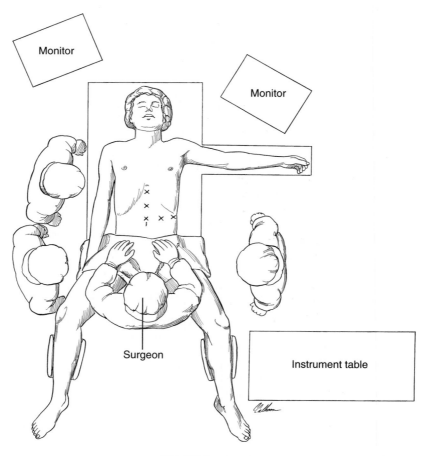

FIGURE 23–1A

VIII. Position of Monitors and Placement and Size of Trocars

FIGURE 23–1A. Two monitors are used, one at each side of the head of the operating table. The patient is placed in a modified lithotomy position with minimal (10 to 15 degree) hip flexion and rotated 30 degrees to the right using a longitudinally oriented roll behind the left thorax/flank. A carbon dioxide pneumoperitoneum (15 mm Hg) is achieved through the umbilicus using either an open or closed technique.

FIGURE 23–1B. Port size is dictated by the size of the available instruments. A subxiphoid retraction port is placed in the midline under direct visualization. A second retraction port is placed later midway between the subxiphoid and the umbilical ports if additional retraction is needed. Two working ports are placed in the left subcostal region in the midclavicular and anterior axillary lines at or above the level of the umbilicus. In general, ports are placed 10 cm apart or more. Avoid placing the working ports too low in patients with long torsos.

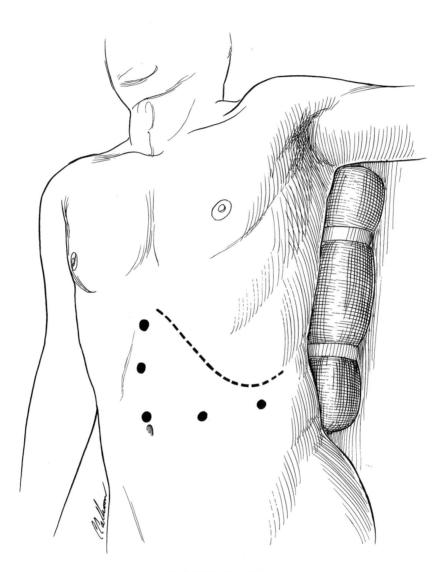

FIGURE 23–1B

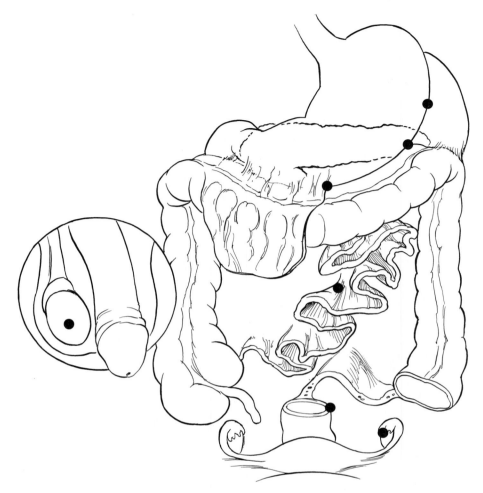

FIGURE 23-2

IX. Narrative of Surgical Technique

FIGURE 23-2. The procedure commences with a thorough exploration of the abdomen and pelvis including the greater omentum in a search for accessory splenic tissue. Their typical locations are shown in the figure. Exploration of the lesser sac is deferred until the short gastric vessels have been divided except in staging operations. The perihilar area is surveyed once it is exposed.

FIGURE 23-3A. *Exposure.* Following the survey for accessory splenic tissue, the operating table is rotated to the right to approximate a right lateral decubitus position. This allows gravity to provide medial retraction of the spleen. After the splenocolic ligament is divided, the lower pole of the spleen is exposed through both caudal retraction of the colon at the splenic flexure, using either a fan retractor or, more often, an atraumatic grasper, and medial retraction of the spleen. The attachments between the colon and the spleen are often vascular and require ligation with clips, a Harmonic Scalpel, or a linear stapling device before they are divided.

FIGURE 23-3B. *Ligation and division of the inferior pole attachments.* The lower pole vasculature varies from nonexistent to two or three significant vessels. These are exposed and then ligated and divided utilizing any available technique.

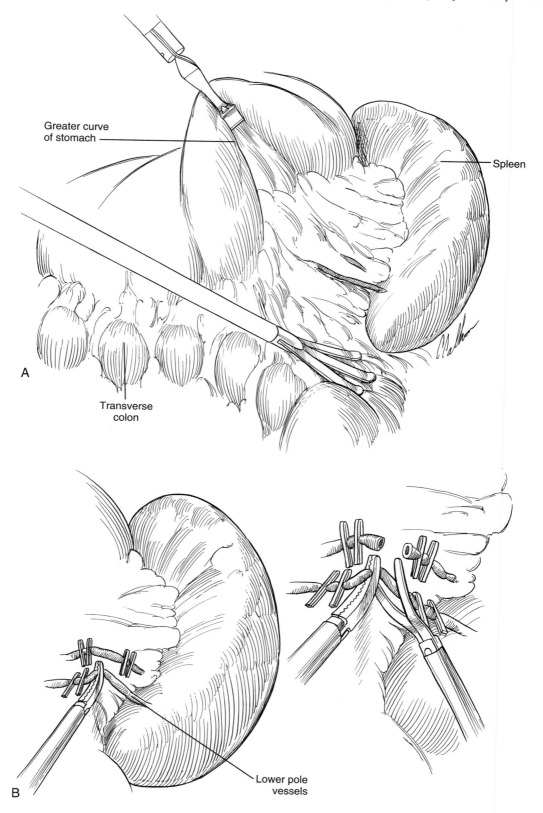

Greater curve
of stomach

Spleen

Transverse
colon

A

Lower pole
vessels

B

FIGURE 23–3A and B

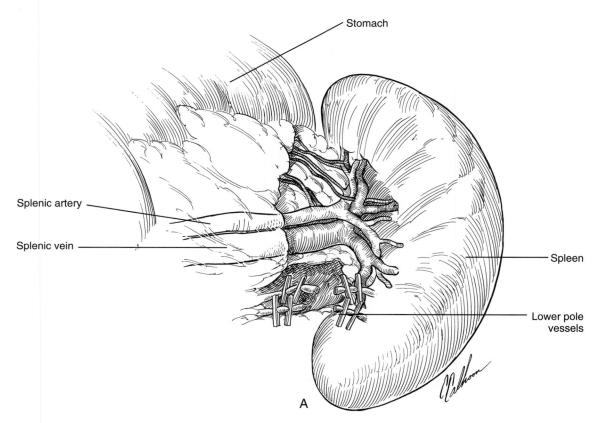

FIGURE 23-4A

FIGURE 23-4A. *Exposure of hilum after dividing the inferior pole.* Following division of the lower pole vessels, the splenic hilum is exposed. The lateral attachments are normally left intact to provide lateral countertraction and secure the spleen. Partial division of these lateral attachments inferiorly is occasionally required to provide circumferential exposure of the splenic hilum.

FIGURE 23-4B. *Exposure of the splenic vessels.* The location of the hilar vessels, often obscured by peritoneum and fatty tissue, is located by identification of the splenic artery pulsations. A blunt 5-mm instrument is passed behind the hilum to elevate it away from the head of the pancreas and expose the hilar vessels.

FIGURE 23-4C. *Division of splenic vessels with a linear laparoscopic stapling device.* The splenic artery and vein may be dissected separately or divided en masse using a linear stapling device with a vascular staple load. This dissection must be performed under direct visualization to avoid life-threatening hemorrhage. This device provides rapid division with excellent hemostasis and does not appear to increase the incidence of arteriovenous fistulas. Other methods of ligation such as clips or ties may also be used.

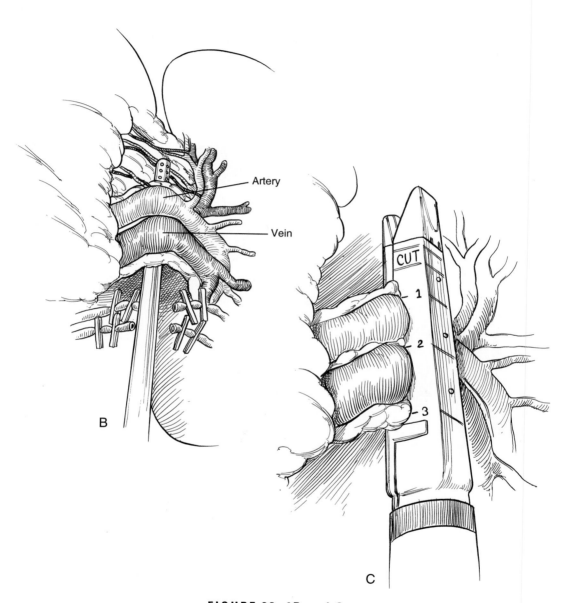

FIGURE 23–4B and C

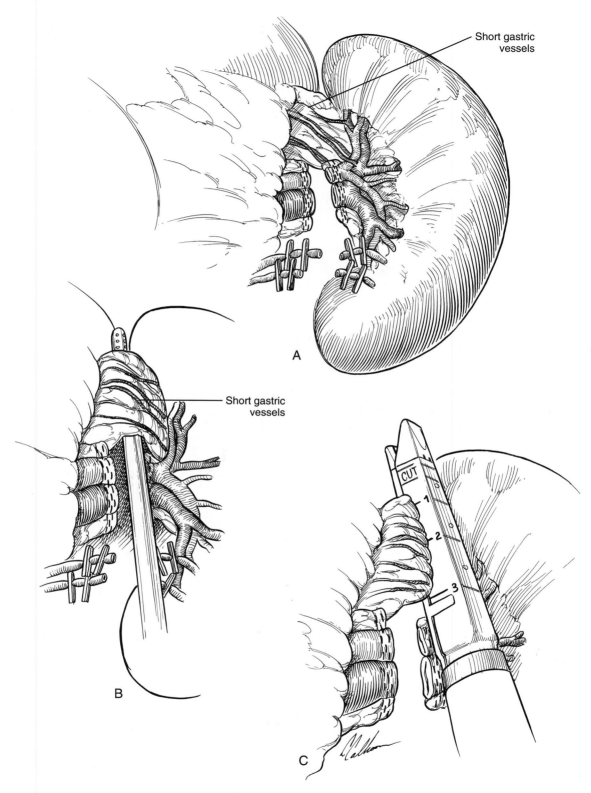

Short gastric
vessels

A

Short gastric
vessels

B

CUT

C

FIGURE 23–5 A–C

FIGURE 23–5A. *Exposure of the short gastric vessels.* Following hilar division, the only remaining medial attachments are the short gastric vessels in the gastrosplenic ligament.

FIGURE 23–5B. *Suction instrument behind the short gastric vessels.* A blunt 5-mm instrument is passed behind the short gastric vessels to elevate them off the greater curvature of the stomach.

FIGURE 23–5C. *Division of the short gastric vessels.* The short gastric vessels are divided next using a linear stapling device, vascular clips, or ultrasonic dissector. Care is taken to avoid injury to the stomach wall during this step. The ultrasonic dissecting shears may also be used for this step. Following short gastric division, the lesser sac is surveyed for accessory splenic tissue.

FIGURE 23–6. *Division of remaining lateral attachments.* The remaining lateral attachments (splenophrenic ligaments) are divided using endoscopic scissors or an ultrasonic dissector.

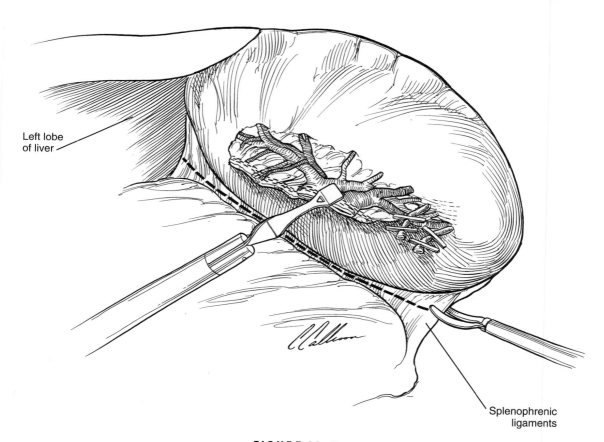

FIGURE 23–6

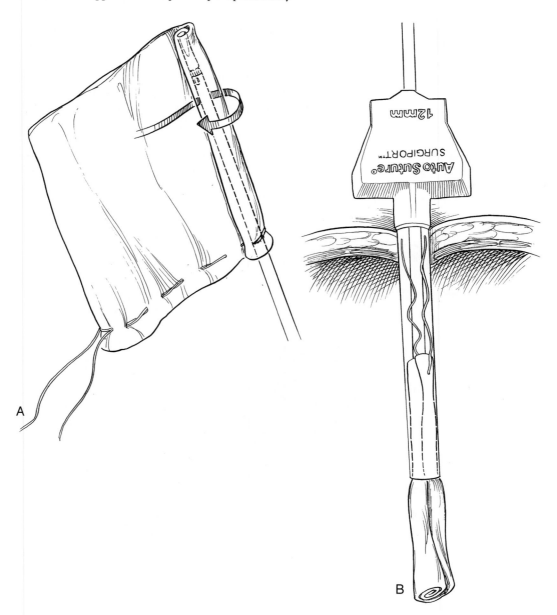

A

B

12mm

AutoSuture®
SURGIPORT™

FIGURE 23–7A and B

FIGURE 23–7A and B. *Insertion of extraction sack.* A large (over 750 ml), heavy nylon extraction bag is rolled and inserted through a 12-mm trocar.

FIGURE 23–7C. *Placement of the spleen into the sac.* Three instruments are used to open the extraction bag in the left upper quadrant or, optionally, the left pelvis. Rotating the table back to the left and reducing the Trendelenburg positioning facilitates this step. A piece of umbilical tape placed around the spleen aids manipulation.

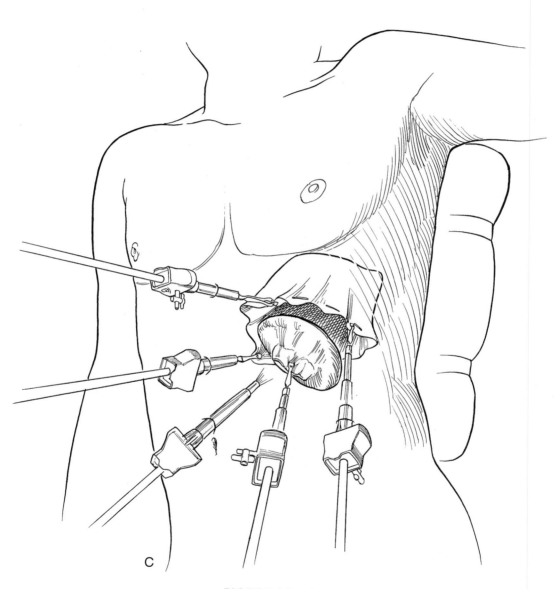

FIGURE 23–7C

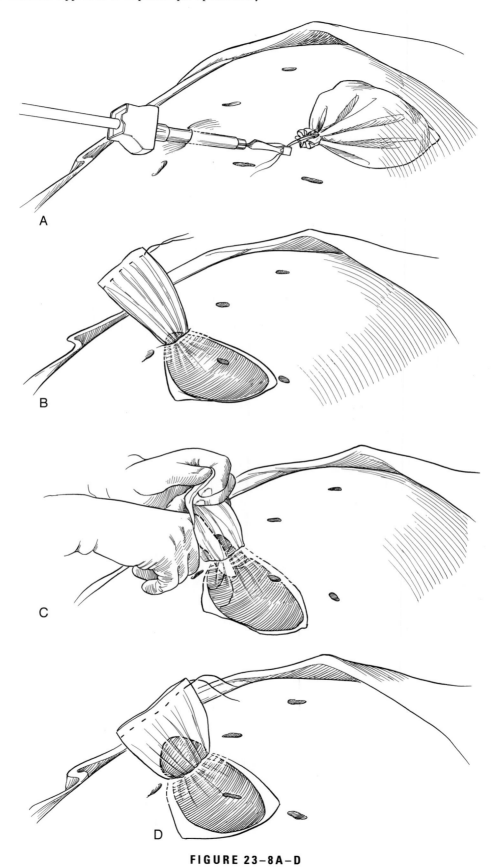

FIGURE 23-8A-D

FIGURE 23-8A-C. *Extraction and morcellation.* The extraction bag is brought out of the abdomen at one of the 12-mm trocar sites once the spleen is secure. The spleen is then removed piecemeal using digital fracture and a blunt clamp or ringed forceps to morcellate the spleen. Extension of the fascial incision facilitates morcellation.

FIGURE 23-8D. *Extraction of an intact spleen.* Extraction of an intact spleen is accomplished by extending the skin and fascial incisions. An incision of 6 to 8 cm is usually large enough to extract even very large spleens with minimal damage.

Heavy absorbable suture is used to close the fascia at all port sites larger than 5 mm.

X. Postoperative Medications

A. Analgesics: Patient-controlled analgesia (narcotic infusion pump) is required in some patients for the first 24 to 36 hours. Oral narcotics or nonsteroidal anti-inflammatory drugs may be used initially in other patients according to pain tolerance.
B. Antiemetics are given as needed.
C. Corticosteroids: Medications are tapered according to underlying diagnosis and duration of therapy in consultation with a hematologist.
D. Antibiotic prophylaxis is given for 24 hours in patients with hematologic malignancies (optional).

XI. Advancement of Diet

A. Clear liquids are given when patient is awake and alert
B. Diet is advanced as tolerated on the morning of postoperative day 1.

XII. Determinants of Discharge

A. Afebrile; no evidence of sepsis
B. Hemodynamically stable
C. Ambulating
D. Tolerating liquids or regular diet
E. Stable hematocrit

XIII. Return to Employment and Normal Activity

A. Normal activity (driving, housework): 7 to 14 days.
B. Employment: 14 to 21 days, longer in patients who perform heavy labor.

Chapter 24

Laparoscopic Adrenalectomy

MICHEL GAGNER, M.D.

I. Indications

A. Pheochromocytoma
B. Nonfunctional adenoma
C. Aldosterone-secreting tumors (Conn's syndrome)
D. Cortisol-secreting tumors (Cushing's adenoma)
E. Cushing's disease
F. Paraneoplastic hypercortisolism
G. Metastasis
H. Macronodular hyperplasia
I. Angiomyolipoma
J. Virilizing and feminizing tumors
K. Cyst

II. Contraindications

A. Invasive adrenal carcinoma, because it is a cancer operation that can become complex and extensive: Removal of the kidney en bloc with the perinephric fat, sometimes a more extensive node dissection on the right side, and liver resection may be necessary.
B. Coagulopathy that cannot be controlled preoperatively.
C. Patients with malignant pheochromocytoma may have multiple periaortic nodes, and an open technique may be more desirable in these patients, especially when the MIBG nuclear scan shows that nodes are present in the periaortic chain or close to the bladder.
D. Relative contraindications include suspected metastasis to the liver or an adjacent organ in patients with malignant pheochromocytoma.

III. Factors Important in Patient Selection

Several factors may make the dissection more difficult. These should be avoided during one's early experience:
A. Previous surgery in the area, such as nephrectomy and splenectomy, or trauma to this area that may create dense adhesions, making it more difficult to expose the space.

B. On the right side, a previous hepatectomy, particularly if it involves the posterior and superior segment of the liver, may make the dissection difficult, as will also a right nephrectomy.

C. Diaphragmatic hernias on the left side may make dissection difficult because the splenic flexure of the colon may be elevated toward the diaphragm.

D. Another relative contraindication is a mass of any kind that is 10 cm or larger. Such a mass will make dissection difficult, and the time needed for dissection depends on the surface area of the lesion. A 10-cm lesion requires much more time, and exposure is more difficult because the lesion reduces the space available to work around the adrenal mass. Often these masses are surrounded by multiple vessels that connect to the retroperitoneal space, so many clips must be applied to control these masses. Only those surgeons with extensive laparoscopic experience should attempt to perform resection of larger masses.

IV. Preoperative Preparation

This varies with the specific diagnosis of the patient.

V. Choice of Anesthesia

General anesthesia is required.

VI. Accessory Devices

A. Nasogastric tubes are not used.
B. Urinary catheter
C. Pneumatic compression stockings

VII. Instruments and Telescopes

A. Veress needle
B. 30-degree 10-mm telescope
C. Hasson retractors (doubles)
D. Laparoscopic electrocautery scissors
E. Laparoscopic ultrasonic dissector (shears)
F. Laparoscopic curved dissector
G. Laparoscopic Dorsey bowel forceps
H. Laparoscopic hook cautery
I. Laparoscopic fan or paddle retractor
J. Laparoscopic surgical clips (medium to large)
K. Laparoscopic Nezhat-Dorsey suction/irrigation device
L. Laproscopic impermeable nylon bag for extraction of specimen
M. Laparoscopic vascular stapler (30 mm)
N. Laparoscopic ultrasonography

Laparoscopic Left Adrenalectomy

VIII. Position of Monitors and Placement and Size of Trocars

FIGURE 24–1. For a left adrenalectomy, the patient is placed in the lateral decubitus position with the left side up. The surgeon and assistant stand on the side opposite the pathology. To position the patient, the table is flexed, and a flank cushion is positioned under the patient's right side.

FIGURE 24–2. The left side should be hyperextended so that the space between the costal margin and the iliac crest is exposed maximally. The left arm is extended and suspended.

The surgical area is prepared and draped; the area from the umbilicus to the vertebral column

and from the nipple down to the superior anterior iliac crest should be exposed. Next, carbon dioxide insufflation up to a pressure of 15 mm Hg is initiated in the left subcostal area using a Veress needle. Or one can use an open technique using Hasson retractors. The needle is inserted under the costal margin at the anterior axillary line and lateral to the rectus muscle through three layers of muscle. A saline test is performed to ensure that no organs have been injured by the needle penetrating the abdominal wall. One 11-mm trocar is then inserted in the left subcostal area at the level of the anterior axillary line, and a 30-degree, 10-mm laparoscope is inserted through it. Diagnostic laparoscopy is performed then in the decubitus position. The ligament suspending the splenic flexure of the colon is inspected as well as the descending colon, the left adnexal area in women, and the femoral area for possible hernias. The spleen, the indentation of the inferior

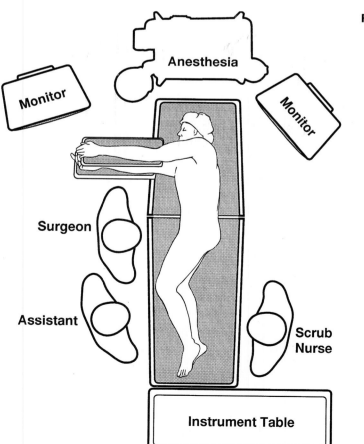

FIGURE 24–1

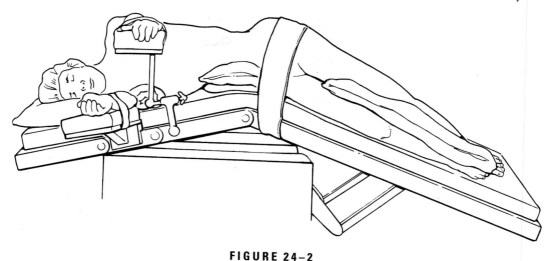

FIGURE 24-2

pole of the left kidney, the lateral portion of the left liver (mainly segments two and three), the diaphragm, and the greater curvature of the stomach are also inspected.

FIGURE 24-3. If the inspection is satisfactory, two more 11-mm trocars are inserted under direct vision in the flank, one under the eleventh rib and one slightly more anterior and medial to the first trocar. All trocars should be at least 5 cm apart, and at best are 8 to 10 cm apart. The laparoscope is then inserted into the most anterior trocar, and the surgeon works laterally using a two-handed technique through the other two trocars. Laparoscopic reducers are positioned (11 mm to 5 mm) for the insertion of a pair of laparoscopic scissors with cautery, either straight or curved (for the right hand), and a laparoscopic curved dissector (for the left hand) that can gently grasp the tissue.

FIGURE 24-3

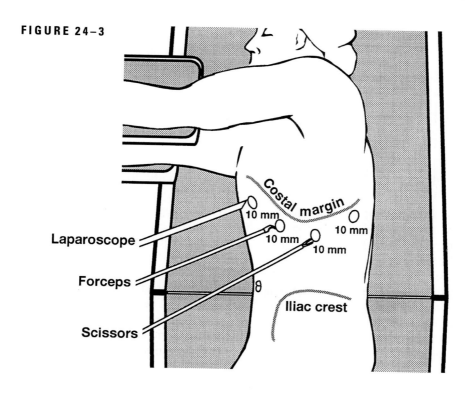

FIGURE 24–4A

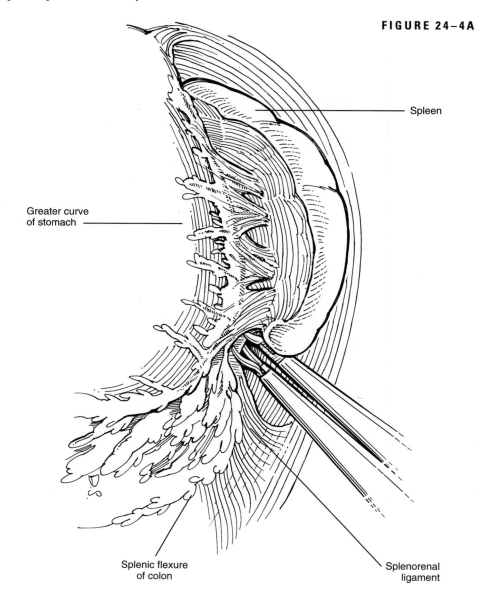

Spleen

Greater curve
of stomach

Splenic flexure
of colon

Splenorenal
ligament

IX. Narrative of Surgical Technique

FIGURE 24-4. Mobilizing the colonic flexure usually is necessary to open the retroperitoneal space and move the colon from the inferior pole of the adrenal gland. Mobilization allows instruments to be inserted more easily and helps prevent inadvertent trauma to the colon during instrument insertion. In the first plane of dissection, the lateral dissection of the spleen at the splenorenal ligament, approximately 1 cm of peritoneal covering lateral to the spleen is in-

cised (A). With graspers in the left hand, the ligament is grasped and dissected to open the space between the spleen and the kidney. The dissection is carried up to the diaphragm, very close to the greater curvature of the stomach or the fundus and close to the short gastric vessels. Once the spleen is fully mobilized (B), it will fall medially, and this space will open by itself like a book. The lateral edge and anterior portion of the adrenal gland will become visible in the perinephric fat, superiorly and medially.

The dissection of the adrenal gland can be

FIGURE 24–4B

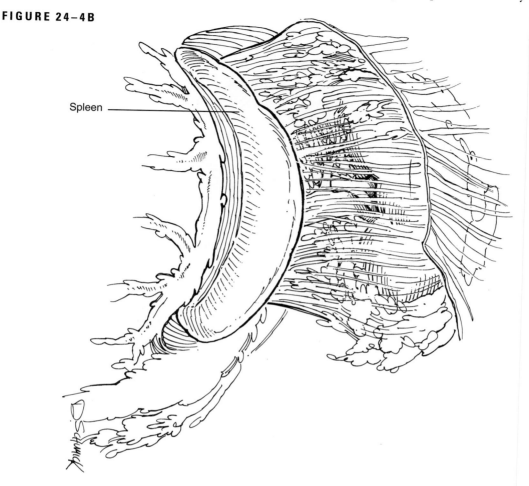

Spleen

easy or difficult depending on the type of peri-nephric fat that is present. Two main types have been encountered: the soft, nonadherent, areo-lar fat that is easy to dissect using laparoscopic scissors with cautery, and the dense, adherent fat that contains multiple small veins coming from the retroperitoneum. To avoid fracture of the adrenal capsule, I use the hook cautery to dissect the adrenal gland from the surrounding tissue, or one can use the ultrasonic dissector (endoshears, 5 or 10 mm). This dissection is much slower, and one has to be patient to avoid bleeding or fracture of the adrenal tissue.

Once the lateral portion of the adrenal gland has been exposed, the patient is moved to the Fowler position to permit further downward migration of the bowel loops and the spleen.

Any saline irrigation, bleeding, or oozing in this area will flow downward. A fourth trocar may be necessary to retract the spleen further and open the space or to push the left kidney or the surrounding fat downward to better expose the inferior pole and lateral edge of the adrenal gland. If this fourth trocar is needed, it is in-serted in the costovertebral angle dorsally. Also, this trocar should always be inserted after the previous three because the splenorenal ligament must be exposed first to allow this trocar to pass over the lateral and superior borders of the kidney. If this ligament is not exposed, the tro-car may inadvertently be inserted into the kid-ney. A retractor or Babcock clamp is then used to retract the lateral border of the splenorenal ligament, as discussed earlier.

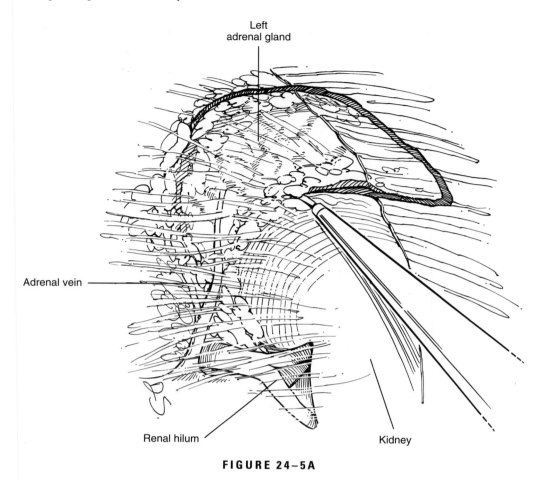

Left
adrenal gland

Adrenal vein —

Renal hilum

Kidney

FIGURE 24–5A

FIGURE 24-5A-C. The dissection can be continued inferiorly so that the left adrenal vein can be clipped, or it can be started superiorly, working down medially to clip the adrenal vein at the end. The direction depends on the exposure gained after the spleen has been dissected, the type of pathology, and the size of the adrenal mass. If a very large adrenal mass (5 to 10 cm) must be dissected, the left adrenal vein may be more difficult to visualize. In such cases, dissecting the lateral and superior adrenal poles first will allow better mobilization and make it easier to clip the adrenal vein. In most smaller tumors (less than 5 cm in diameter), dissecting

and clipping the adrenal vein is feasible and easy. Most left adrenal veins are about 8 to 10 mm in diameter and can be clipped with a medium to large titanium clip placed with a single-application clip applier. With a right-angle dissector, the adrenal vein is dissected from its insertion into the left adrenal gland; it is not necessary to then identify the junction between the adrenal vein and the renal vein. The adrenal vein is then clipped about 1 cm from the renal vein; two or three clips are placed proximal to the gland, and two clips are positioned distally (C).

FIGURE 24–5B

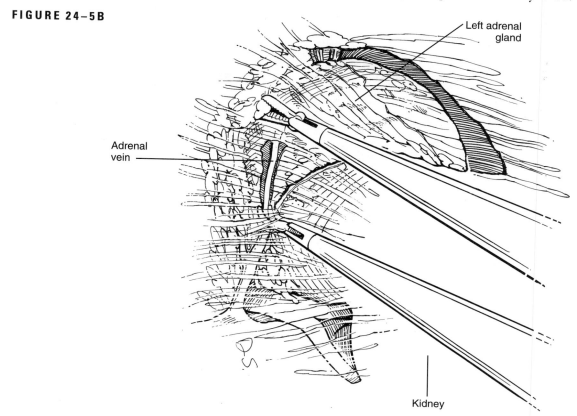

Left adrenal
gland

Adrenal
vein

Kidney

FIGURE 24–5C

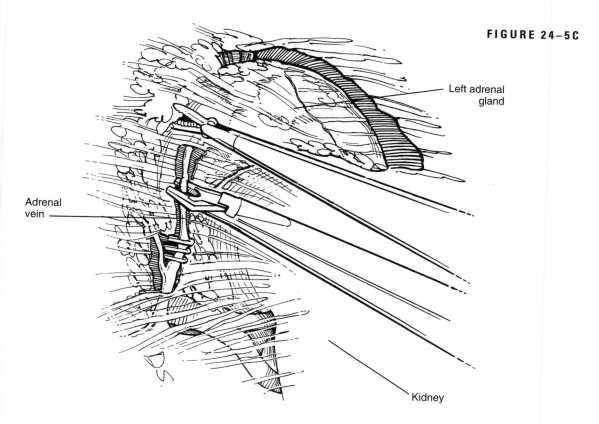

Left adrenal
gland

Adrenal
vein

Kidney

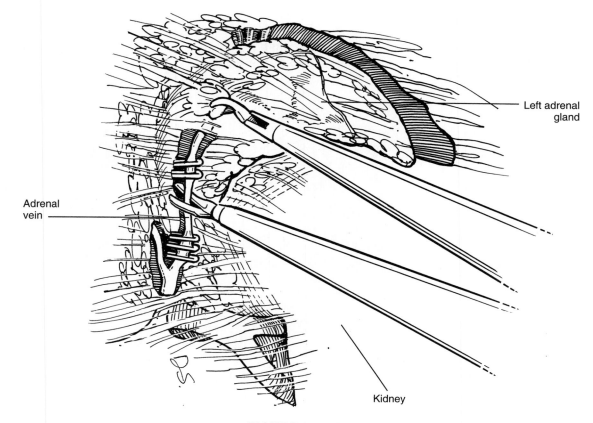

Left adrenal
gland

Adrenal
vein

Kidney

FIGURE 24–6A

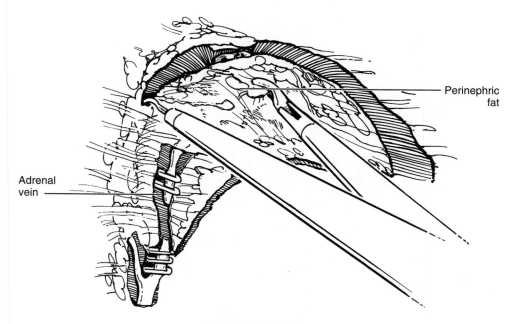

Perinephric
fat

Adrenal
vein

FIGURE 24–6B

FIGURE 24-6A and B. The vein is divided with the laparoscopic straight scissor. At this point, adrenal mobilization is easy because the gland is grasped on the perinephric fat with the left hand grasper; it is then pushed upward and laterally to permit dissection of the medial and superior portions. This dissection is done with the hook cautery, and anything that offers resistance should be examined and then cauterized or clipped. One must remember that the inferior phrenic arterial branches may be ligated as one approaches the superior pole of the left adrenal gland.

FIGURE 24-7. Once the adrenal gland is free, hemostasis is verified by irrigation aspiration using the Nezhat-Dorsey apparatus. The entire gland is extracted after it has been placed in a 10 × 10 cm sterile nylon bag (A), but a variety of other sizes should be available because the lesion may be larger or smaller than expected. This bag should be fairly rigid so that it will not rupture during extraction, which would lead to adrenal cell seeding of the wound or abdominal cavity. The bag is removed through the most anterior trocar with minimal spreading of the oblique muscles using a Kelly clamp (B).

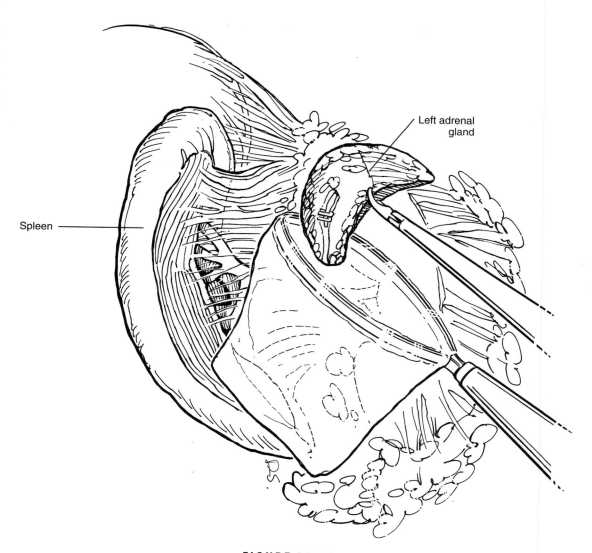

FIGURE 24-7A

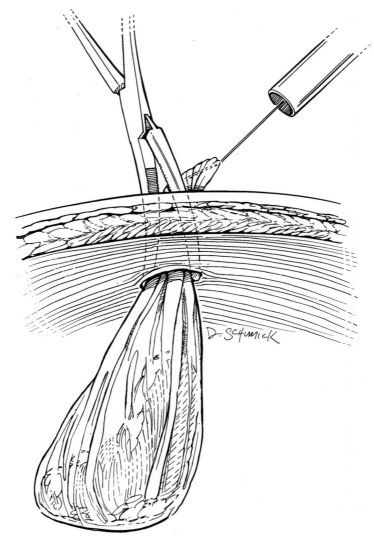

FIGURE 24–7B

The incision may be enlarged if the lesion is larger than 4 cm. Usually the incision size must be about half the original dimension of the lesion. Drainage is seldom necessary, and we have abandoned it in our most recent cases. Initially, we used a Jackson-Pratt drain. It was left in place overnight to drain excess peritoneal fluid in the lower abdomen and right side that accumulated as a result of using the Fowler position. Also, if the patient goes into the recovery room in the dorsal position, leakage often occurs from the posterior trocar incisions. If one has used a minimal amount of irrigation, the drain can be avoided. An attempt is made to close all fascial incisions with 2–0 absorbable sutures. The skin incisions are closed with 4–0 absorbable sutures.

Laparoscopic Right Adrenalectomy

VIII. Position of Monitors and Placement and Size of Trocars

FIGURE 24-8. All patients are placed in the lateral decubitus position with the right side up. Pneumoperitoneum is established in the same way as for a left adrenalectomy, using a Veress needle inserted in the subcostal area. The Veress needle must be inserted very carefully to avoid injuring the liver parenchyma because bleeding may occur, or, if carbon dioxide insufflation is initiated in the liver parenchyma, gas emboli may develop. The insertion of the Veress needle is performed with careful palpation to avoid the liver edge about 2 cm below the costal margin and the anterior axillary line. Alternatively, Hasson retractors can be used (open technique). Pneumoperitoneum is maintained at 15 mm Hg during the procedure. An 11-mm trocar is inserted, and diagnostic laparoscopy is performed using a 30-degree laparoscope to inspect the right hepatic lobe, triangular liga-

ment, diaphragm, descending colon, hepatic flexure of the colon, and the right half of the transverse colon. In both men and women, the right inguinal area is inspected for hernia; in women, the right adnexal area is also inspected for possible pathology. If inspection is satisfactory, three more 11-mm trocars are necessary, for a total of four 11-mm trocars. Under direct vision, the second trocar is inserted in the right flank, just above the right hepatic flexure of the colon. The hepatic flexure of the colon seldom needs to be dissected. The third trocar is then inserted in the most anterior position of the subcostal area between the epigastrium and the anterior axillary line. The last trocar is inserted at the costovertebral subcostal angle after the peritoneal reflection of the lateral edge of the right kidney has been dissected to avoid injury to the right kidney. Four trocars are necessary because the right lobe of the liver must be retracted to expose the most medial aspect of the right adrenal gland. It is, therefore, critical that the liver retractor is inserted in the anterior trocar under direct vision so that the right hepatic lobe can be lifted and pushed medially.

FIGURE 24-8

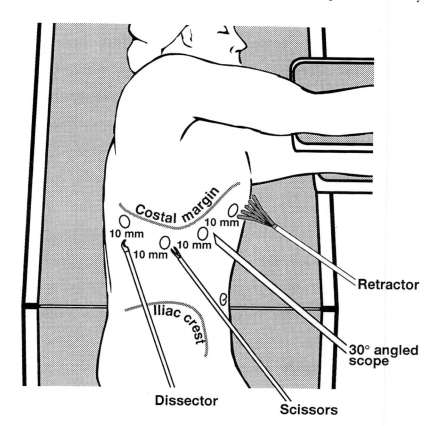

The laparoscope is removed from the first trocar and inserted in the second trocar, and the surgeon works with the two most lateral trocars. The camera can be positioned dorsally, and the surgeon will work with the two trocars in the middle to obtain another view of the dissection field, primarily the superior aspect.

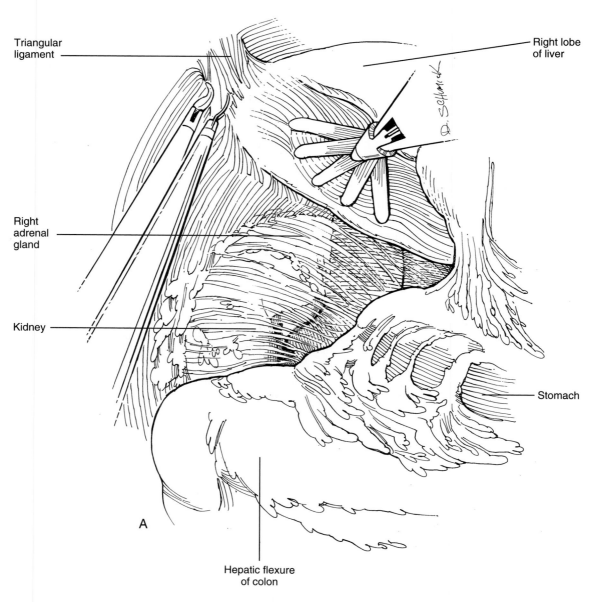

Triangular ligament

Right lobe of liver

Right adrenal gland

Kidney

Stomach

A

Hepatic flexure of colon

FIGURE 24–9A

IX. Narrative of Surgical Technique

FIGURE 24–9A and B. The liver often must be mobilized to obtain the best exposure of the junction between the adrenal gland and the inferior vena cava. I prefer to create a right-angle plane between the anterior aspect of the right kidney and the lateral portion of the liver. This plane provides enough space to work and to intervene if bleeding occurs. Takeda et al. have used the ultrasonic aspirator to permit bet-ter dissection of the gland around the perinephric fat, especially in patients with Cushing's syndrome. They also advocate using the argon beam coagulator for a right adrenalectomy if the adrenal gland is embedded in the surrounding liver; the coagulator makes partial liver resection and coagulation easier in this area. Therefore, using laparoscopic scissors, the right triangular ligament of the liver is dissected from the diaphragm as far as necessary. This dissection permits more effective retraction to push the liver medially.

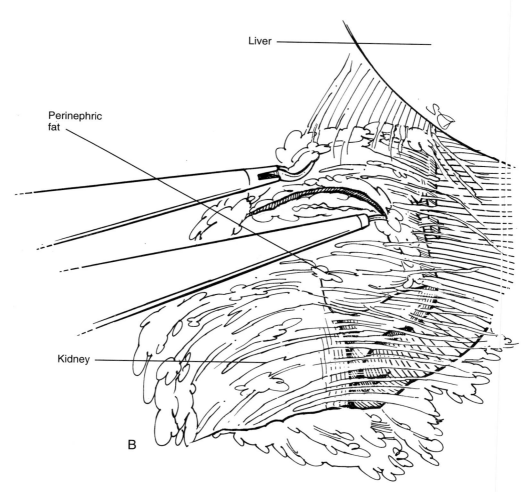

Liver

Perinephric fat

Kidney

B

FIGURE 24–9B

FIGURE 24–10A–C. The right adrenal gland is dissected next. If the mass is less than 4 cm in diameter, access to the right adrenal vein (A) can be gained initially, which makes dissection of the rest of the adrenal gland easier. The inferior portion is then dissected using the hook cautery or the laparoscopic 5-mm curved scissors with the curved dissector in the other hand. The dissection proceeds medially and upward, along the lateral edge of the vena cava. The right renal vein should be visible; this is the most inferior portion of the dissection. As one dissects along the vena cava, one will encounter the right adrenal vein. This vein is often short and is sometimes broad. Usually the vein can be clipped with medium to large titanium clips (B), at least two of which should be positioned on the vena cava side. If there is not enough space for clips, then the cartridge of a 30-mm or 35-mm laparoscopic stapler (Endo GIA, United States Surgical Corporation, Norwalk, CT, or Ethicon, Cincinnati, OH) is positioned to divide the right adrenal vein (C). Smaller veins may be encountered superiorly; these should be clipped to prevent bleeding.

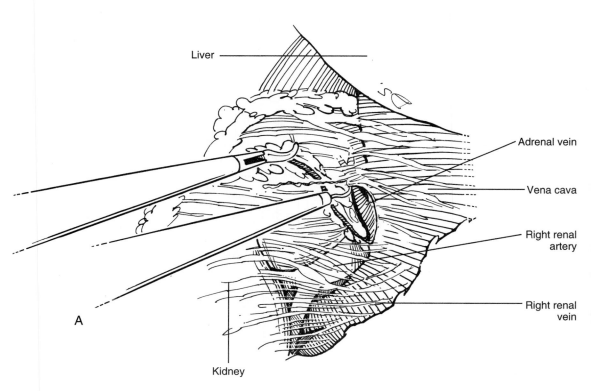

FIGURE 24–10A

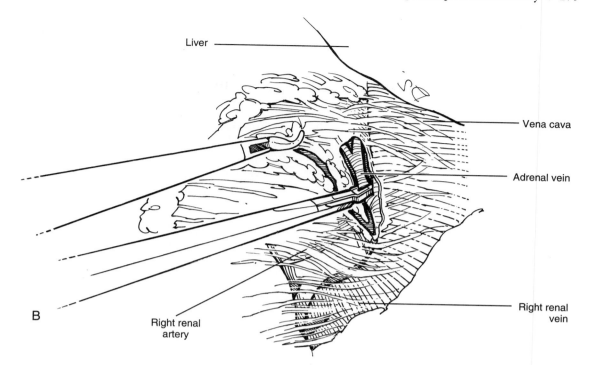

Liver

Vena cava

Adrenal vein

Right renal
artery

Right renal
vein

B

FIGURE 24–10B

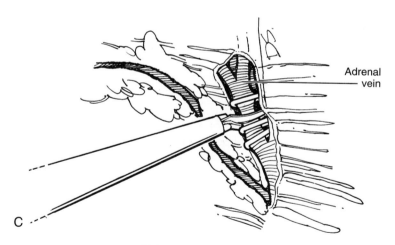

Adrenal
vein

C

FIGURE 24–10C

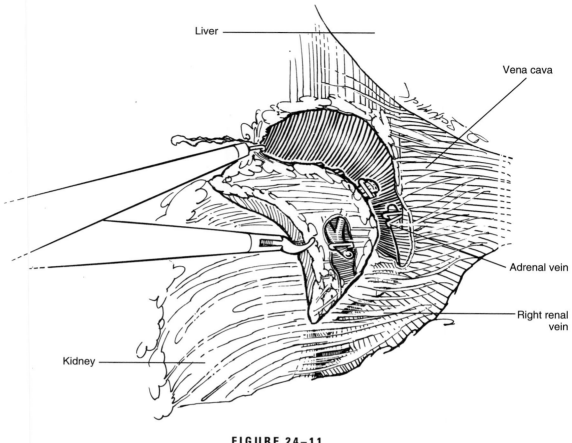

Liver

Vena cava

Adrenal vein

Right renal vein

Kidney

FIGURE 24-11

FIGURE 24-11. The superior pole of the adrenal vein is dissected next, and small branches from the inferior phrenic vessels can be clipped or cauterized with hook cautery. Again, a Fowler position permits all fluid to migrate downward. The lateral adrenal gland is then dissected from the perinephric fat using the same 5-mm laparoscopic hook or with the Harmonic ultrasonic dissector (shears). Meticulous dissection close to the gland will prevent tearing of the lateral branches of the vena cava and other vessels from the retroperitoneum. If a large mass is encountered, we prefer to dissect laterally and superiorly first and then move down along the vena cava to reach the adrenal vein.

Once the mass has been dissected free, it is placed in a sterile nylon bag, usually 10 × 10 cm, and removed through the most anterior trocar site. All wounds are closed as described for the left adrenalectomy. The fascia from the fourth trocar (dorsal) often is not closed because of the depth of this wound.

Laparoscopic Bilateral Adrenalectomy

Bilateral laparoscopic adrenalectomy is needed infrequently. In the lateral decubitus position, the left side is usually dissected first. Because the left side is easier, the chances are greater that the patient will benefit from a laparoscopic technique. Once all wounds have been closed on the left, the patient is repositioned and redraped to expose the right side, which requires a 15- to 20-minute turnover time. This may not be necessary if one uses an anterior technique with trocars in the anterior subcostal left and anterior subcostal right areas. Nonetheless, because in the lateral decubitus position gravity helps to make adrenalectomy easier, I prefer to do the left side or use the lateral decubitus position first, and then complete the right side. In all the cases in which we have followed this sequence, we have successfully performed bilateral laparoscopic adrenalectomy within a reasonable amount of time.

X. Postoperative Medications

A. Intravenous or intramuscular narcotics are administered for 12 to 24 hours after surgery.
B. Most patients require only oral codeine for pain after 24 hours.

XI. Advancement of Diet

A. Nasogastric tubes are not required in these patients.
B. Oral fluids are started on the day of surgery.

XII. Determinants of Discharge

A. Most patients are discharged on the first or second postoperative day.
B. Discharge may be delayed in patients who require substantial hormonal support or adjustments in antihypertensive medication.

XIII. Return to Normal Activities

Postoperative recovery is very similar to that following laparoscopic cholecystectomy. Patients resume normal activities as tolerated, usually within 1 to 2 weeks.

Part VI

LAPAROSCOPIC SURGERY OF THE LOWER GASTROINTESTINAL TRACT

Chapter 25

Laparoscopic Appendectomy

PHILIP F. CAUSHAJ, M.D.

I. Indications

A. Patients who present with the typical picture of acute appendicitis

B. Patients who present with a confusing clinical picture with right lower quadrant pain.

C. Right lower quadrant pain in women during their child-bearing years. The visualization of the pelvis, fallopian tubes, and ovaries obtained through a laparoscope is vastly superior to that obtained through a right lower quadrant incision.

D. Patients over the age of 50 who have right lower quadrant pain. Laparoscopic assessment in these patients can help to distinguish among acute appendicitis, perforated cecal carcinoma, solitary cecal diverticulitis, and acute sigmoid diverticulitis. Once the correct diagnosis is established, the feasibility of treating the condition with laparoscopic techniques or a traditional operation can be judged. If it proves necessary to proceed with an open operation, the surgeon can use the incision he favors for the appropriate operation rather than attempting to operate through a right lower quadrant incision.

II. Contraindications

A. Abdominal distention due to adynamic ileus or intestinal obstruction.

B. Severe cardiovascular disease that precludes general anesthesia.

C. Severe restrictive pulmonary disease that may prevent the anesthesiologist from ventilating excess carbon dioxide from the pneumoperitoneum.

III. Factors Important in Patient Selection

A. Distention of the small bowel because of adynamic ileus or obstruction makes it difficult to initiate the pneumoperitoneum and expose the appendix adequately.

B. Laparoscopic appendectomy is more easily accomplished in thin women than in obese men. Men tend to store more of their fat in the bowel mesentery. This makes dissection of the appendix more difficult.

IV. Preoperative Preparation

A. Counseling of the patient about the possibility of converting to an open appendectomy as deemed necessary by the surgeon is important.

B. All patients receive a preoperative dose of a second-generation cephalosporin.

V. Choice of Anesthesia

General endotracheal anesthesia

VI. Accessory Devices

A. Nasogastric tube
B. Urinary catheter
C. Pneumatic compression stockings

VII. Instruments and Telescopes

A. 10-mm, 0-degree telescope
B. Veress needle
C. Two 5-mm atraumatic grasping instruments
D. 5-mm laparoscopic scissors
E. Pre-tied laparoscopic suture loops or laparoscopic Endo GIA 30
F. Impermeable laparoscopic bag

VIII. Positioning of Monitors and Placement and Size of Trocars

FIGURE 25–1. The patient is placed in the supine position. After endotracheal intubation has been achieved, all patients undergo bladder and gastric decompression with appropriate catheters. The abdomen is prepared and draped widely should conversion to open laparotomy be required. The positions of the video monitor, surgeon, assistant, and scrub nurse are shown. This arrangement allows the surgeon to operate in a comfortable position. In this set-up, the movements of the assistant surgeon are generally reversed on the video monitor. This is slightly inconvenient, but once exposure of the appendix is established, the assistant remains relatively static. It is often easier for the surgeon to position the instruments of the assistant since the motions of the surgeon are not reversed on the monitor. Alternatively, some surgeons prefer to place the monitor at the patient's feet.

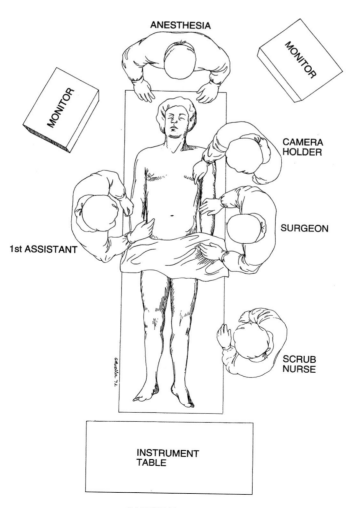

ANESTHESIA

MONITOR

MONITOR

CAMERA HOLDER

1st ASSISTANT

SURGEON

SCRUB NURSE

INSTRUMENT TABLE

FIGURE 25–1

FIGURE 25-2. The carbon dioxide pneumoperitoneum is insufflated. A 10-mm trocar is inserted into the abdomen in the umbilical position. A 10-mm forward viewing laparoscope is passed through the trocar, and the peritoneal cavity is inspected. If acute appendicitis is noted or visualization of the appendix cannot be achieved, a 12-mm trocar is placed midline in the suprapubic region below the "bikini line," and a 10-mm trocar is placed either in the right upper or right lower quadrant. We prefer the upper quadrant placement because it allows better cecal retraction. These ports allow manipulation and mobilization of the cecum and perhaps the right colon in order to visualize the appendix, especially if the appendix is retrocecal. If a normal appendix is noted, further inspection of other organs is required. This can be generally accomplished by placing a second 10-mm trocar in the suprapubic position.

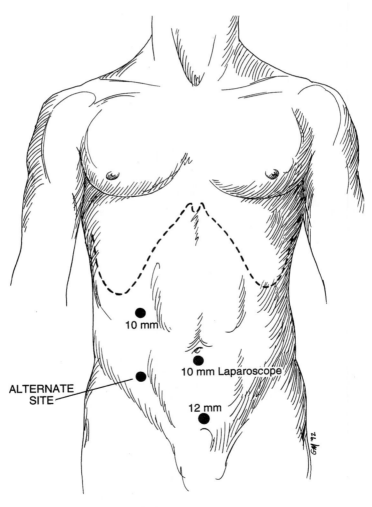

FIGURE 25-2

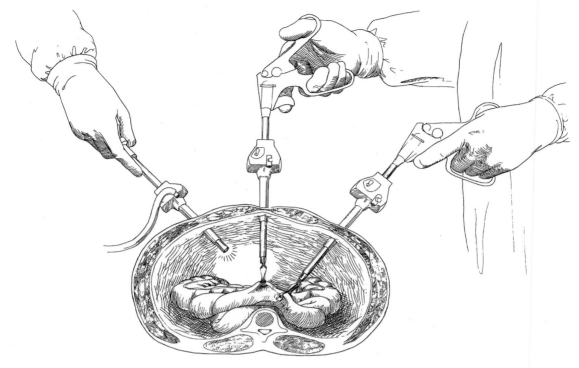

FIGURE 25-3

IX. Narrative of Surgical Technique

FIGURE 25-3. After placing the patient in the Trendelenburg position, a 10-mm periumbilical skin incision is made. The Veress needle is inserted through the incision into the abdominal cavity. Its position is confirmed by the "saline drop test" and by the initially low pressures achieved with insufflation. The peritoneal cavity is insufflated with carbon dioxide to a pressure of 14 to 15 mm Hg. After adequate pneumoperitoneum has been achieved, a 10-mm trocar is introduced.

Placing the patient right side up in the Trendelenburg position facilitates inspection of the right lower quadrant, including the appendix, cecum, distal small bowel, ovaries, tubes, and uterus. An atraumatic grasping instrument or simply a blunt probe is inserted through the suprapubic port. This is used to push the small bowel out of the pelvis. With the patient in a deep Trendelenburg position, the small bowel generally slides up toward the stomach and re-mains out of the way. The sigmoid colon is displaced first toward the left side and then toward the right side. The grasping instrument or probe can be used to elevate the uterus anteriorly and thereby improve the exposure of the pelvis, fallopian tubes, and ovaries. Alternatively, the uterus can be retracted anteriorly with the transvaginal placement of a uterine sound. The grasping instrument can be used to examine the small bowel. This is most easily accomplished by starting at the ileocecal valve and running the bowel back toward the ligament of Treitz. In some patients, it may prove necessary to insert a second trocar so that two grasping instruments can be used to grasp the bowel in sequence.

Laparoscopy also affords an opportunity to inspect the upper abdomen. This is best accomplished with the patient in a reverse Trendelenburg position. With the head up, the liver, gallbladder, spleen, stomach, and proximal small bowel are readily visualized.

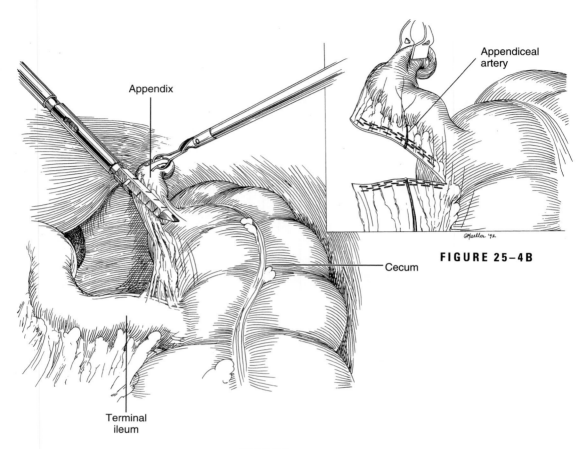

Appendix

Appendiceal
artery

FIGURE 25–4B

Cecum

Terminal
ileum

FIGURE 25–4A

FIGURE 25–4A. After mobilizing the appendix, the diagnosis of acute appendicitis is made by direct inspection. Removal of the appendix begins with the exposure and ligation of the mesoappendix. The appendiceal tip is retracted using an atraumatic grasper or Surgi-Tie to "tent" the mesoappendix.

FIGURE 25–4B. The mesoappendix can be ligated using the Endo GIA 30 after a small fenestration has been fashioned at the base of the appendix with a blunt instrument.

FIGURE 25-5. Alternatively, the mesoappendix can also be dissected with electrocautery or laser energy after titanium clips or Surgi-Ties have been used to ligate the appendiceal artery. Dissection can start at the tip or the base, depending on the position of the appendix or associated adhesions. The mesoappendix should be divided as close to the appendix as possible. This allows better hemostasis and less bulk on the appendix for easier extraction.

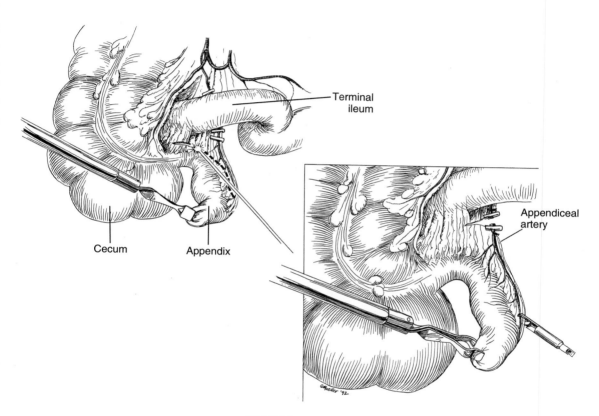

Terminal
ileum

Cecum   Appendix

Appendiceal
artery

FIGURE 25-5

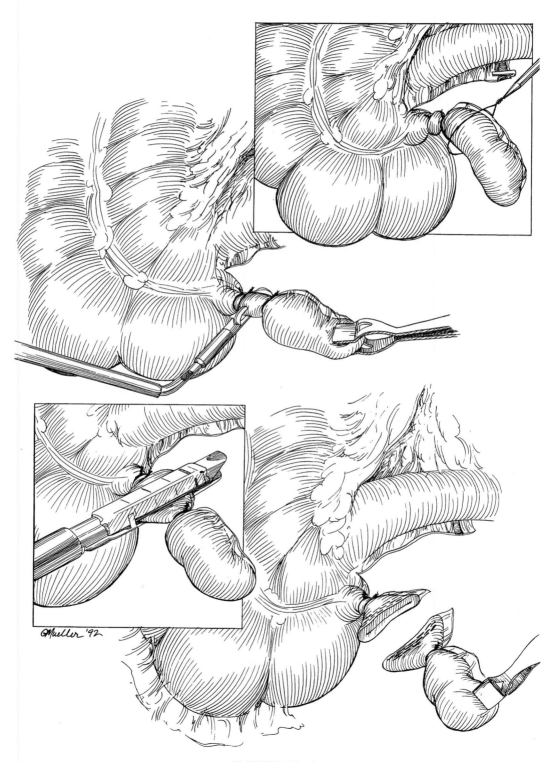

FIGURE 25-6

FIGURE 25-6. After skeletonizing, the base of the appendix is exposed, and two to three chromic Surgi-Ties are secured on the proximal cecal portion of the appendix. An additional Surgi-Tie is placed distally. The appendix can then be ligated with scissors, laser, or electrocautery. Alternatively, the Endo GIA 30 may be used to transect the appendix from the cecum. After transection by either method, inspection of the appendiceal stump as well as the mesoappendix is mandatory. Titanium clips, electrocautery, or Surgi-Ties may be used to secure hemostasis. The appendiceal stump may be cauterized as well.

Invagination of the appendiceal stump is not performed routinely. This is technically more challenging and has been shown to be unnecessary. Occasionally, the base of the appendix or cecum is so inflamed that simple ligation of the appendiceal stump may not be secure. It is in this situation that stump invagination is useful. As described by Semm, either a purse-string or Z stitch suture is used to invaginate the stump. The suture is tied extracorporeally, using an atraumatic grasper to "dunk" the base.

Occasionally an appendix may be so inflamed or gangrenous that a retrograde approach may be useful. This approach begins with dissection, ligation, and division of the appendiceal base. Used as a retractor, the appendix is systematically dissected free from its mesentery and adhesions using laser or electrocautery in sharp and blunt dissection. If an appendiceal abscess is encountered and the surrounding tissue is too inflamed and friable to allow a safe appendectomy, laparoscopic directed drainage and irrigation is performed. A closed suction drain is placed in the abscess cavity and brought out through the right trocar site. An interval appendectomy, either laparoscopic or open, is performed at a later date.

Once ligated, the appendix is removed through the 12-mm suprapubic trocar site. If the appendix is exceedingly inflamed or bulky, a 15-mm trocar can be placed. An additional technique is to encase the appendix in a sterile condom or bag such as the Endo-Catch before extracting it. This prevents rupture of the appendix and contamination of the peritoneum and abdominal wall.

After the appendix has been removed, the patient is placed in the right side down, reverse Trendelenburg position and irrigation with copious amounts of heparinized Ringer's lactate solution is performed, followed by aspiration. A drain may be left in the right lower quadrant and brought out through the right trocar site in patients with a localized collection or phlegmon. The cecum, mesoappendix, and stump are inspected once more for security and hemostasis. The trocars are removed under direct visualization, and the pneumoperitoneum is released. The wounds are irrigated and closed with either metal staples or a 4–0 Vicryl subcuticular suture and dressed with Steri-Strips. The Foley catheter and nasogastric tube are removed postoperatively in the operating room.

X. Postoperative Medications

Postoperatively, the patient may receive antibiotic therapy, depending on the degree of inflammation or purulence and the individual surgeon's preference.

XI. Advancement of Diet

In most patients the diet can be advanced after 8 to 12 hours, and the patient is ambulatory soon after surgery.

XII. Determinants of Discharge

Patients can be discharged as early as 24 hours after surgery.

XIII. Return to Normal Activity

Patients are permitted to resume normal activities as tolerated. Young patients typically return to their normal activities very quickly. Older patients require 1 to 3 weeks to recover their usual zest and vitality.

Laparoscopic Assisted Ileocolectomy for Inflammatory Bowel Disease

AVRAM COOPERMAN, M.D.

I. Indications

Patients with documented Crohn's disease of the ileum or ileocecal region or other segmental areas of the small bowel who require surgical resection for:
A. Obstruction
B. Bleeding
C. Abscess with perforation

II. Contraindications

Complicated Crohn's disease: Complicated Crohn's disease implies that an abscess, fistula, inflammatory mass, or adherent ureter has complicated the segment of bowel involved in Crohn's disease. When such complications are present laparoscopic dissection may be more difficult. If the cecum and ileum are fixed to the right retroperitoneum (usually because a perforation has occurred), dissection may be more difficult because the mesentery may have enlarged nodes, a fistula, or an abscess. Because freeing the ureter or encompassing nodes in the dissection may interfere with the blood supply to a proximal area of nondiseased bowel, great care during dissection must be taken to avoid risking devascularization of the more proximal normal bowel. In this circumstance, it is safer and wiser to open the abdomen and continue the operation rather than risk injury to a retroperitoneal ureter or proximal bowel.

III. Factors Important in Patient Selection

A. Complete evaluation of the gastrointestinal tract from the esophagus to the rectum is performed prior to any resection.
B. A CT scan of the abdomen and pelvis is essential to exclude an inflammatory mass because this helps to determine how much of the surgery can be done safely and easily through the laparoscope. Identification of the right ureter by contrast CT scan or intravenous pyelogram may identify extrinsic compression due to an inflammatory mass and avoid uncomfortable intraoperative moments.

IV. Preoperative Preparation

A. The patient is admitted the evening before surgery (if the patient's health maintenance organization allows it) to facilitate hydration and bowel preparation.
B. Assuming that no acute obstruction is found, 3 to 4 ounces of citrate of magnesium and intramuscular broad-spectrum antibiotics are administered 2 hours prior to surgery.

V. Choice of Anesthesia

General endotracheal anesthesia without nitrous oxide.

VI. Accessory Devices

A. Orogastric tube (removed at end of operation)
B. Urinary catheter
C. Pneumatic compression stockings

VII. Instruments and Telescopes

A. 10-mm, 0-degree telescope
B. 10-mm, 30- or 45-degree telescope
C. Laparoscopic suction/irrigation device
D. Veress needle
E. Harmonic Scalpel (Ethicon Endo-Surgery, Cincinnati, OH), electrocautery hook, or electrocautery scissors
F. Atraumatic laparoscopic graspers
G. Laparoscopic Babcock clamps
H. Laparoscopic clips or laparoscopic stapling device
I. GIA stapling device

VIII. Position of Monitors and Placement and Size of Trocars

FIGURE 26-1. Position of patient: The patient is placed in a supine or lithotomy position. The table should have the capability for a Trendelenburg or reverse Trendelenburg position. The position of the monitor should be in the line of dissection so that the surgeon's eyes and instruments directly face and work toward the monitor. Working with a mirror image or with the monitor opposite or behind the plane of dissection creates confusion for the surgeon and/or assistant.

Port position: Four to five trocars are placed. In the absence of previous surgery, closed needle insertion may be done safely through or below the umbilicus. If any difficulty is encountered passing the Veress needle or if previous surgery has been done, open trocar placement is used. A 10-mm sheath is placed after an adhe-

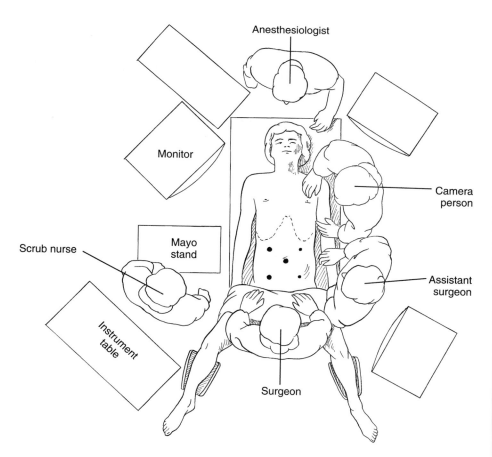

FIGURE 26-1

sion-free area through which a 10-mm laparoscope can be inserted has been ensured. A 0-degree, 30-degree, or 45-degree laparoscope may be needed to visualize all the viscera and the diseased bowel, particularly in the right lower quadrant. Tradition and experience have limited most surgeons to the 0-degree scope, but an angled telescope may provide better exposure, particularly when an inflammatory mass is present.

A second trocar (5 mm) is placed in the left lower quadrant lateral to the rectus muscle. This will provide traction on the ileocecal re-

gion and segments of small bowel. The third trocar (10 mm) is inserted in the right upper quadrant or right lower quadrant depending on the site of the monitor and the angle of dissection. My personal preference is to place the monitor in the right upper quadrant and the dissecting trocar in the right lower quadrant. Mobilization of the ileocecal region begins at the cecum and works toward the hepatic flexure. Other surgeons prefer to start the dissection at the hepatic flexure and work toward the ileocecal valve.

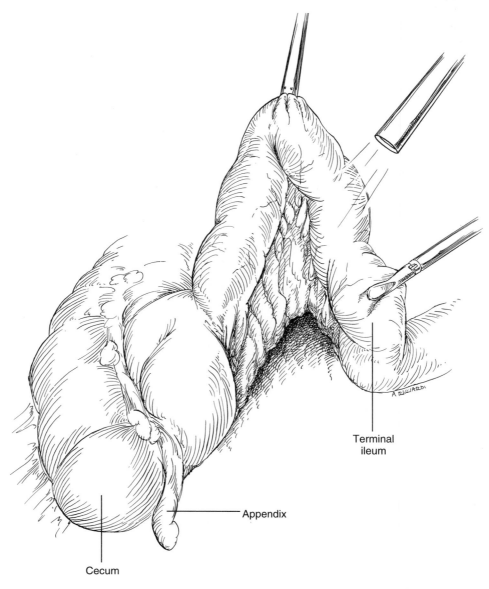

Terminal
ileum

Appendix

Cecum

FIGURE 26-2

IX. Narrative of Surgical Technique

FIGURE 26-2. The entire small bowel is examined from the ileocecal valve to the duodenojejunal ligament. This examination is facilitated by placing a suction probe against the bowel (with the suction channel open) while a clamp or second suction probe secures the bowel proximally. The entire small bowel is examined from distal to proximal, alternating the position of the clamps.

Crohn's disease causes transmural changes in the bowel, and the diseased segments are easily recognized. They are thickened, erythematous, and frequently obstructed by the time surgery is performed.

FIGURE 26-3. If after thorough exploration the disease is found to be confined to the terminal ileal or ileocecal region, it will be necessary to mobilize this segment of bowel through a port placed in the left lower quadrant; a 5-mm clamp is used to provide countertraction.

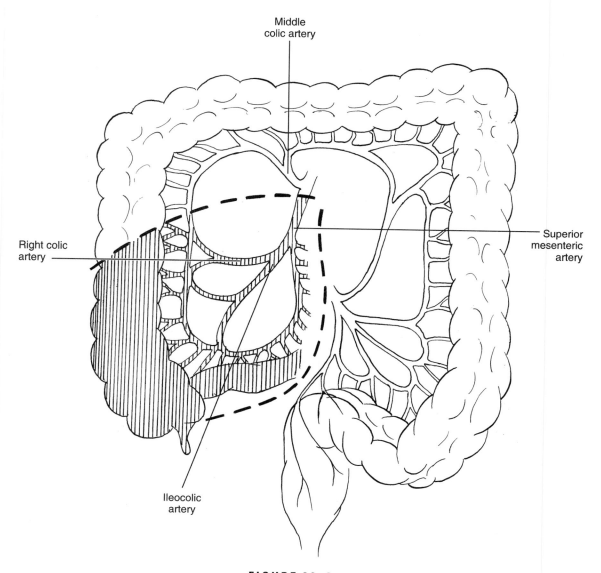

FIGURE 26-3

FIGURE 26–4. The cecum is grasped gently and retracted to the left. A Harmonic Scalpel (hook or scissors), or scissors with a cautery attachment, is used to incise along the avascular plane up to the hepatic flexure and around the ileocecal valve and distal ileum. This exposes and mobilizes the terminal ileum, cecum, and ascending colon. In Crohn's disease the line of resection is proximal and distal to the grossly diseased bowel, and a formal right hemicolectomy with the distal line of resection at the transverse colon is not required unless the disease extends to this point.

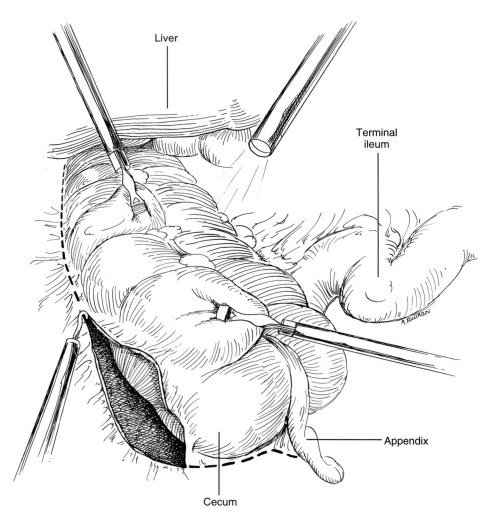

FIGURE 26–4

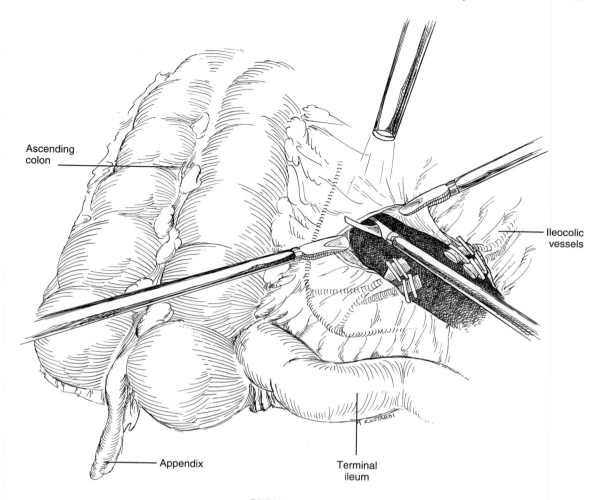

Ascending colon

Ileocolic vessels

Appendix

Terminal ileum

FIGURE 26-5

FIGURE 26-5. There are two options once the bowel is mobilized: (1) One can deliver the bowel outside the abdomen through a small extension of the right lower quadrant or midline incision. This incision can be 1 to 2 inches in length. The mesentery can be divided and ligated easily outside the abdomen, the bowel can be transected and reapproximated and the mesenteric defect closed, and the bowel can then be replaced and the incision closed. (2) The second alternative is to ligate and divide the mesentery using clips, a stapling device, or a Harmonic Scalpel in the abdomen.

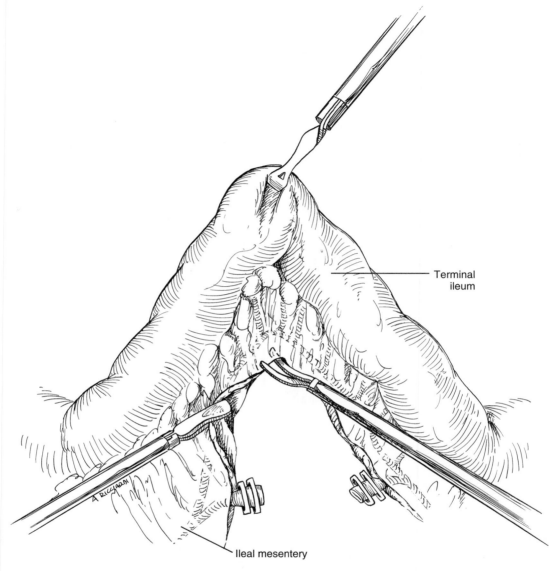

Terminal
ileum

Ileal mesentery

FIGURE 26–6

FIGURE 26–6. The line of division can be kept close to the bowel unless large nodes, an abscess, or matted loops of bowel are present.

FIGURE 26–7. The bowel may now be transected and joined intracorporeally or brought outside, divided, and joined.

X. Postoperative Medications

Patients receive only analgesics as needed.

XI. Advancement of Diet

Patients are given liquids the day after surgery and advanced to a regular diet as tolerated.

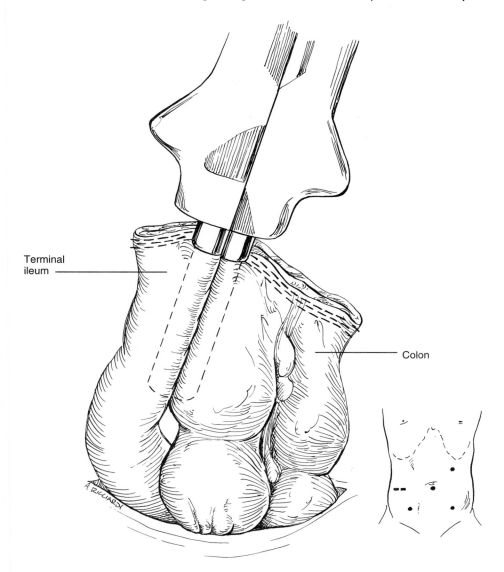

Terminal ileum

Colon

FIGURE 26-7

XII. Determinants of Discharge

A. The patient is tolerating the diet.
B. The patient is having bowel movements.
C. The incision is healing.
D. Oral analgesics are controlling pain.

XIII. Return to Normal Activity

Patients can return to normal activities as tolerated, usually within 7–10 days.

Chapter 27

Laparoscopic-Assisted Right Hemicolectomy for Malignancy

DAVID OTA, M.D.

I. Indications

A. Sessile benign polyps of the cecum and ascending colon not amenable to colonoscopic polypectomy
B. Carcinoma of the cecum and ascending colon

II. Contraindications

Large bulky lesions that require large incisions for extraction

III. Factors Important in Patient Selection

Patients with severe obstructive pulmonary disease may tolerate carbon dioxide pneumoperitoneum poorly.

IV. Preoperative Preparation

A. Patients are admitted on the day of surgery.
B. Patients undergo standard mechanical and antibiotic bowel preparation at home.

V. Choice of Anesthesia

General endotracheal anesthesia is required.

VI. Accessory Devices

A. A nasogastric tube is inserted at the beginning of the procedure and then removed at the end.
B. A urinary catheter is inserted at the beginning of the procedure and removed when the patient is ambulatory.
C. Pneumatic compression stockings are used in all patients.

VII. Instruments and Telescopes

A. 10-mm, 0-degree telescope
B. Electrocautery spatula
C. Laparoscopic Babcock clamps
D. Laparoscopic scissors
E. Laparoscopic surgical clips
F. GIA stapling device
G. TA stapling device
H. 0 chromic endo-loop

VIII. Position of Monitors and Placement and Size of Trocars

FIGURE 27–1. The positioning of the monitor and the distribution of the operating team are shown. The surgeon stands by the patient's left hip. The monitor is placed directly in front of the surgeon. The assistant surgeon stands by the patient's left shoulder. This leaves the right side of the patient free for the scrub nurse.

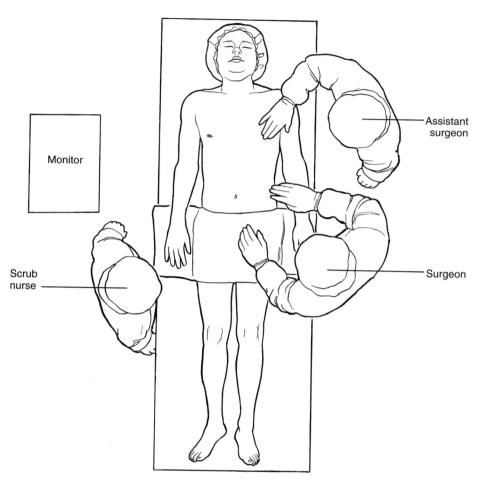

FIGURE 27–1

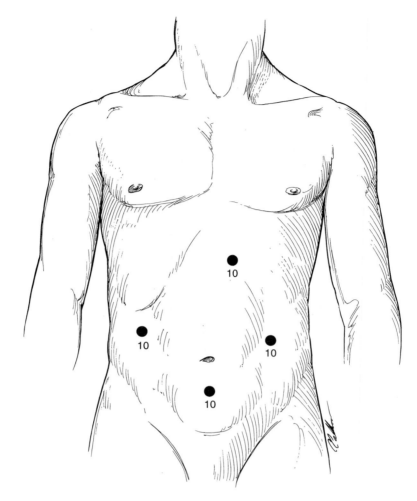

FIGURE 27-2

FIGURE 27-2. Four 10/11-mm trocars are used during a laparoscopic right hemicolectomy. The telescope is inserted through the left upper quadrant trocar. The right and left trocars are used for retraction. Dissection is accomplished using an electrocautery spatula inserted through the hypogastric port.

IX. Narrative of Surgical Technique

FIGURE 27-3. View from the left upper quadrant port. The greater omentum has been placed cephalad, exposing the transverse colon.

FIGURE 27-4. The cecum and terminal ileum are retracted cephalad with the Babcock clamps.

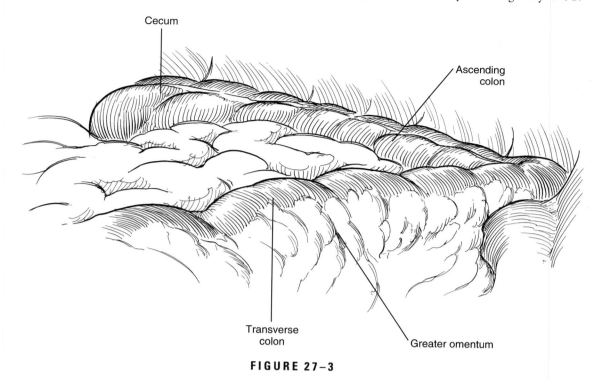

Cecum

Ascending
colon

Transverse
colon

Greater omentum

FIGURE 27–3

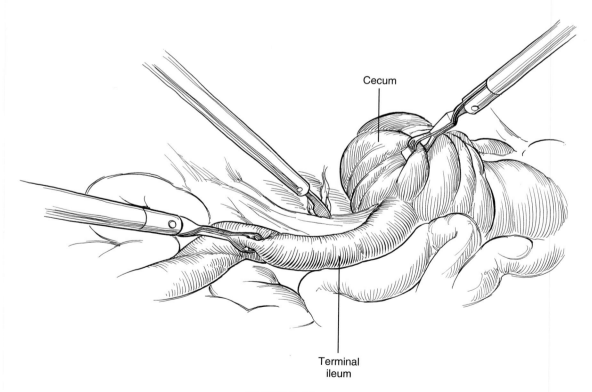

Cecum

Terminal
ileum

FIGURE 27–4

FIGURE 27–5. The cautery spatula is in the infraumbilical port and is incising the peritoneum at the base of the terminal ileal mesentery. Babcock clamps in the right and left port are retracting the cecum and terminal ileum cephalad. The lateral peritoneal attachment is incised with the cautery.

FIGURE 27–6. The variable anatomy of the ileocolic and right colic arteries. In the vast majority of cases the right colic artery is a distal branch of the ileocolic artery. For this reason, in the laparoscopic right colon resection only one artery and vein must be secured.

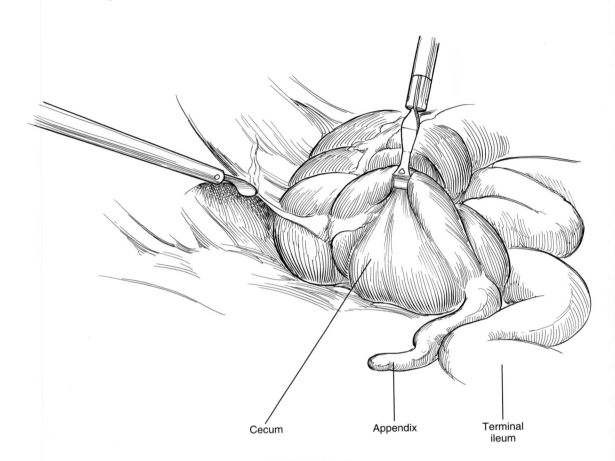

Cecum   Appendix   Terminal ileum

FIGURE 27–5

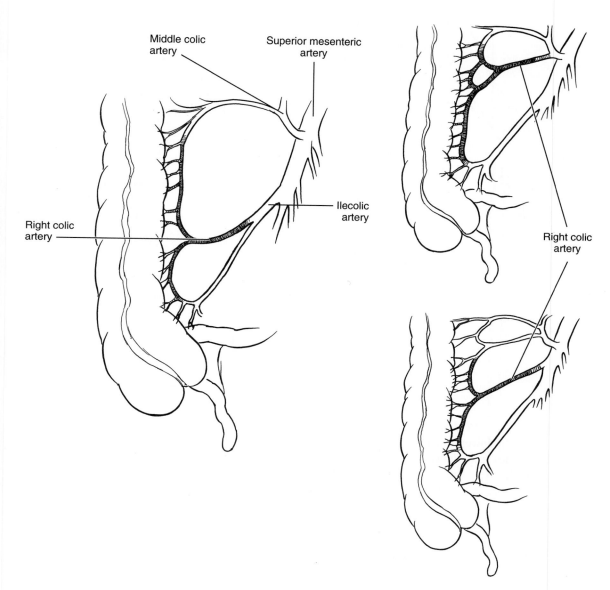

FIGURE 27–6

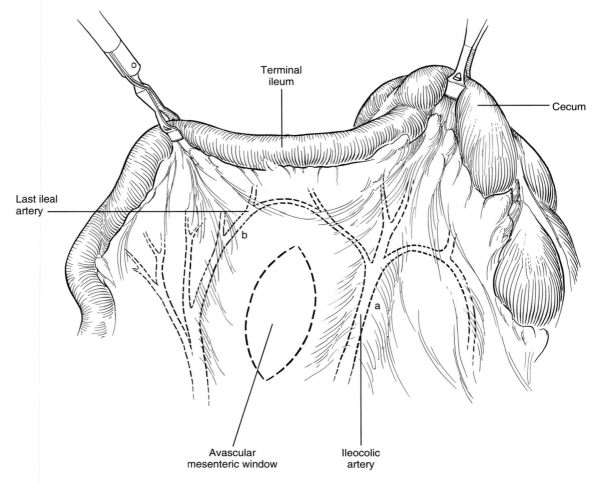

Terminal
ileum

Cecum

Last ileal
artery

b

a

Avascular
mesenteric window

Ileocolic
artery

FIGURE 27–7

FIGURE 27–7. The ileum and cecum are held up in the right lower quadrant, and the bow-string identifies the ileocolic artery (a). The arterial arcade from the last ileal artery to the ileocolic artery is shown (b). The avascular mesenteric window (dotted line) is shown adjacent to the ileocolic artery.

FIGURE 27–8. The window is opened from the ileal arterial arcade to the base of the ileocolic vessels.

FIGURE 27–9. The ileocolic artery and vein are dissected out at the base of the right colon mesentery. Double L clips are placed proximally and distally. The vessels are transected, and a 0-chromic endo-loop is placed on the arterial stump.

FIGURE 27-8

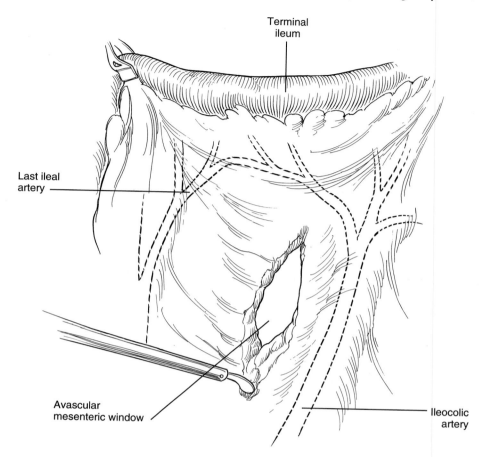

Terminal
ileum

Last ileal
artery

Avascular
mesenteric window

Ileocolic
artery

FIGURE 27-9

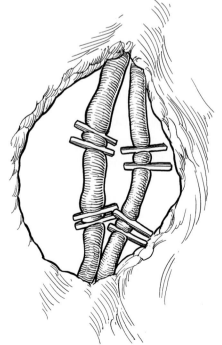

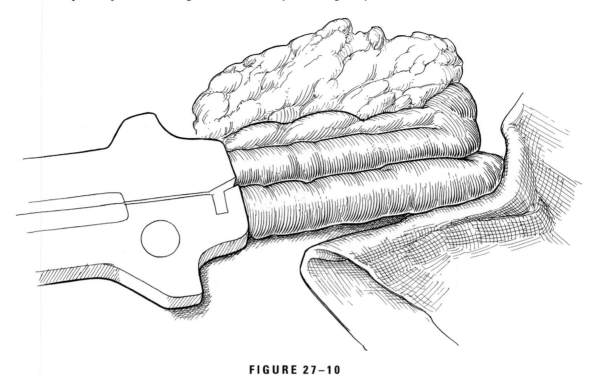

FIGURE 27–10

FIGURE 27–10. A 5- to 7-cm transverse incision is made at the right port, and the specimen is brought out to the exterior. An intestinal stapler is used to transect the ileum and transverse colon. A side-to-side ileotransverse colostomy anastomosis is constructed. The defect in the mesentery is left open.

X. Postoperative Medications

Patients are given parenteral and oral narcotics as required.

XI. Advancement of Diet

A. Patients are given clear liquids on the day after surgery.

B. They are advanced to a regular diet as tolerated in 2 to 4 days.

XII. Determinants of Discharge

A. Patients are tolerating a regular diet.
B. Pain is controlled by oral pain medicines.
C. Bowel movements have occurred.
D. Social conditions allow an acceptable level of care at home.

XIII. Return to Normal Activity/Work

Patients are encouraged to return to normal activities as tolerated (in 2 to 3 weeks).

Chapter 28

Laparoscopic Right Hemicolectomy with Intracorporeal Anastomosis

JOSEPH F. UDDO, JR., M.D.

I. Indications

A. Angiodysplasia
B. Solitary cecal diverticulitis
C. Cecal volvulus (after spontaneous or colonoscopic reduction)
D. Benign neoplasms
E. Colon cancer

II. Contraindications

Intestinal obstruction due to intestinal distention

III. Factors Important in Patient Selection

Colon cancer with metastatic disease may be handled laparoscopically without fear of compromising the resection. However, not everyone agrees that confined colon cancer should be removed through the laparotelescope. Concern that an "adequate cancer operation" cannot be performed successfully through the laparotelescope keeps this disease process a debatable indication for laparoscopic colectomy. However, once one has become familiar with laparoscopic colon procedures, it is apparent that the same resection can be performed laparoscopically and by the open technique. High ligation of the vessels is possible, and adequate margins and adequate mesenteric dissection can be performed. Long term follow-up of confined colon

cancers treated laparoscopically will be the only way to put this issue to rest.

IV. Preoperative Preparation

A. When surgery is required for a benign or malignant colonic neoplasm, a preoperative barium enema should be performed. This confirms the position of the lesion and facilitates planning for the procedure.
B. Because the laparoscopic approach eliminates the ability to palpate, it is helpful to obtain a preoperative computed tomographic scan of the abdomen. This is particularly helpful for evaluating the liver and retroperitoneum.
C. Special attention should be given to the consent process. All patients must consent to an open procedure in the event that the laparoscopic procedure is not successful. It is not reasonable for a patient to limit consent to a laparoscopic procedure only.
D. Bowel preparation:
   1. Clear liquids are started the day prior to surgery.
   2. A bowel preparation of 4 liters of a polyethylene glycol electrolyte solution is given over 4 hours the day before surgery.
   3. Erythromycin base 1 g and neomycin 1 g are given orally at 1, 2, and 11 PM the day prior to surgery.

4. A bisacodyl suppository is given the evening before surgery.
E. Most patients are admitted the morning of surgery.
F. Preoperative intravenous antibiotics are given.
G. Some form of deep venous thrombosis prophylaxis is used (support hose, subcutaneous heparin, or intermittent compression devices).

V. Choice of Anesthesia

General anesthesia is used.

VI. Accessory Devices

A. A nasogastric tube and Foley catheter are placed once the patient is asleep.
B. A urinary catheter is also inserted.

VII. Instruments and Telescopes

A. Laparotelescopes: Two 10-mm, 0-degree laparotelescopes are used. A 10-mm, 30-degree laparotelescope and a 5-mm laparotelescope should be available.
B. Video equipment: Two full camera systems with individual light sources are used, plus three or four monitors.
C. Insufflation device: A rapid automatic insufflation device with a smoke evacuator is preferred.
D. Electrocautery: monopolar electrocautery device with an assortment of wands
E. Instruments
   1. Four noncrushing bowel graspers
   2. Probes and retractors

3. Endoscopic clip applier
4. Endoscopic loop ties
5. Endoscopic needle holder, knot pusher, and suture material
6. Curved endoscopic scissors capable of conducting electrocautery
7. An assortment of endoscopic dissectors capable of conducting electrocautery
F. Endoscopic stapling devices
   1. Endoscopic GIA 30 or endoscopic GIA 60
   2. Endoscopic hernia stapler
   3. Endoscopic TA 60

VIII. Position of Monitors and Placement of Trocars

FIGURE 28–1. The patient's position depends on where the lesion is and how the anastomosis is to be accomplished. For a laparoscopic right hemicolectomy with intracorporeal anastomosis, the supine position with both arms at the patient's side has been the position of choice. If the lesion may require intraoperative localization with a colonotelescope, the patient's legs have to be placed in a low stirrup position. However, if the lesion can be confidently localized preoperatively, the supine position offers more latitude in manipulation of instruments.

Use of an electric table facilitates intraoperative positioning of the patient. During the procedure, it is helpful to lower one side or the other of the patient to allow the small intestines to fall away from the operative site. An electric table expedites this process.

Three or four video monitors are helpful in decreasing potential stress during these cases. A minimum of two monitors, placed at either side of the patient's head, is required. A third and fourth monitor on either side of the patient's feet allows an adequate view of the operative field from almost any position around the table. If only three monitors are available, placing the third monitor at the end of the table will accomplish nearly the same effect as four monitors.

Because laparoscopic colon resection may require frequent moves from one side of the table to the other, it is essential that the surgeon not get "roped in" by cables and tubing. All video cables and suction/irrigation tubing should be placed to allow free movement around the table without having to disconnect and reconnect equipment. This is easy to accomplish if proper attention is paid to the placement of equipment. The room layout shown in Figure 28–1 has been successful.

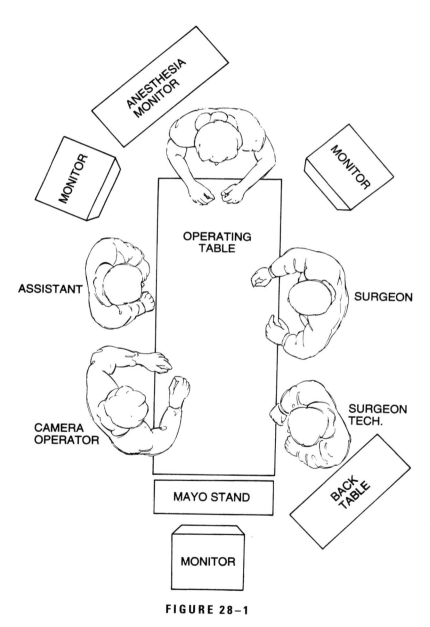

FIGURE 28–1

FIGURE 28-2. Unlike laparoscopic cholecystectomy, in which there are well-established approaches to trocar placement, there is no consensus on the number and location of trocars to be used in laparoscopic colon resection. In general, it is most useful to begin with an umbilical 10-mm port plus a 10-mm port in each quadrant of the abdomen. This affords full access to the abdominal contents and allows placement of a 10-mm telescope and laparoscopic Babcock clamps from any direction. This is particularly important when two telescopes are employed.

Because the endoscopic stapling device requires large ports, an additional 12-mm port (for the Endo GIA 30 device) or 15-mm port (for the Endo GIA 60 or TA 60 device) will be needed to accomplish the intracorporeal anastomosis. Placement of this port is crucial, and its position should be chosen just prior to performing the anastomosis when, after evaluating the position of the colon and terminal ileum, the most appropriate site can be determined.

Once the 12-mm or 15-mm port site has been determined, a telescope placed behind it and slightly to one side will provide the best visualization for the anastomosis. To complete the anastomosis, the umbilical 10-mm port should be changed to a 12- or 15-mm cannula. Alternatively, a 12- or 15-mm port can be placed in the umbilicus initially.

To perform a laparoscopic right hemicolectomy with intracorporeal anastomosis, at least five 10-mm trocars and two 12- or 15-mm trocars are needed. Five-millimeter trocars for additional retractors should be used as needed. There is no evidence that the cumulative length of the trocar incision or an increased number of trocars leads to significantly increased postoperative pain or prolonged ileus.

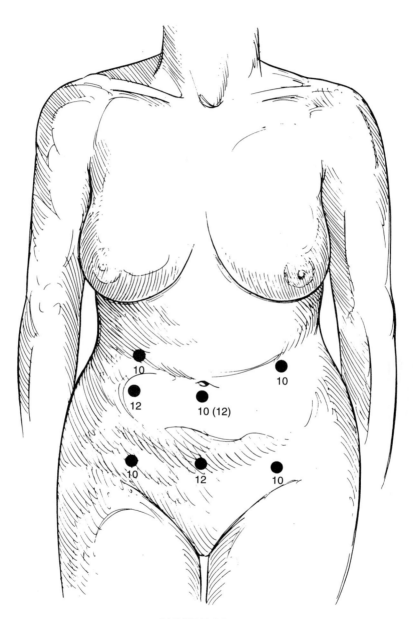

FIGURE 28–2

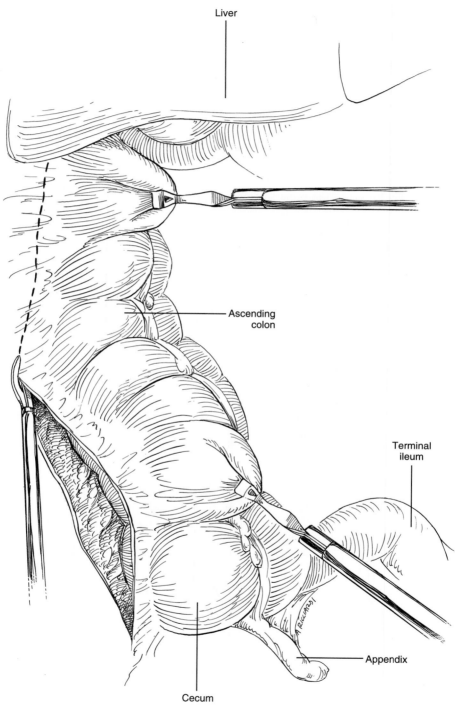

FIGURE 28–3A

IX. Narrative of Surgical Technique

FIGURE 28–3A and B. The peritoneal cavity is insufflated using the surgeon's technique of choice. Veress needle insufflation is considered successful. If the patient has had prior surgery, a site away from the old incision is chosen for Veress needle insertion. The insufflator is preset to 15 mm Hg, but occasionally higher settings may be required. A 10-mm port is placed, and a telescope is introduced. A brief survey of the abdomen is made. If there is no obvious contraindication to continuation of the laparoscopic procedure, an additional 10-mm port is placed in each abdominal quadrant as noted. The abdomen is then fully explored. The small bowel, colon, omentum, peritoneum, and liver are inspected.

Once the exploration is complete, attention is turned to the right colon. The right colon is grasped proximally and distally with atraumatic bowel graspers and pulled to the left. Although laparoscopic bowel graspers are atraumatic, if not handled properly, most bowel clamps available at this time can still damage the intestinal serosa and possibly cause full thickness tears. Consequently, when manipulating the bowel, it is important to try to place graspers on the portion of bowel to be removed. The surgeon must be as gentle as possible when manipulating the remainder of the bowel.

With the colon retracted to the left, a dissector (scissors or electrocautery) is placed through the lower quadrant port. The attachment of the colon to the parietal peritoneum ("white line of Toldt") is dissected. The colon is drawn to the left, and the colon mesentery is dissected using blunt and sharp dissection. Use of electrocautery scissors and laparoscopic kittners facilitate the mobilization of the right colon. The right ureter can be identified as mobilization of the mesentery is completed.

FIGURE 28–3B

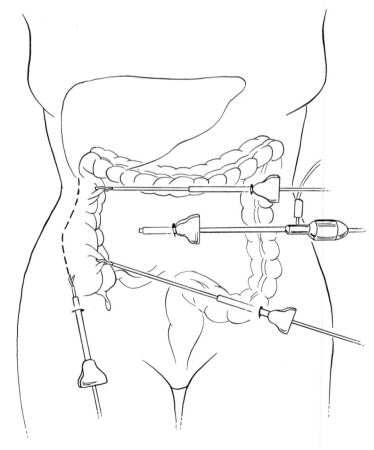

FIGURE 28-4. The hepatic flexure is then mobilized. The hepatocolic ligament is divided. Division of the white line is continued around the hepatic flexure, and the gastrocolic ligament is dissected to the point of division of the transverse colon. The hepatic flexure can then be swept off the duodenum using blunt dissection. Occasionally, we have found that "flipping" the omentum cephalad is helpful at this point. Mobilization of the hepatic flexure is the most difficult phase of this operation.

The right colon, now fully mobilized, is grasped and held anterior and to the right. This exposes the medial side of the colon mesentery. Electrocautery scissors are used to score the mesentery along the line of dissection. The mesentery is then divided along this path. Blunt dissection and dissection with electrocautery aids in this process. A second telescope placed behind the mobilized right colon transilluminates the mesentery and helps to identify the vessels. The light source on the first camera has to be dimmed to appreciate the transillumination of the mesentery.

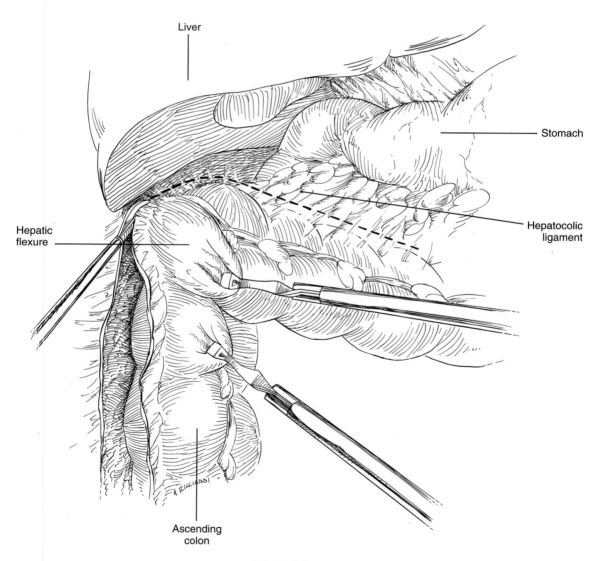

FIGURE 28-4

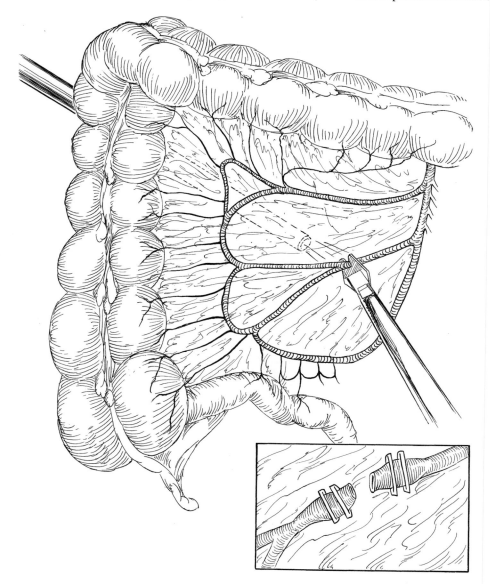

FIGURE 28-5

FIGURE 28-5. As small vessels are encountered, they can be clipped and divided. Larger vessels can be clipped, ligated with endoscopic ties, or divided using the endoscopic GIA stapler with a vascular cartridge in place. A full mesenteric dissection can be accomplished laparoscopically with great precision and minimal blood loss because of the enhanced visualization.

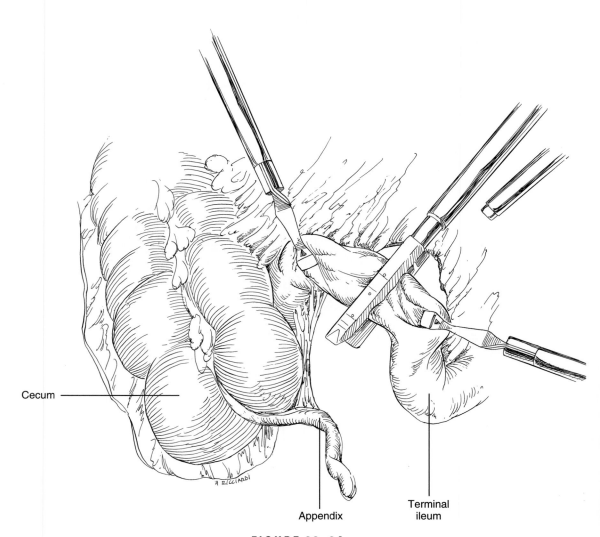

Cecum

Appendix

Terminal
ileum

FIGURE 28–6A

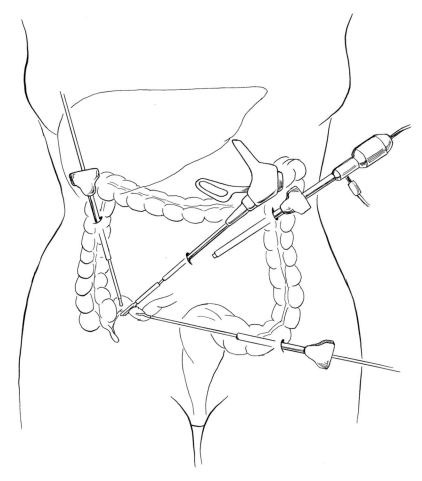

FIGURE 28–6B

FIGURE 28–6A and B. A window in the mesentery is created at the point of transection of the terminal ileum. The endoscopic GIA stapler is then placed through the umbilical port, and the ileum is divided. An opening in the trans-verse mesocolon is made at the site of transection. The omentum may be divided to this point. The gastrocolic ligament has previously been opened and should not pose a problem.

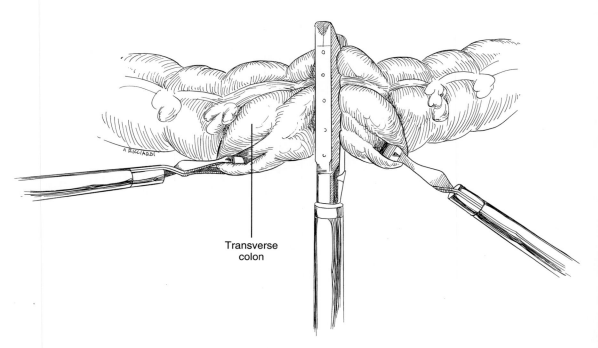

Transverse
colon

FIGURE 28–7A

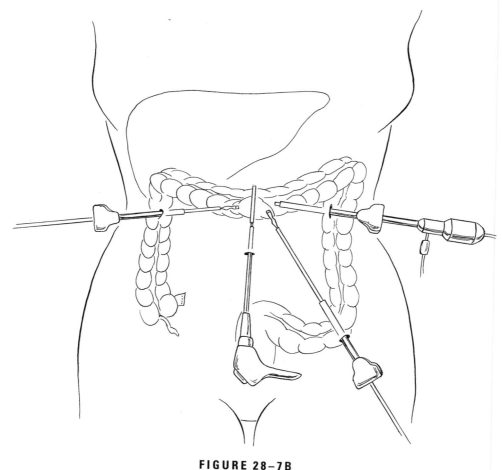

FIGURE 28–7B

FIGURE 28–7A and B. The endoscopic GIA stapler is again placed through the umbilical port and used to divide the transverse colon. Each time the endoscopic GIA device is used, it is helpful to place a second telescope 90 degrees to the first. This essentially adds depth perception to the otherwise two-dimensional perspective of one camera. The second telescope allows complete visualization to the ends of the stapling device with minimal manipulation of bowel and confirms the stapler's position before it is fired.

Once the specimen has been completely freed from all attachments, it can be placed in the pelvis to be extracted at the completion of the procedure. Both ends of the specimen are securely stapled, and spillage from the specimen should not be a concern. The specimen is not removed at this point because the required enlargement of the umbilical incision makes retention of pneumoperitoneum difficult.

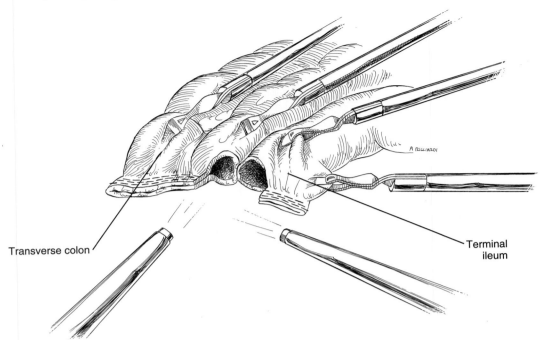

Transverse colon

Terminal ileum

FIGURE 28–8A

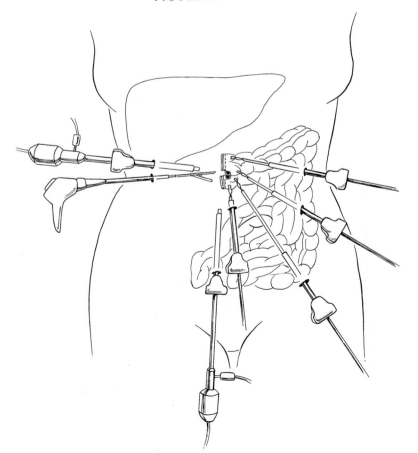

FIGURE 28–8B

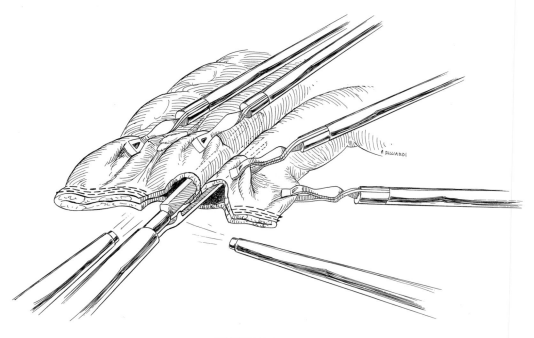

FIGURE 28–8C

FIGURE 28–8A–C. The midtransverse colon and distal ileum are then prepared for anastomosis. A functional end-to-end anastomosis using the endoscopic GIA stapler is performed. Each limb of bowel is controlled with two graspers. A small enterotomy using the electrocautery scissors is made in each limb. Alignment of the bowel for anastomosis is crucial. The bowel ends are placed side by side with the enterotomies aligned. At this point the second 12-mm or 15-mm port is placed; its position is determined by assessing the position of the limbs of bowel. Adequate distance from the bowel is required for manipulation of the stapling device. A second telescope behind and just to the side of the stapling device aids in introduction of the endoscopic GIA into the enterotomies by giving a "straight on" view.

The first camera is placed through one of the lower abdominal ports to gain a 90-degree view of the introduction of the endoscopic GIA stapler. The stapling device is placed in the abdomen, opened, and inserted into the enterotomies. Care must be taken to ensure adequate placement; confirmation that both limbs of the stapling device are in the bowel is essential. The stapler is then closed and fired. If the 30-mm device is used, two or three firings will be required. However, with the 60-mm device, one firing should be adequate.

The anastomosis is then inspected through the second telescope, which looks directly into it. Both sides of the anastomosis and bleeding from the staple lines can be easily evaluated in this fashion.

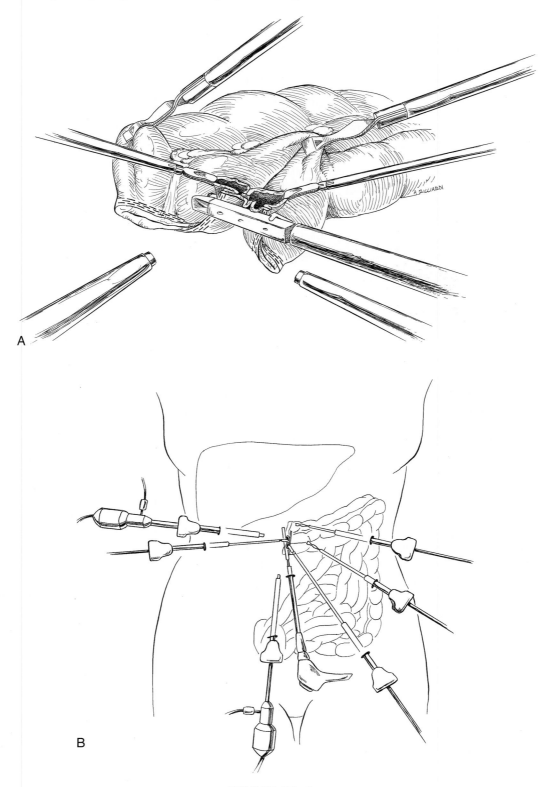

FIGURE 28-9

FIGURE 28–9A and B. A stapling device is then placed through the umbilical port and used to close the enterotomies. The bowel is held securely by graspers from the right and left. Again, the second telescope can be helpful in determining proper placement of the stapling device. The endoscopic TA 60 device is ideal for this purpose. The endoscopic GIA 30 has worked well for closure of the enterotomies thus far. Once the position of the stapling device across the enterotomies is confirmed, the stapler is fired, and the staple line is then inspected.

The mesenteric defect can be closed by suturing or by using an endoscopic hernia stapler. The abdomen is irrigated, and the fluid is removed. In preparation for removal, the specimen is securely grasped and positioned near the umbilicus. The umbilical incision is enlarged 2 to 3 cm, and the specimen is removed. It may be necessary to insert a suction device into the specimen to allow its collapse and removal.

Closure

The fascial incision at the umbilicus is closed with interrupted absorbable sutures. An attempt to place one fascial stitch at each of the 10-mm sites is made. In obese patients this is often not possible. Skin incisions are closed with staples or subcutaneous stitches. The Foley catheter is removed in the recovery room or the next morning.

X. Postoperative Medications

A. Antibiotics are continued for 48 hours.
B. Minimal postoperative pain control is required.

XI. Advancement of Diet

A. A nasogastric tube is left in place until the first signs of bowel function return. This usually occurs on the first or second postoperative day.
B. Clear liquids are started shortly after the nasogastric tube is removed. The patients stay on clear liquids until they have a strong desire for something more or until full bowel function has returned.

XII. Determinants of Discharge

A. Patients are discharged when they:
1. Tolerate liquids with no nausea or vomiting.
2. Can ambulate without difficulty.
3. Have had a bowel movement.
B. Discharge usually takes place within 3 to 5 days.

XIII. Return to Normal Activity/Work

Patients can return to unrestricted activity on the fifth to seventh postoperative day.

Chapter 29

Laparoscopic-Assisted Sigmoid Colectomy for Benign Disease

GARTH H. BALLANTYNE, M.D.

I. Indications

A. Sigmoid diverticulitis
   1. Recurrent attacks of sigmoid diverticulitis
   2. Sigmoid stricture from chronic diverticulitis
B. Benign polyp of the sigmoid colon
C. Sigmoid volvulus
D. Crohn's sigmoid colitis
E. Ischemic sigmoid stricture

II. Contraindications

A. Severe restrictive pulmonary disease
B. Recent myocardial infarction
C. Previous lower abdominal incision that was closed with mesh
D. Severe bleeding disorder

III. Factors Important in Patient Selection

Factors that make operation more difficult:
A. Obesity
B. Men are more difficult than women.
C. Previous abdominal operations

IV. Preoperative Preparation

A. Patients are admitted on the day of surgery.
B. Patients accomplish their mechanical and antibiotic bowel preparation at home. This typically includes:
   1. Drinking a gallon of GoLYTELY over 3 hours the day before surgery (e.g., noon to 3 PM).
   2. Taking three doses of 1 g each of erythromycin and neomycin after drinking all of the GoLYTELY (e.g., at 4 PM, 7 PM, and 10 PM).
C. Patients are given Zofran 4 mg intravenously when they are first brought into the operating room.
D. Patients are given one dose of a cephalosporin intravenously prior to the operation.

V. Choice of Anesthesia

All patients receive general anesthesia. The trocar sites and specimen extraction site are injected with Marcaine prior to making the incisions and again at the end of the procedure.

VI. Accessory Devices

A. Nasogastric tubes are inserted in all patients.
B. Urinary catheters are used in all patients.
C. Pneumatic compression stockings are placed on the legs of all patients.
D. An infrared lighted ureteral stent is advanced up the left ureter in patients in whom a difficult pelvic dissection is anticipated.

VII. Instruments and Telescopes

A. 10-mm 0-degree telescope
B. Electrocautery scissors
C. Atraumatic grasper
D. Laparoscopic Babcock clamps
E. Endo GIA 30 linear stapling device with vascular and blue staple cartridges
F. EEA-type circular stapling device
G. Purse-string device
H. Luminal sizing devices (25 mm, 28 mm, and 31 mm)
I. Rigid sigmoidoscope

VIII. Position of Monitors and Placement of Trocars

FIGURE 29–1. The patient is placed in a modified Lloyd-Davies position with legs in Allen stirrups. The thigh must be straight; any flexion of the thighs will limit the excursion arcs of the laparoscopic instruments. The principal monitor is placed between the patient's legs. The secondary monitor is positioned by the patient's left shoulder. During one's early experience, a five-trocar technique facilitates the procedure, and this is the technique illustrated in this chapter. With this technique, the surgeon stands on the patient's left side, and the assistant surgeon stands on the patient's right. The camera person stands by the patient's right shoulder, and the scrub nurse stands by the patient's left leg. With experience, this operation can be accomplished by a single surgeon with a robot, Aesop 3000 (Computer Motion, Santa Barbara, CA), holding the video telescope.

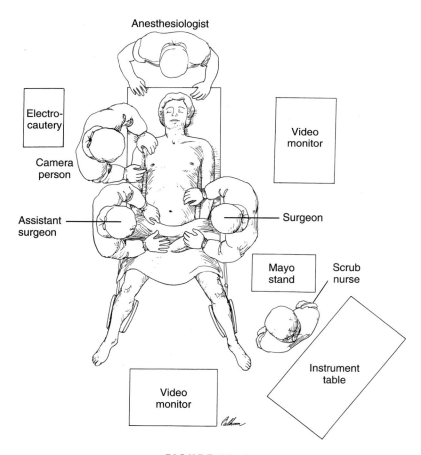

FIGURE 29–1

FIGURE 29–2. The 10-mm, 0-degree video telescope is inserted through the supraumbilical 10/11-mm trocar. With the five-trocar technique, two 10/11-mm trocars are placed in the left lower quadrant and two (one 12-mm and one 10/11-mm) in the right lower quadrant. These are inserted lateral to the rectus sheath.

The surgeon initially uses the two trocars on the patient's left side, and the assistant surgeon uses the two on the right side. When the surgeon is more experienced, he or she can accomplish the procedure using a three-trocar technique, the two right lower quadrant trocars and the supraumbilical one.

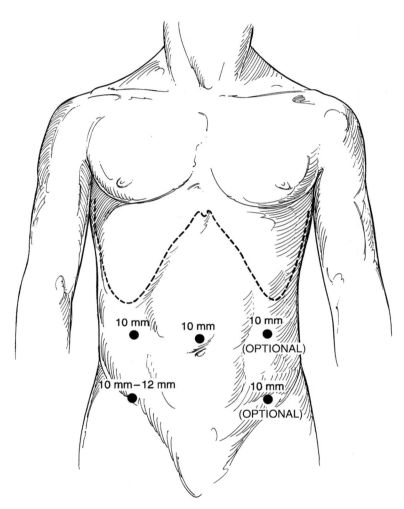

FIGURE 29–2

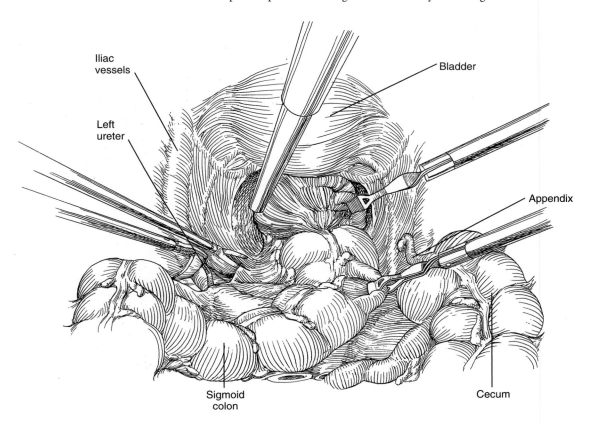

Iliac vessels

Left ureter

Bladder

Appendix

Sigmoid colon

Cecum

FIGURE 29–3

IX. Narrative of the Procedure

FIGURE 29–3. After the induction of anesthesia, the rectum is irrigated through the rigid sigmoidoscope. The pneumoperitoneum is insufflated using either a Veress needle or the Hasson technique. The trocars are inserted, and the patient is dropped into a very deep Trendelenburg position. Once a sufficiently deep angle is reached, the small bowel will slide out of the pelvis. The left side of the table is then rolled up. The assistant surgeon retracts the sigmoid and rectosigmoid colon anteriorly and medially. If an infrared ureteral stent was inserted in the left ureter, the flashing red light should now become visible. The surgeon exerts countertraction using the grasping instrument in the left hand. The posterior parietal peritoneum is incised over the left iliac vessels, and this incision is extended down into the pelvis. The mesorectum and mesosigmoid are swept medially with the blunt curved side of the laparoscopic scissors. The left ureter is identified. The assistant then reapplies the Babcock clamps more proximally on the colon. The peritoneum of the left lateral gutter is incised, and the colon is swept medially. The ureter is then followed up toward the left kidney until the mesosigmoid is freed from the retroperitoneum medially to the aorta.

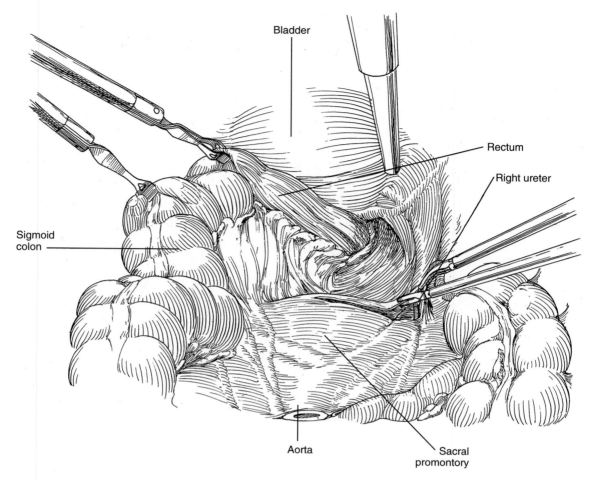

FIGURE 29-4

FIGURE 29-4. The surgeon moves to the right side of the patient, and the assistant moves to the left. The assistant again provides anterior and medial traction on the sigmoid and rectosigmoid. The right ureter is usually visible as it passes over the right iliac vessels. The surgeon palpates the sacral promontory with the tip of the laparoscopic scissors and then opens the peritoneum over the sacral promontory. The incision in the peritoneum is extended cephalad and anterior to the aorta. The inferior mesenteric artery is visible as an arch extending from the aorta along the lower portion of the meso-sigmoid.

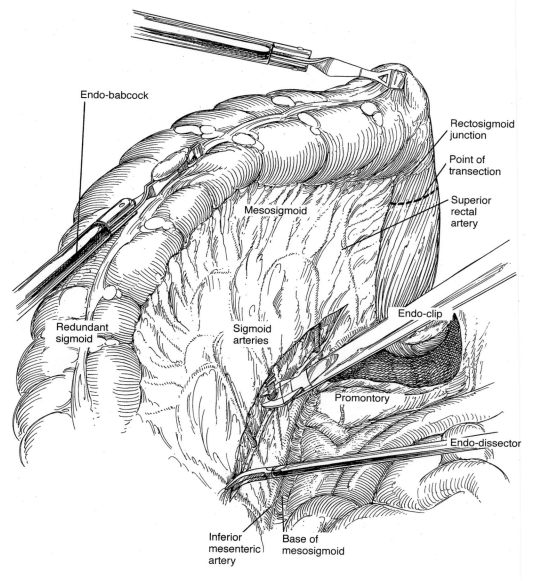

Endo-babcock

Rectosigmoid
junction

Point of
transection

Superior
rectal
artery

Mesosigmoid

Redundant
sigmoid

Sigmoid
arteries

Endo-clip

Promontory

Endo-dissector

Inferior
mesenteric
artery

Base of
mesosigmoid

FIGURE 29–5

FIGURE 29–5. The inferior mesenteric vessels are preserved to ensure an excellent blood supply for the anastomosis. The individual sigmoid branches are divided between surgical clips as shown. These vessels can also be divided using the laparosonic coagulating shears (LCS), or Harmonic Scalpel (Ethicon Endosurgery, Cincinnati, OH) or the Endo GIA 30 stapler (United States Surgical Corporation, Norwalk, CT) using the vascular cartridges.

FIGURE 29-6. The rectosigmoid junction is identified as the point where the taenia coli coalesce into a complete longitudinal muscle layer of the rectum. The Endo GIA 30 stapler armed with a blue cartridge is inserted into the abdomen through the right lower quadrant 12-mm trocar. It is applied across the rectum just distal to the rectosigmoid junction from the antimesenteric side toward the mesenteric side and is fired, opened, and withdrawn. Generally a second and sometimes a third application is required to fully transect the rectum.

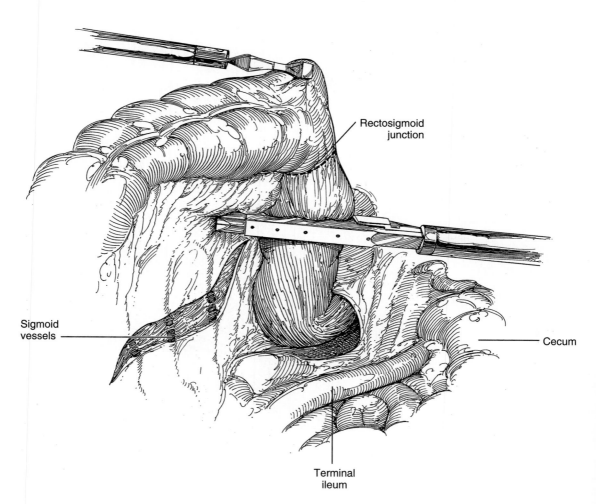

Rectosigmoid
junction

Sigmoid
vessels

Cecum

Terminal
ileum

FIGURE 29-6

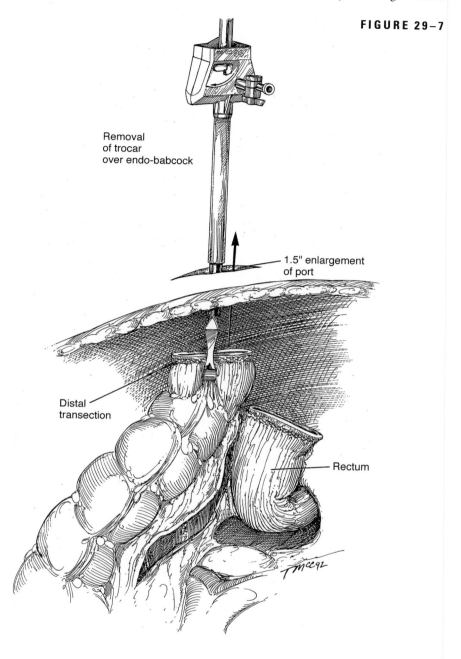

Removal
of trocar
over endo-babcock

1.5" enlargement
of port

Distal
transection

Rectum

FIGURE 29-7. The sigmoid colon is now fully mobilized. The planned site of transection is pulled down toward the rectal pouch. If the proximal bowel does not easily reach the rectum without tension, additional descending colon is mobilized. If necessary, the splenic flexure is mobilized.

The specimen is now extracted from the ab-domen. A Babcock clamp is inserted through the caudad left lower quadrant trocar and used to grasp the stapled closure of the specimen. The trocar site is enlarged to about 2 inches. The trocar, the Babcock, and the end of the colon are withdrawn. When a three-trocar technique is used, the specimen is withdrawn through a suprapubic incision.

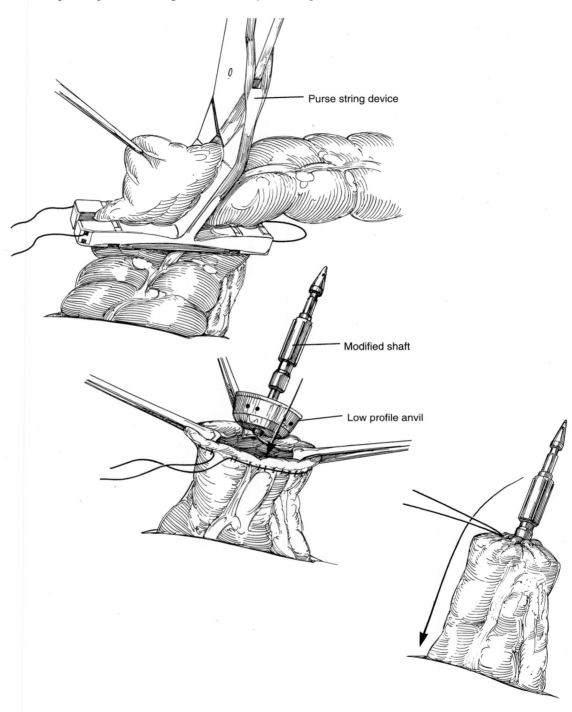

FIGURE 29–8

FIGURE 29–8. The proximal site of resection is selected. In patients with diverticulitis or Crohn's disease, a point is selected where the bowel wall is no longer thickened. The automatic purse-string device is applied and fired. A Kocher clamp is placed across the specimen side. The specimen is then transected along the edge of the purse-string device. The specimen is opened on a side table and examined. The edges of the proximal colon are grasped with Babcock clamps, and the caliber of the lumen is measured with the sizers. The largest possible EEA stapling device is selected, and the anvil shaft assembly of the circular stapling device is secured in position with the purse string. The colon is then dropped back within the abdomen. The shaft is positioned so that it points down into the pelvis. The fascial defect of the extraction site is then closed using a continuous monofilament suture.

FIGURE 29–9. The anus is dilated to admit four fingers. The EEA stapling device is advanced up the rectum and is pressed up against the stapled closure of the rectum. The white trocar is unscrewed and aligned so that it penetrates the center of the previous staple line; this trocar is then retrieved and withdrawn through a trocar. The shaft of the anvil-shaft assembly is grasped with a Babcock clamp and inserted into the central rod of the EEA device. The taenia coli of the colon is followed proximally to ensure that the bowel has not been twisted. Also, the bowel is checked for any tension on the anastomosis. The EEA stapler is screwed closed and fired and then is partially opened, twisted, and removed from the rectum. The donuts are checked. The pelvis is then filled with irrigation fluid. The anastomosis is examined with the rigid sigmoidoscope, and the rectum is insufflated. The pool of water is then observed for escaping bubbles.

The abdomen is again checked for hemostasis. The pneumoperitoneum is partially deflated and the trocar sites are again checked for bleeding. Finally, the pneumoperitoneum is deflated, and the trocars are removed. The fascial defects of the trocar sites are closed with simple sutures using an absorbable suture material. The skin edges of the trocar sites and extraction site are approximated with subcuticular sutures.

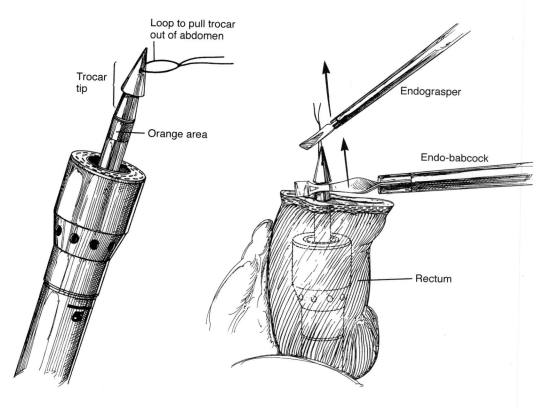

FIGURE 29–9

X. Postoperative Medications

A. Patients are given parenteral narcotics as required.
B. Oral pain agents are started when the patient is taking liquids by mouth.

XI. Advancement of Diet

A. The nasogastric tube is left in place overnight.
B. The patient is given clear liquids the morning after surgery.
C. The patient is advanced to a regular diet on the second day after surgery.

XII. Determinants of Discharge

Patients are generally discharged when they are tolerating a regular diet, their pain is controlled with oral agents, and they have passed flatus.

XIII. Return to Normal Activity

Wounds reach 90 per cent of their ultimate strength within 10 to 14 days. Consequently, I limit patients to walking and jogging for a 2-week period. They may resume more vigorous exercise after this time period. They may return to sedentary jobs as tolerated.

Chapter 30

Laparoscopic Left Hemicolectomy

WILLIAM E. KELLEY, JR., M.D.

I. Indications

A. Colonic polyps not amenable to colono-
   scopic polypectomy
B. Diverticulitis
C. Crohn's colitis
D. Colon cancer (controversial)

II. Contraindications

A. Absolute contraindications:
   1. Patient is unable to tolerate general anes-
      thesia.
   2. Large bulky cancer or inflammatory mass
B. Relative contraindications (based on level of
   surgeons' experience):
   1. Colonic obstruction
   2. Colonic perforation
   3. Curative resection for colorectal cancer

III. Factors Important in Patient Selection

A. Factors that may make an operation easier
   to accomplish:
   1. A taller individual provides a larger peri-
      toneal volume within which to work than
      a shorter patient.
   2. Among patients of similar size, females
      are easier to operate on than males be-
      cause the female mesocolon contains less
      fatty tissue to impede dissection of the
      vessels and because there is less paracolic
      fat in women.

B. Factors that may make the operation more
   difficult to complete:
   1. The thickened omentum characteristic of
      obese patients also makes the dissection
      and mobilization of the splenic flexure
      considerably more difficult in these indi-
      viduals.
   2. A history of multiple prior abdominal
      operations should alert the surgeon that
      extensive adhesions may increase the dif-
      ficulty of the operation and prolong op-
      erating room time.
   3. Subacute diverticulitis or inflammatory
      bowel disease may result in local in-
      flammation or scarring that could make
      dissection more difficult.
   4. A large diverticular mass of the left colon
      may increase operative risks because of
      local adhesion to the ureter.

IV. Preoperative Preparation

A. Clinical indications for surgical intervention
   must be every bit as strict for laparoscopic
   surgery as they are for traditional operations.
B. Localization of the pathology: Laparotomy
   by videolaparoscopy is primarily a visual and
   surface-oriented procedure. The ability to
   palpate the deep structures and parenchymal
   lesions and to identify subtle masses in the
   colon is very limited. Therefore, an accurate
   preoperative colonoscopic evaluation is of
   critical importance in identifying synchro-

353

nous lesions and accurately charting their location. If the laparoscopic surgeon does not perform the colonoscopy personally, or if there is any question about the exact location of the salient pathology after colonoscopy has been completed, a barium enema should be performed. The proximal extent of diverticulosis cannot be accurately assessed laparoscopically. Small neoplasms and even relatively large polyps cannot be identified with confidence by the laparoscopic technique. The surgeon must therefore be confident of the colonic pathology preoperatively and must have a relatively precise plan for the anatomic resection that he or she will perform. Although a barium enema is often considered redundant and imprecise, it frequently provides the surgeon with added certainty about the anatomic relationships of colonic pathology. The added cost of a barium enema is very rapidly made up in cost savings for the operating time needed to confirm the location of a neoplasm, to resect extra colon to obtain an adequate margin, or to resect additional diverticular disease.

C. Preoperative colonoscopy with tattooing of the colon is very helpful in localization of polyps and small cancers. Tattoos should be placed at three separate circumferential locations to ensure that the mark will be visible to the laparoscope. Nonabsorbable dye such as India ink should be used.

D. Preoperative computed tomography (CT) scan: A more liberal use of CT scans should also be considered in the preoperative evaluation of laparoscopic colectomy. Since the liver cannot be accurately palpated, deep parenchymal liver metastases may be missed in operations for malignancy. This may have important prognostic significance and may indicate a more conservative operation. CT evaluation of a diverticular mass is often helpful in predicting the degree of local inflammation, involvement of the left ureter, and involvement of adjacent structures such as the bladder or small bowel. Less experienced laparoscopic surgeons should know these details in advance and factor them into the decision matrix for patient selection. Additional studies such as barium enemas and CT scans should certainly not be considered standard in the preoperative evalua-

tion for laparoscopic hemicolectomy. They should be used liberally, however, especially during a surgeon's early experience.

E. Mechanical bowel preparation:
1. Liquid diet starting on the morning of the first preoperative day.
2. The patient takes one 10-mg tablet of metaclopramide at supper the night before surgery.
3. Beginning 1 hour later, 2 to 3 liters of GoLytely bowel preparation solution are consumed over a 2-hour interval.
4. Two to three hours before surgery, the patient is given a Fleet's enema to empty the distal colon of any residual fluid.

F. Oral antibiotic bowel preparation: Neomycin and erythromycin base are given together in four doses at 3-hour intervals, beginning at 2 PM on the day prior to surgery.

G. A single dose of a second-generation cephalorsporin is given intravenously (IV) in the holding area preoperatively. If there is any unexpected contamination during the procedure, the IV antibiotic is continued at appropriate intervals for an additional 24 hours.

V. Choice of Anesthesia

General endotracheal anesthesia is required.

VI. Accessory Devices

A. Nasogastric tube
B. Urinary catheter
C. Ureteral stent(s) in selected patients

VII. Instruments and Telescopes

A. A 10-mm, 0-degree videolaparoscope is used throughout the procedure in the majority of left hemicolectomies.
B. Often a 10-mm, 30-degree laparoscope is useful to improve visualization during mobilization of the splenic flexure.
C. A second laparoscope and light source may be helpful for transilluminating the mesocolon to assist in identification of blood vessels. The 30-degree laparoscope can be used quite efficiently for this purpose.
D. Atraumatic grasping forceps
E. Nondisposable Glassman and DeBakey forceps

F. Atraumatic Babcock forceps, preferably with a flattened, rounded grasping surface
G. Disposable or sharp electrocautery scissors
H. Diamond jaw laparoscopic needle holders
I. Endoscopic linear stapling devices with both vascular and bowel cartridges
J. An ultrasonic scalpel may be used to divide the omentum, mesentery, and secondary vessels.
K. Laparoscopic surgical clip appliers
L. Fan retractor

VIII. Position of Monitors and Placement and Size of Trocars

FIGURE 30–1. Two video monitors are used during a left colectomy. At the beginning of the procedure, one monitor is positioned on each side of the patient. The monitor to the patient's left begins at the patient's iliac crest. As the dissection moves toward the splenic flexure, this left side monitor is moved to the level of the patient's shoulder. This adjustment improves the surgeon's orientation as he or she proceeds with the dissection.

The assistant's monitor is positioned behind the surgeon. It is usually placed in a neutral position at the level of the patient's umbilicus. The camera operator begins the operation at the surgeon's left side, next to the patient's right shoulder. The scrub nurse is positioned between the patient's legs during most of the procedure.

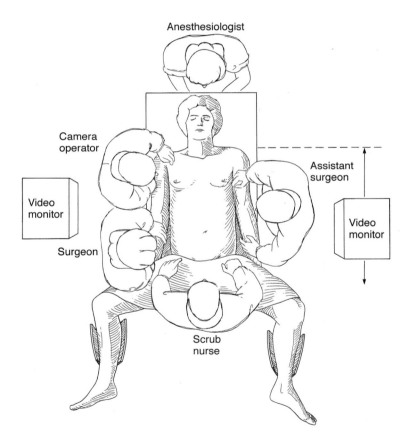

FIGURE 30–1

FIGURE 30–2. Typically, five trocars are used during the procedure. Two 10-mm ports are inserted in the left midclavicular line, one just below the costal margin, and one just below the iliac crest. These ports provide access for the atraumatic grasping forceps or for endo-Babcock clamps during most of the procedure. Three 12-mm ports are inserted, one at the umbilicus and two just medial to the right midclavicular line. The right-sided ports are positioned somewhat closer together than the left-sided ports to permit the surgeon to use both hands in concert for a two-handed dissecting technique. The videolaparoscope is positioned at the umbilical port during most of the procedure but can be moved to the left lower quadrant or to the right upper quadrant port, if necessary, to improve exposure. Any of the 12-mm ports can be used for application of the 30-mm linear stapler for transection of blood vessels or division of the bowel. When the 60-mm stapler is used, a 15-mm port may be substituted for the right lower quadrant trocar site. The cost of disposable kits can be reduced by using all 12-mm ports with five sleeves and one sharp trocar. Patient recuperation is affected very little by the use of 12-mm ports.

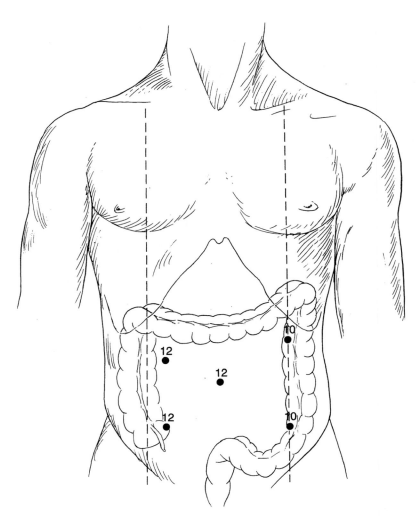

FIGURE 30–2

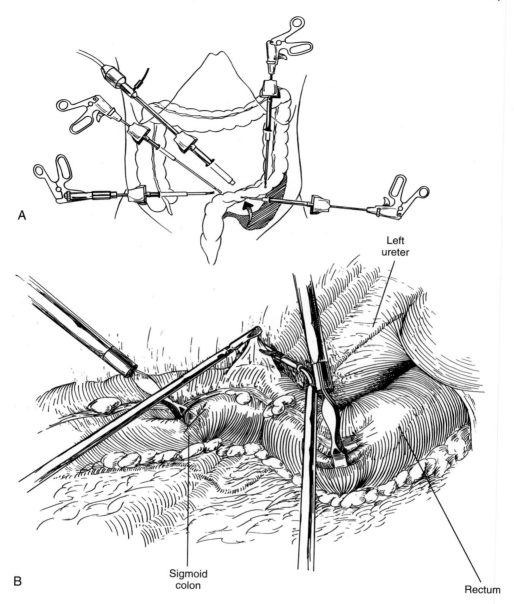

A

Left
ureter

Sigmoid
colon

B

Rectum

FIGURE 30-3

IX. Narrative of Surgical Technique

FIGURE 30-3. The patient is rotated 20 to 40 degrees to the right during most of the procedure. After the abdomen has been thoroughly explored, the table is rotated to the right and placed in a steep Trendelenburg position. The sigmoid colon is retracted medially using atraumatic grasping forceps or endo-Babcock clamps inserted through the left upper quadrant and left lower quadrant ports. The sigmoid is then immobilized along the white line of Toldt using cautery scissor dissection or the ultrasonic scalpel. Cautery should never be used in the vicinity of the ureter. The videolaparoscope is positioned through the umbilical port, and the surgeon operates through the two right-sided ports.

As the dissection develops, the left ureter is identified crossing the iliac artery. The ureter is followed distally as the mobilization of the sigmoid continues toward the peritoneal reflection.

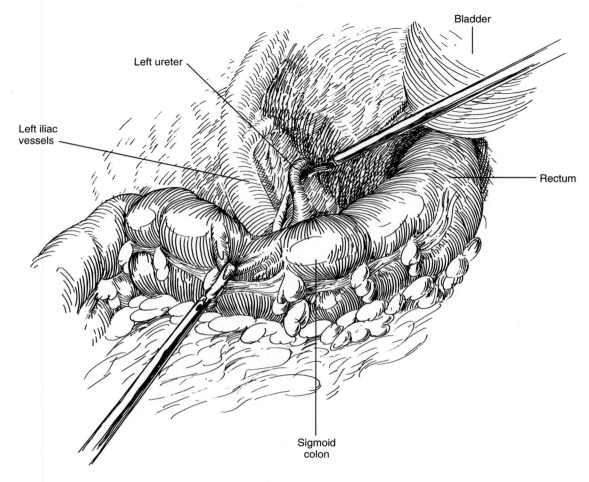

Bladder

Left ureter

Left iliac
vessels

Rectum

Sigmoid
colon

FIGURE 30-4

FIGURE 30-4. The ureter must always be identified. When an inflammatory mass is anticipated in the area of the ureter, it may be advisable to pass a left ureteral stent preoperatively. The stent can usually be palpated with the dissecting forceps early in the course of the dissection to facilitate identification. A lighted stent, if available, can be even more helpful in difficult cases. By dimming the laparoscope light source, the light from the ureteral stent can readily be seen after the colon is reflected medially.

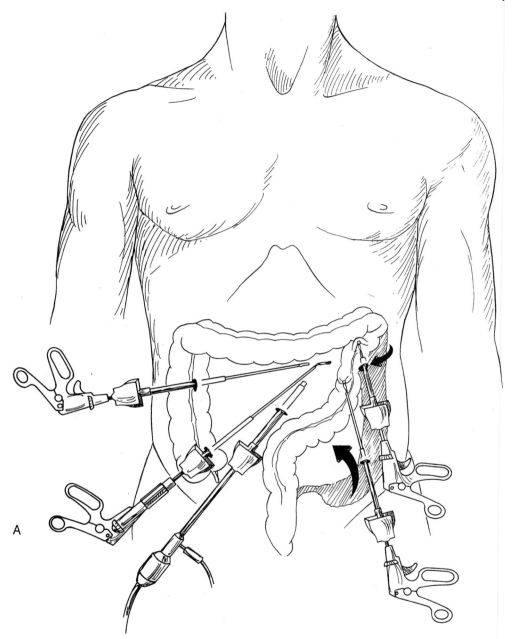

A

FIGURE 30-5A

FIGURE 30-5. After the distal dissection has been completed, the descending colon is mobilized in the same fashion, progressing toward the splenic flexure. The table is changed to the reverse Trendelenburg position to improve exposure. The monitor on the patient's left is moved cephalad at this time to improve the surgeon's orientation. It is sometimes helpful to

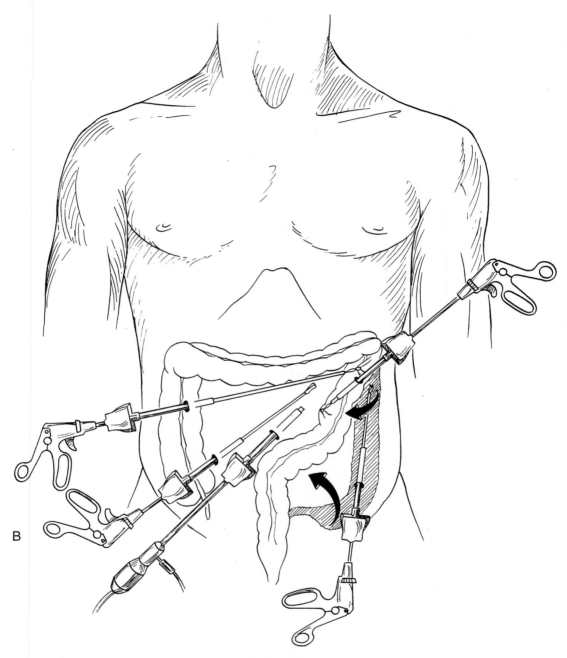

FIGURE 30–5B

change the position of the laparoscope to the left upper quadrant port and to dissect from the left lower quadrant port while retracting through the umbilical port as the proximal descending colon is mobilized. The surgeon must be very flexible in the use of the ports. The laparoscope port is often changed several times during the procedure to provide better visualization. Occasionally, an additional suprapubic port is inserted to introduce the linear stapler in order to divide the rectosigmoid colon or proximal rectum for a low resection.

FIGURE 30–6. As the splenic flexure is approached, attention is directed to the left transverse colon. The omentum is dissected free from the transverse colon in the avascular plane using cautery scissor dissection or the ultrasonic scalpel. The dissection begins well proximal to the anticipated level of transection of the colon and progresses in the direction of the lienocolic ligament. Unless a malignancy of the splenic flexure is expected, it is advisable to stay close to the bowel as the splenic flexure is approached. The linear stapler or Harmonic Scalpel are very helpful in completing the dissection at the lienocolic ligament.

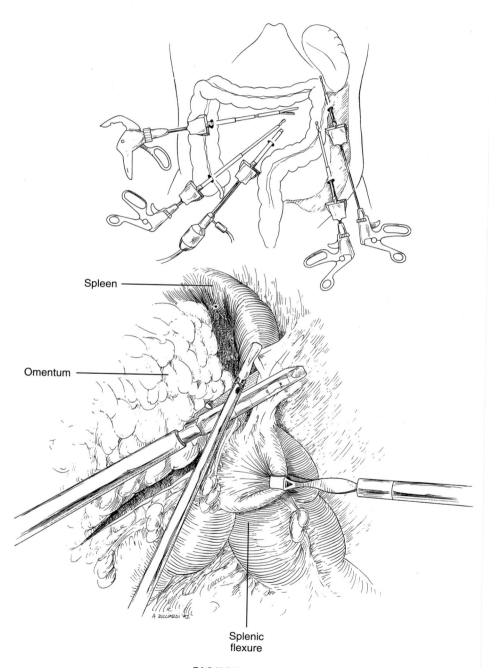

Spleen

Omentum

Splenic
flexure

FIGURE 30–6

FIGURE 30–7. It is sometimes helpful to transfer the videolaparoscope to the right upper quadrant port as the splenic flexure is approached.

For malignant lesions of the splenic flexure, a more radical resection of the gastrocolic omentum is carried out. In this case, the omentum is mobilized at the level planned for transection of the transverse colon. The gastrocolic omentum is then divided, progressing toward the greater curvature of the stomach. This dissection can be carried out in a relatively avascular plane. The omentum is then divided from right to left using Harmonic Scalpel or cautery scissor dissection and endoclips for hemostasis. In obese individuals it is often safest to use the linear stapler liberally during this portion of the dissection to minimize bleeding. The vessels can be somewhat difficult to identify in the thickened omentum of an obese patient.

After the splenic flexure has been mobilized, the descending and left transverse colon is then reflected downward and to the right. The dissection continues on the posterior surface of the mesocolon, leaving the quadratus and psoas muscles and the left ureter exposed. The extent of this dissection depends on the indication for surgery. In patients with a malignant lesion of the left colon, the origin of the left colic artery can be exposed, and the inferior mesenteric artery can be identified and isolated. The surgeon should have gained considerable experience with laparoscopic bowel surgery before proceeding with left hemicolectomy for a malignancy in this area. Curative laparoscopic colectomy for malignancy is considered controversial.

At this point the transection of the mesocolon is initiated. The serosal surface of the mesocolon is scored along the intended line of dissection using either the ultrasonic scalpel or cautery scissors. The vessels can then be dissected free from the fatty tissue and isolated. A second laparoscope and light source can be inserted through the left ports to transilluminate the major vessels. This technique is particularly useful in obese patients and in identifying the takeoff of the left colic and inferior mesenteric arteries.

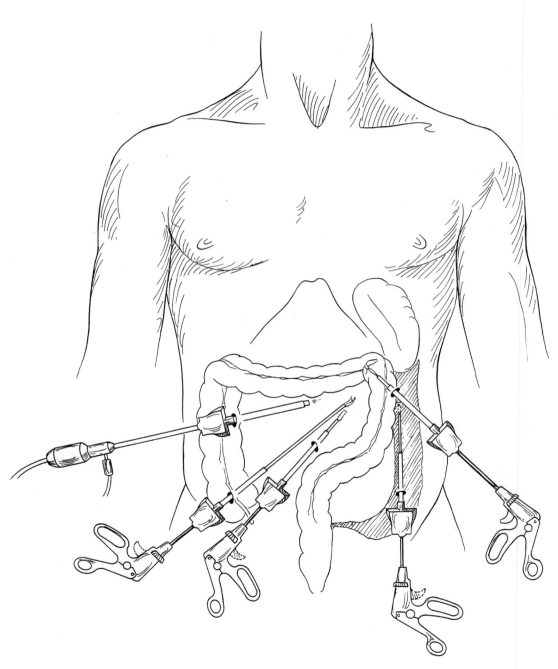

FIGURE 30–7

FIGURE 30-8. The major vessels are ligated and divided using either the linear stapler with 2-mm staples or endoclips. The linear stapler has proved to be a safe and efficient instrument for dividing the major vessels, especially when endoclips appear to be too short to completely ligate the larger blood vessels. When endoclips are used, four clips should be applied, two proximally and two distally. When the vessels are divided, the tissue should be grasped on the arterial side as the linear stapler is released or the scissors are applied. In this fashion, proximal control is ensured if bleeding results. Bleeding at the linear staple line is rare, especially with 2-mm staples, but it can occur. Bleeding through a doubly clipped vessel is also rare. If a bleeding point is encountered, however, the proper technique involves elevation and exposure of the vessel from behind with a grasping forceps. This technique presents the bleeding point and fixes it for prompt ligation by the endoclip applier. If necessary, an endotie or endosuture can be applied to ensure secure hemostasis. Unnamed vessels can be divided with the ultrasonic scalpel, but care should be taken to ensure that the jaws of the ultrasonic scalpel extend beyond the vessel being divided.

An alternative method of transecting the mesocolon involves serial applications of the linear stapler without specifically identifying the vessels. This method can be somewhat faster than performing individual dissection and ligation of each vascular pedicle. It may offer some advantage in obese patients. As the surgeon becomes experienced with laparoscopic bowel surgery, however, the time saving is reduced and the added cost for extra staple cartridges becomes difficult to justify on a routine basis. In many cases, most of the mesocolon dissection can be performed with clamps and ties after exteriorization.

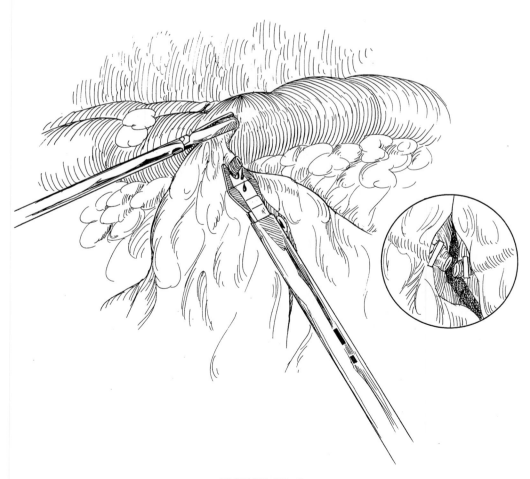

FIGURE 30-8

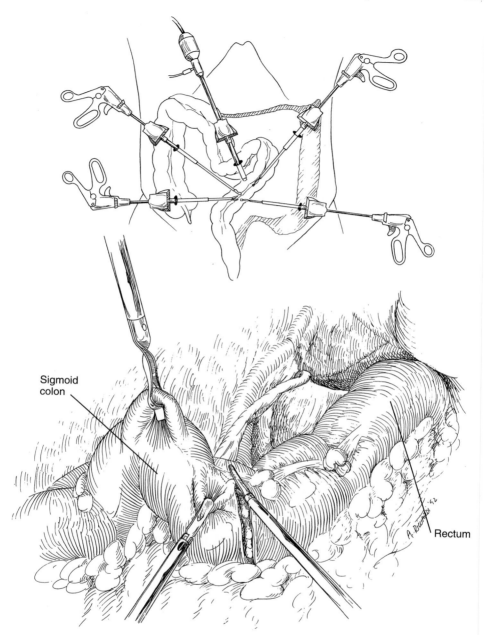

Sigmoid
colon

Rectum

FIGURE 30-9

FIGURE 30-9. After division of the mesocolon has been completed, the transverse colon is
grasped and brought into approximation with
the distal bowel to ensure that sufficient colon
has been mobilized for a tension-free anastomosis. The gastrocolic omentum is further dissected free from the right transverse colon if
necessary. When a full left hemicolectomy with
resection of the sigmoid colon is performed, the
hepatic flexure may also have to be mobilized
to gain sufficient length. In the latter case, the
entire omentum is dissected free from the right
transverse colon, and the dissection is continued
along the hepatic flexure. By staying close to
the antimesenteric surface of the hepatic flexure, the hepatocolic ligament can be divided
readily with cautery scissor dissection or the
Harmonic Scalpel. Only a few endoclips are
needed if the dissection is directed adjacent to
the colon.

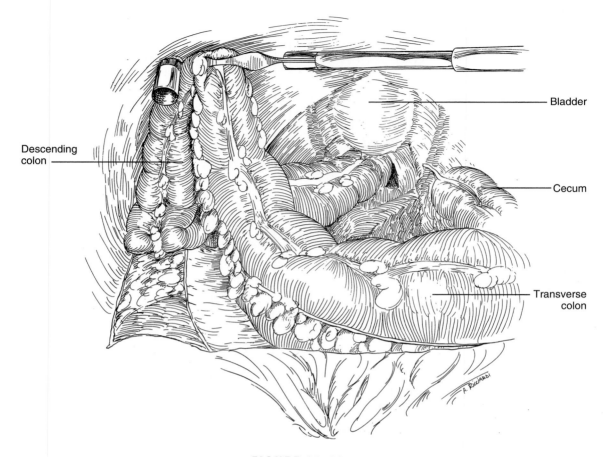

Descending colon

Bladder

Cecum

Transverse colon

FIGURE 30–10

FIGURE 30–10. If most of the sigmoid colon is to be resected, the anastomosis will be carried out using the circular stapling device. The transverse colon is brought up to the abdominal wall at a comfortable location in the left lower quadrant to identify the optimal site for exteriorization. If possible, the exteriorizing incision should incorporate the left lower quadrant trocar site. The sigmoid colon is transected distally using the linear stapler inserted through the right lower quadrant incision with the videolaparoscope inserted through the umbilical port. Frequently, two applications of the 30-mm or 45-mm stapler are required. A single application of the 60-mm stapler is often sufficient. One helpful method for reducing the number of applications of the linear stapler is to close the instrument on the bowel at the transection site and release it without firing. This maneuver is atraumatic and will not injure the bowel but will produce spasm, thus contracting the bowel and making the diameter to be divided smaller. Fewer cartridges are then needed to transect the bowel.

FIGURE 30–11. The proximal cut end of the sigmoid is grasped on the antimesenteric surface with an Endo-Babcock clamp introduced through the right lower quadrant port. The bowel is then positioned just deep to the left lower quadrant port. A left lower quadrant incision is then made, typically 4 to 7 cm in length, depending on the size of the specimen. When possible, the incision begins along the lateral rectus border and extends laterally through the left lower quadrant trocar site. The external oblique aponeurosis is incised, and the oblique abdominis muscle layers are serially separated in the direction of the fibers. The peritoneum is incised, evacuating the pneumoperitoneum. The proximal end of the bowel is then exteriorized by advancing the Endo-Babcock clamp through the incision. If there is a malignant lesion in the specimen, it is placed in a plastic bag before it is drawn through the incision to avoid seeding the abdominal wall with cancer cells and to minimize shedding of cancer cells into the peritoneal cavity.

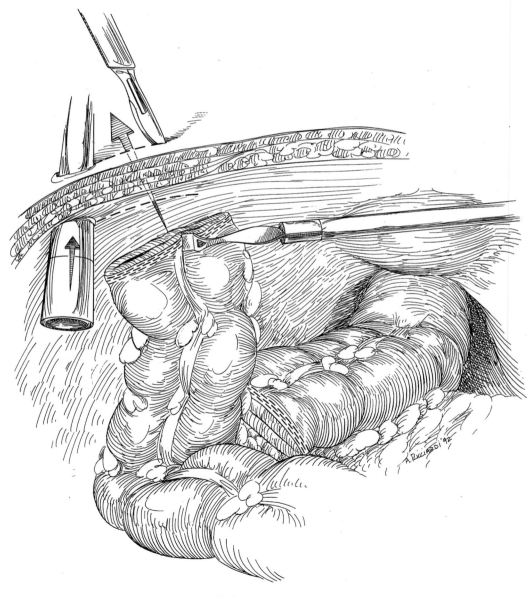

FIGURE 30–11

FIGURE 30–12A. At this point the bowel is divided extracorporeally, and a purse-string suture is applied. A disposable purse-string device can be applied to the skeletonized loop of colon at the level chosen for proximal transection. The instrument is then fired, producing a circumferential row of staples that holds the purse string along the serosal surface. The bowel is transected along the closed stapler, and the specimen is sent to pathology. If the purse-string device is not used, the bowel may be transected between Allen clamps, and a monofilament purse-string suture is then applied by hand.

FIGURE 30–12B and C. The appropriate size circular stapling device is then chosen, the anvil is inserted into the proximal colon, and the purse-string suture is tied. The anvil and the proximal bowel are then returned to the abdominal cavity, and the peritoneum and external oblique aponeurosis are closed separately using running sutures. The pneumoperitoneum is then reestablished with carbon dioxide. The patient is repositioned in the Trendelenburg position, right side down, and the distal staple line is exposed.

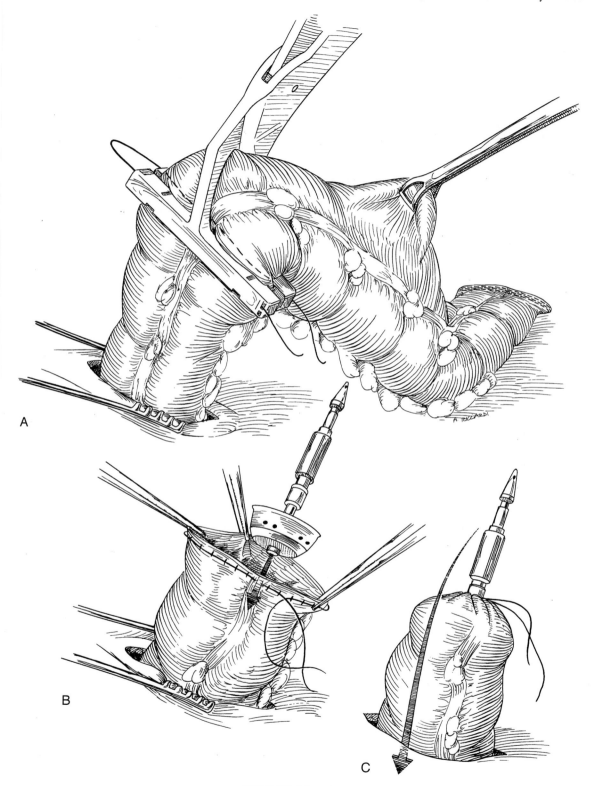

A

B

C

FIGURE 30–12

FIGURE 30-13A. The rectosigmoid pouch is irrigated with Neosporin genitourinary irrigant by gravity through a three-way Foley catheter inserted through the anus. This maneuver reduces the bacterial count and tests the pouch for possible leaks. The circular stapler is then inserted transanally and advanced to the staple line. The stapler trocar is advanced through the staple line at the rectosigmoid. If the trocar cannot be lined up with the staple line, it can be brought out through the anterior surface of the bowel, leaving at least 1 cm between the linear staple line and the proposed circular staples.

FIGURE 30-13B-D. The trocar is then encircled with a tie inserted through the right lower quadrant port. The trocar is then dislodged by pulling on the endotie through the right upper quadrant port. The trocar itself is then grasped and placed in the right lower quadrant port blunt end first and is withdrawn from the abdomen by pulling the tie out through the right lower quadrant port. Alternatively, with the newer staplers, a silk tie can be passed through a hole in the end of the trocar before inserting the stapler. The tie can be grasped through the right lower quadrant port, and the trocar can be dislodged and withdrawn through the port quite easily.

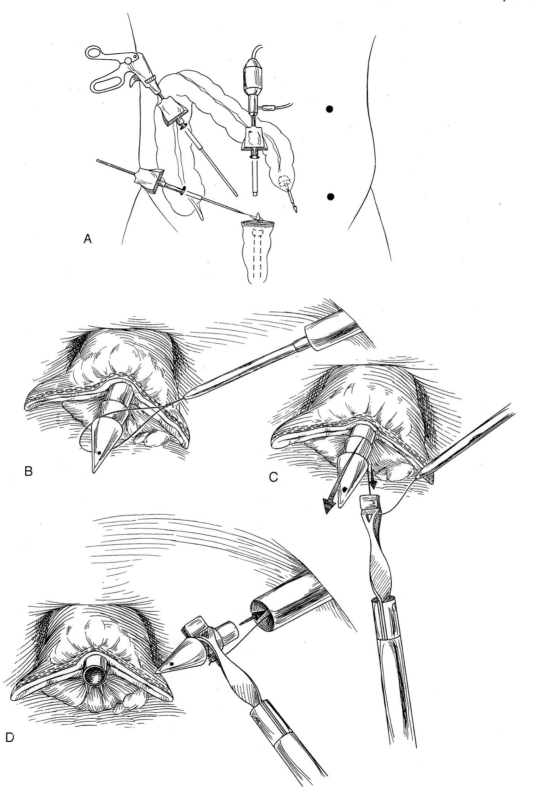

FIGURE 30-13

FIGURE 30–14. The post of the anvil is then grasped with an Endo-Babcock clamp through the right lower quadrant port and is married to the stapler. The stapler is then approximated and fired. The anvil is advanced three half turns and is then withdrawn, along with the stapler, and removed from below. The circular donuts are inspected for continuity. The anastomosis itself is inspected laparoscopically and is then tested.

To test the anastomosis, the pelvis is filled with irrigating solution to a level that just covers the anastomosis. The three-way Foley catheter is reinserted through the anal canal, and the colon is compressed above the anastomosis. The rectum is then inflated with air forced through the Foley catheter while one observes the fluid laparoscopically for bubbles. The absence of air bubbles confirms a satisfactory anastomosis.

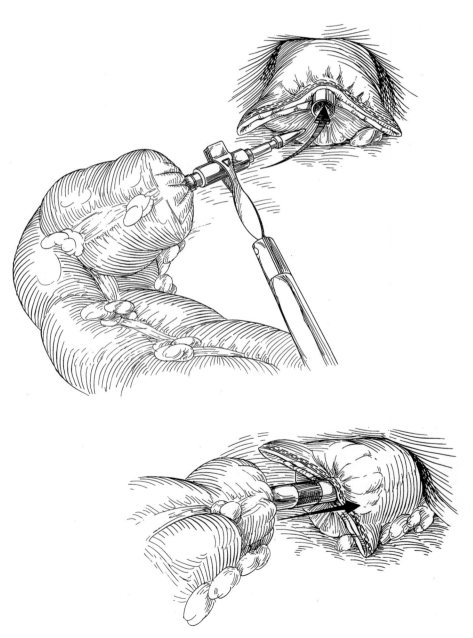

FIGURE 30–14

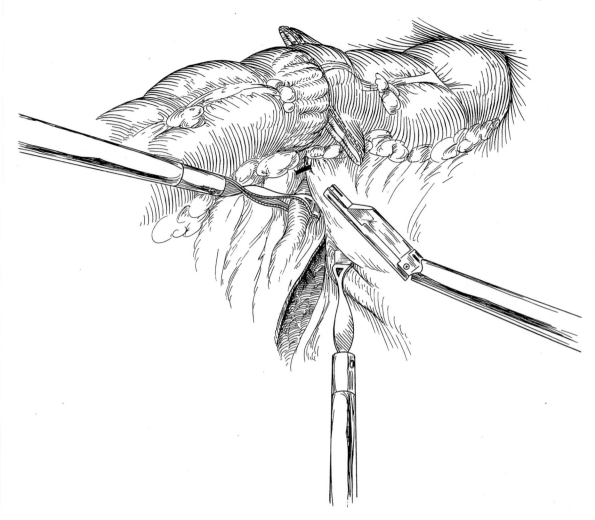

FIGURE 30–15

FIGURE 30–15. The defect in the mesocolon may be closed to prevent formation of an internal hernia. The defect can be closed with an endosuture technique or with a hernia stapler.

Closure

At the conclusion of the procedure, care is taken to evacuate the pneumoperitoneum thoroughly. Evacuating the pneumoperitoneum minimizes the likelihood of diaphragmatic irritation and resultant shoulder pain. The transverse, muscle-splitting incision has already been closed using running absorbable sutures. The 12-mm trocar incisions are closed at this time using interrupted absorbable sutures. A UR-6 needle greatly facilitates suture placement through the narrow incisions. The fascia is also closed in this fashion at the 10-mm trocar sites if a mixture of 10-mm and 12-mm trocars has been used.

X. Postoperative Medications

A. A single dose of a second-generation cephalosporin is administered in the holding area preoperatively. If unexpected contamination is experienced during the operative procedure, the antibiotic is continued at appropriate intervals for 24 hours.

B. If the pathology includes an inflammatory diverticular mass, intravenous antibiotics are continued for 48 hours postoperatively.

XI. Advancement of Diet

A. A nasograstic sump tube is left in place postoperatively and removed on the first postoperative day.

B. If excessive drainage is experienced, the nasogastric tube is left in place for an additional period of time.

C. If the patient begins passing flatus prior to this time, the nasogastric tube is removed after a shorter interval.

D. Sips of clear liquids are ordered for the first or second postoperative day.

E. The diet is gradually advanced in a stepwise fashion as tolerated.

XII. Determinants of Discharge

When the patient is tolerating liquids well, has no nausea, and can void without difficulty, he or she is eligible for discharge. Patients must be afebrile and must be able to tolerate adequate fluids by mouth to sustain a proper state of hydration. It is advisable to monitor patients in the hospital until they successfully pass flatus or move their bowels. Using these criteria, the average time for patient discharge is the third postoperative day for patients under 80 years old, and the fourth postoperative day for patients of all ages.

XIII. Return to Normal Activity

The patient returns to normal activities as tolerated. This generally requires two to three weeks.

Chapter 31

Laparoscopic-Assisted Sigmoid Colectomy for Colon Cancer

SAMUEL P. Y. KWOK, F.R.C.S. (Ed.), F.R.A.C.S., F.H.K. Am. (Surgery)

I. Indications

Various benign and malignant colorectal conditions that require a sigmoid colectomy or a high anterior resection of the rectum are suitable for a laparoscopic resection. The main indications are divided into two categories:

A. Benign disorders
1. Large sigmoid colon polyp
2. Resolved sigmoid volvulus
3. Sigmoid diverticular disease
B. Malignant conditions
1. Low sigmoid tumor
2. Rectosigmoid junction tumor
3. Upper rectal tumor

II. Contraindications

A. General considerations
1. Compromised cardiopulmonary status
2. Previous multiple laparotomies
3. Gross obesity
B. Emergencies
1. Frank bowel obstruction
2. Prolonged large bowel perforation
C. Local conditions of malignancy
1. Large tumor (more than 6 to 8 cm in diameter)
2. Infiltration of tumor to adjacent organs or to abdominal wall
3. Rectal tumor below peritoneal reflection

III. Factors Important in Patient Selection

A. Preoperative localization of tumor, especially for small tumor or polyp
B. Avoid tumors less than 10 cm from anal verge
C. Avoid bulky tumors (check by palpation, ultrasonography, or CT scan)
D. Preoperative laparoscopy is used to exclude locally advanced tumor with tumor infiltration to adjacent organ or abdominal wall.
E. Avoid cases involving intestinal obstruction.

IV. Preoperative Preparation

A. Patient is admitted on the day before operation for assessment and general work-up for general anesthesia.
1. Chest x-ray and electrocardiography are performed in older patients.
2. Hemoglobin and electrolytes are measured.
3. Two units of blood are cross-matched.
4. Prophylactic antibiotics using a cephalosporin and metronidazole are given during induction of anesthesia.
B. Bowel preparation: GoLYTELY (polyethylene glycol) 2 liters is given orally the night before surgery.

V. Choice of Anesthesia

Standard general anesthesia techniques with orotracheal intubation, but avoid nitrous oxide.

VI. Accessory Devices

A. Nasogastric tube
B. Urinary catheter

VII. Instruments and Telescopes

A. 30-degree laparoscope
B. Camera
C. Insufflator
D. Two monitors
E. Trocar and cannulas, 5 mm and 12 mm
F. 5-mm endoscopic shears with insulation
G. 5-mm and 10-mm graspers
H. 5-mm endo-Babcock clamps
I. 10-mm curved forceps
J. 5-mm bipolar diathermy forceps
K. Endo GIA 30 (vascular and bowel) stapling device

L. End-to-end circular stapler 31 mm
M. Standard laparotomy set

VIII. Position of Monitors and Placement and Size of Trocars

FIGURE 31–1. The patient is put in the steep head down and right side down position with the lower extremities spread apart. The thighs are in the same plane as the trunk. The right arm of the patient is placed alongside the trunk. The chief surgeon stands on the right side of the patient, and the camera operator stands to the surgeon's left. The assistant surgeon stands on the left side of the patient.

Four ports are used: one subumbilical 10/11-mm port for the laparoscope, one 12-mm port for the use of right hand and one 5-mm port for the left hand of the chief surgeon on the right side of the abdomen, and one 5-mm port on the left side of the abdomen for the assistant.

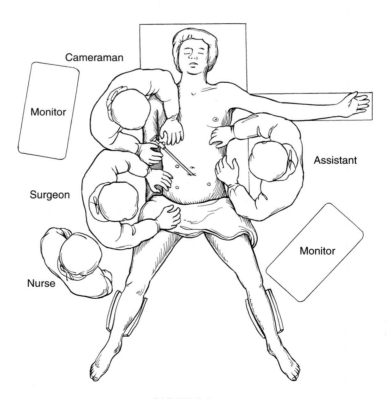

FIGURE 31–1

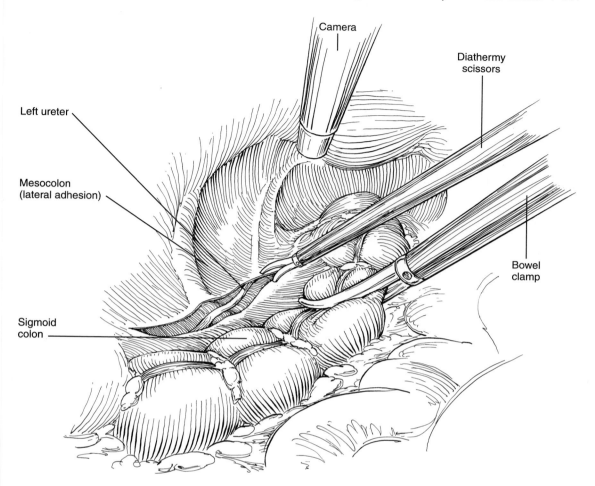

FIGURE 31–2

IX. Narrative of Surgical Technique

FIGURE 31–2. With a grasper applying traction onto the mesosigmoid, the lateral adhesions and the root of the mesosigmoid are incised with endoscopic diathermy scissors. The incision is extended cephalad to the splenic flexure and caudad to the left side of the upper rectum. The gonadal vessels and the left ureter are then exposed. The dissection of the root of the mesentery is extended to the midline of the sacral promontory.

FIGURE 31-3

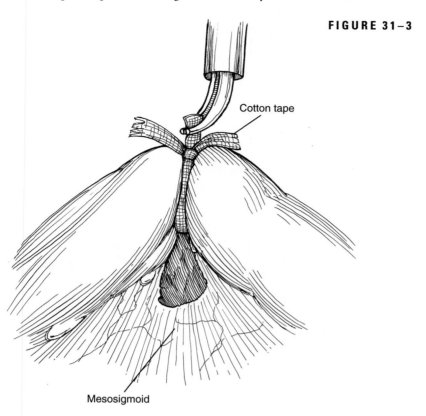

Cotton tape

Mesosigmoid

FIGURE 31-3. The sigmoid colon is lifted up, and the mesosigmoid is fenestrated. Cotton tape is tied around the sigmoid colon. The sigmoid colon is manipulated by holding onto the cotton tape, and multiple clamping of the colon itself is avoided.

FIGURE 31-4. With the sigmoid colon retracted to the left, the medial leaf of the mesosigmoid is incised at the root of the mesentery. A through-and-through window is then made at the root of the mesentery to effectively free the mesentery from the whole of the sacral promontory. With the assistant's atraumatic grasper holding onto the inferior mesenteric lymphovascular pedicle with a lifting action, the dissection in the avascular plane is extended cephalad to the origin of the inferior mesenteric artery.

FIGURE 31-5. The course of the left ureter can be visualized through the retromesosigmoid window. The left colonic artery can also be seen coming off the inferior mesenteric artery at this stage. With the use of a right-angled grasper, the inferior mesenteric vascular pedicle can be delineated and divided with an Endo GIA stapler either at its origin or just below the left colic artery, whichever is appropriate.

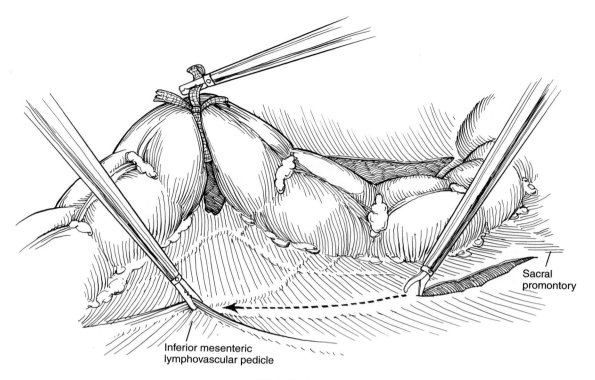

Sacral
promontory

Inferior mesenteric
lymphovascular pedicle

FIGURE 31–4

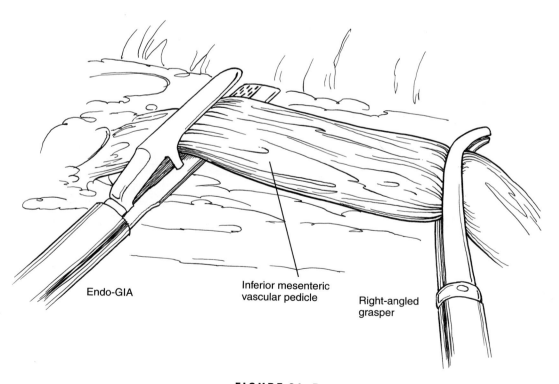

Endo-GIA

Inferior mesenteric
vascular pedicle

Right-angled
grasper

FIGURE 31–5

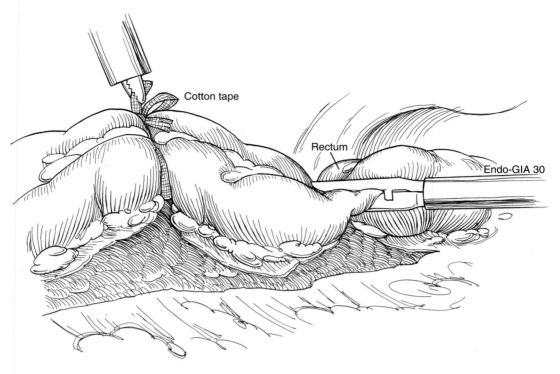

FIGURE 31−6

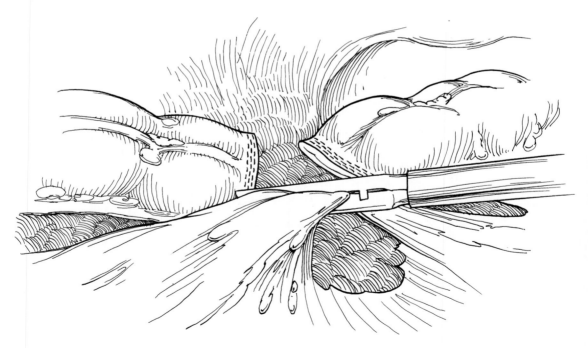

FIGURE 31−7

FIGURE 31-6. A second cotton tape is then tied around the sigmoid colon and its mesentery just below the tumor. A cytocidal rectal washout can be done at this stage. A plane is developed between the upper rectum and its mesorectum. With the sigmoid colon held up at the distal cotton tape and maintaining an adequate distal safety margin, the upper rectum is transected below the distal cotton tape using an Endo GIA 30 fired once or twice.

FIGURE 31-7. The mesorectum can be transected similarly at the same level with an Endo GIA or dissected with endoscopic scissors.

FIGURE 31-8. The left side port is then extended to the estimated cross-sectional diameter of the tumor. A zippered plastic bag cut to form a plastic sleeve is inserted so that the semirigid end is inside to protect the wound when the specimen is retrieved. Cotton tapes are tied distal and proximal to the tumor together with the plastic sleeve as the specimen is drawn out of the wound to totally enclose the tumor within the plastic covering.

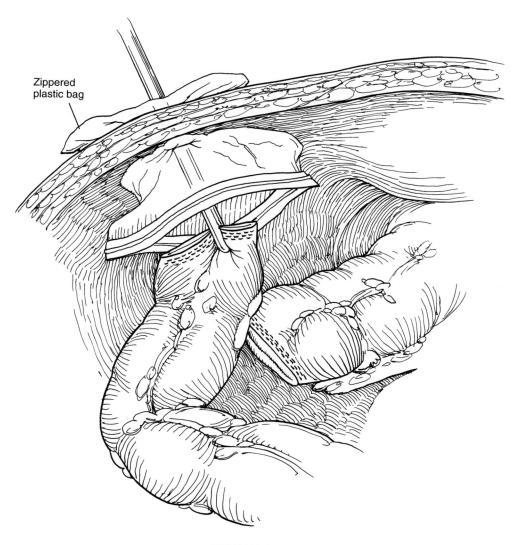

Zippered plastic bag

FIGURE 31-8

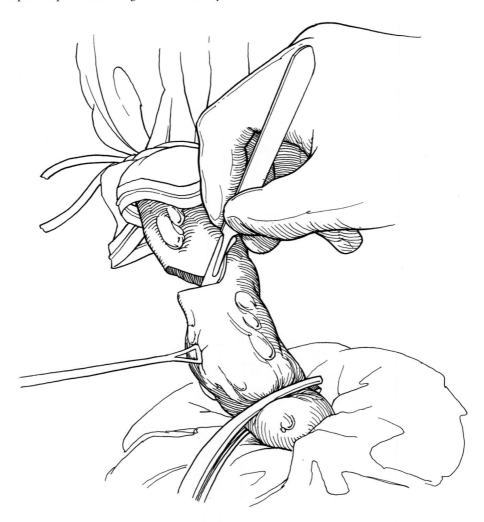

FIGURE 31–9

FIGURE 31–9. The sigmoid colon is then excised with the associated mesentery extracorporeally.

FIGURE 31–10. The anvil of the endoscopic circular stapler is secured in the proximal cut end of the colon with a 2–0 polypropylene purse-string suture. The colon end is then returned to the peritoneal cavity, and the wound is closed.

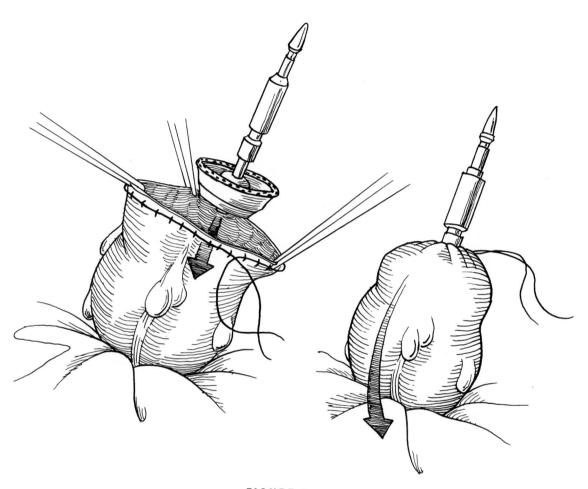

FIGURE 31–10

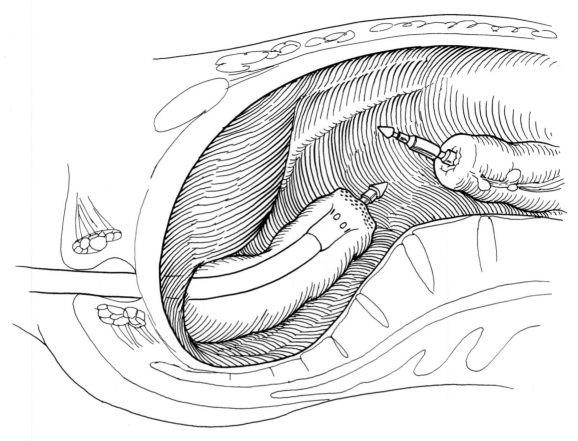

FIGURE 31–11

FIGURE 31–11. After reinsufflation of the peritoneal cavity, the endoscopic circular stapler is inserted to the rectal stump transanally. The spike of the stapler is made to penetrate the rectal stump at the linear staple line made by the endo GIA stapler.

FIGURE 31–12. The descending colon is checked to be sure it is not twisted by inspecting the bowel and its mesentery. With the use of a locking clamp to hold the shaft of the anvil, it is made to engage with the stapler, and the colorectal anastomosis can be fashioned under laparoscopic guidance.

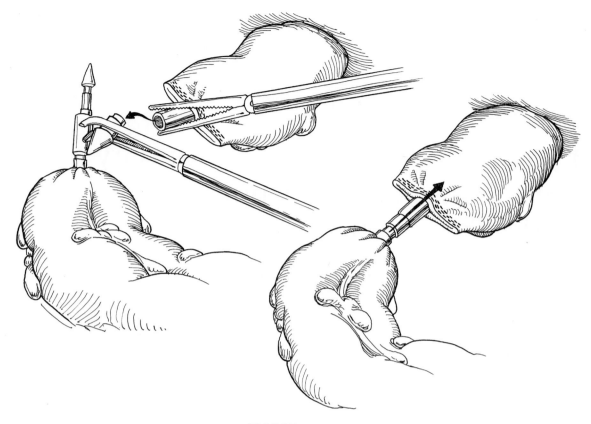

FIGURE 31–12

X. Postoperative Medications

Patient-controlled analgesia using morphine or pethidine

XI. Advancement of Diet

Fluids are started on postoperative day 1. Solid food is given when bowel sounds resume.

XII. Determinants of Discharge

A. Mobility of patient
B. Normal vital signs after the third day
C. Toleration of solid food
D. No signs of complications

XIII. Return to Normal Activity/Work

Normal activities are resumed depending on the condition of the patient and the nature of the work. Sedentary work may be resumed in 7 to 10 days. Manual work may be resumed after 2 weeks.

Chapter 32

Laparoscopic Left Hemicolectomy with Transanal Extraction of the Specimen

MORRIS E. FRANKLIN, JR., M.D., and JOSÉ ANTONIO DÍAZ-E., M.D.

I. Indications

Indications for laparoscopic left colectomy are basically the same as those for an open left hemicolectomy and can be divided into two categories—namely, those of benign and malignant disease.

A. Benign
  1. Quiescent diverticulitis
  2. Polyps or multiple polyps of the left colon
  3. Ischemic left colon
  4. Arteriovenous malformations of the left colon
  5. Segmental Crohn's colitis of the left colon
B. Malignant
  1. Carcinoma of the mid and proximal rectum
  2. Carcinoma of the sigmoid colon
  3. Carcinoma of the descending colon up to and including the splenic flexure

II. Contraindications

A. Contraindications
  1. Noncorrectable cardiovascular disease
  2. Patients who cannot tolerate general anesthesia
  3. Noncorrectable bleeding disorders
  4. Inadequately trained surgeon

  5. Unprepared operating room team
B. Noncontraindications
  1. Multiple abdominal operations in the past
  2. History of perforation of the colon from, for example, diverticulitis
  3. Obesity

III. Factors Important in Patient Selection

The same factors that are important in patient selection for open surgery are present in laparoscopic surgery with several notable exceptions.

A. Particular attention must be paid to the cardiovascular status of the patient, particularly to the patient's cardiac reserve. Placement of the patient in a severe Trendelenburg position and creation of a pneumoperitoneum produce stress on the cardiovascular system. This must be taken into account when a patient is being considered for a laparoscopic or open procedure for colonic disease.
B. Presence or absence of bleeding dyscrasias
C. The number of prior operative procedures that a patient has had. While we have been able to perform numerous laparoscopic procedures in patients with prior operative procedures, the presence of multiple incisions

should alert one to the possibility that severe adhesions may be present, and the patient may indeed be at higher risk for conversion to an open procedure.

D. Body habitus of the patient. Although obesity is not a contraindication to these surgical procedures, it certainly creates a problem that may hamper one's ability to perform this procedure laparoscopically.

E. Extremely thin patients also create certain problems for laparoscopy. Exceptionally thin elderly patients are also susceptible to profound temperature loss and a much more rapid drop in the body core temperature than that occurring in a patient who has adequate subcutaneous tissue. Additionally, trocars tend to be more readily displaced in extremely thin patients, and carbon dioxide leaks occur more frequently, thus increasing the chance of the so-called chimney effect as well as more rapid cooling of the patient during a given laparoscopic procedure.

F. Patients with a rigid abdomen. Nondistensibility of the abdomen creates certain space relationship problems that can hamper the performance of a laparoscopic procedure.

IV. Preoperative Preparation

Generally speaking, the same preoperative preparations that are necessary for open procedures are required in laparoscopic surgery. The bowel must be prepared. The patient must be adequately informed, and the team must be oriented toward the prospect of a laparoscopic procedure. The patient should always be informed that there is always a possibility that a laparoscopic procedure may have to be converted to an open procedure. Close localization of the tumor should have been established preoperatively by means of a barium enema, colonoscopy, and a CT scan when indicated.

A. Same day admission or admission the night before surgery. This is certainly a controversial area, but for the most part admission can be accomplished without extreme difficulty if an adequate system of complete bowel preparation can be ensured. Our experience with this has been somewhat clouded because many of our patients tend to be elderly and do not comply well with bowel preparations, particularly the use of

GoLYTELY and similar harsh bowel preparatory agents. Therefore, we have tended to avoid trying to prepare these patients totally as outpatients.

B. Preoperative medications including medication patches. We very rarely use medication patches on any of our patients except for those needed for cardiac care and/or antihypertensive agents and have no problem whatsoever using these compounds. Our bowel preparation includes oral medications that, if an adequate support system is present, can very readily be given at home as part of the chemical preparation of the bowel.

C. Bowel preparation. Another issue is that of immediate bowel preparation versus bowel preparation lasting several days. We have tended to drift away from GoLYTELY and similar substances because of problems with patient compliance as well as the fact that GoLYTELY leaves a large amount of liquid in the small bowel and frequently results in inadequate preparation of the colon. For this reason, we have gone to a 5-day preparation, in which all fiber is removed from the patient's diet 5 days prior to surgery, but totally absorbed food materials such as baked chicken, baked fish, mashed potatoes without peelings, tomato soup, and so on are continued. Three days preoperatively, the patient changes to essentially a full liquid diet, and milk of magnesia 60 ml is added twice a day. The day prior to surgery, Fleet's phospho-Soda, 30 ml, or magnesium citrate, 120 ml, is given in the morning followed by a saline enema, and this is repeated in the afternoon. Additionally, neomycin, 1g, and erythromycin base, 500 mg, are given three times at 11 AM, 7 PM, and 11 PM the day before surgery. We have been very satisfied with this preparation and have found that, for the most part, the colon is clean and the small bowel is decompressed and not distended with fluid as is commonly seen with the GoLYTELY-type of preparation.

V. Choice of Anesthesia

General anesthesia is used almost uniformly for patients undergoing laparoscopic surgery. Rarely do we use epidural anesthesia because these procedures tend to be longer, and the patients are unable to keep up with the increased carbon dioxide absorption and the increased respiratory rate this type of anesthesia demands of these patients. Therefore, we use general anesthesia almost exclusively. Since the patient is in a steep Trendelenburg position most of the time, we believe that mechanical ventilation is much better at controlling the carbon dioxide than asking the patient to control it. Additionally, on occasion we use postoperative epidural anesthesia if the patient is expected to be particularly pain sensitive, but this is not used routinely and is secondary to various medical requirements.

VI. Accessory Devices

A. Sequential compression devices for the legs
B. Nasogastric tube
C. Urinary catheter
D. Central venous line if the patient is elderly or has cardiac problems or if the procedure is anticipated to last more than 45 minutes
E. Arterial line if the patient has chronic obstructive pulmonary disease
F. Warming blanket
G. Bear-hugger across head and face
H. Warmed irrigation fluid
I. Betadine irrigation for trocar sites

The accessory devices needed for a given laparoscopic colon resection, of course, depend on the site of the colon resection. In patients requiring a steep Trendelenburg position, pneumatic stockings are often not needed, and TED hose seem sufficient. This has not been proved, however, and at the current time we continue to use sequential compression devices on all patients undergoing laparoscopic surgery of any type. We believe that this helps in venous return, offsetting the pneumoperitoneum that has been created. We also routinely use a nasogastric tube, Foley catheter, and central venous line, particularly if the patient is elderly or has cardiac problems or if the procedure is expected to last more than 45 minutes. An arterial line is also readily used, particularly if the patient has chronic obstructive pulmonary disease or if there is any doubt whatsoever about oxygenation or carbon dioxide build-up. Other accessory devices include a warming blanket and a bear-hugger across the head and face. Additionally, we have installed devices to warm the inspired air and irrigation fluids if increased irrigation is anticipated. We routinely use Betadine irrigation of trocars and trocar sites in our patients and frequently have Betadine irrigation available for intra-abdominal irrigation.

VII. Instruments and Telescopes

The instrumentation used for laparoscopic low anterior and left colon resection with transanal extraction is essentially the same as that used for standard laparoscopic left colon resection.

A. 10-mm, 30-degree telescope
B. Three-chip video camera
C. EEA stapler; in patients with higher lesions, a longer one can be useful, but this is decided on a case-by-case basis.
D. A ring forceps for transanal extraction is extremely convenient.
E. Colonoscope. Intraoperative colonoscopy is performed in each patient and is used not only to localize the lesion but also to correct any inadequacy in bowel preparation.
F. During the past 5 years we have moved more and more toward nondisposable instrumentation except for working port trocars, scissors, and stapling devices.

VIII. Position of Patient and Trocars

FIGURE 32-1. After satisfactory general endotracheal anesthesia has been obtained, and with the patient in the supine position, the abdomen is prepared and draped to allow an adequate working area and anal access. A nasogastric tube and Foley catheter are inserted. Sequential compression devices are generally placed on the legs, which are placed in Lloyd-

Davis stirrups for easy anal access. The patient is secured to the table usually with either a bean bag around the pelvis or with 4-inch adhesive tape on the shoulders to prevent unnecessary slippage. We specifically avoid using braces on the shoulders because these can result in brachial plexus injuries. The arms of the patient are always placed at the side and are tucked into a safe position. All exposed nerves, joints, and extremities are protected from metal surfaces on the table.

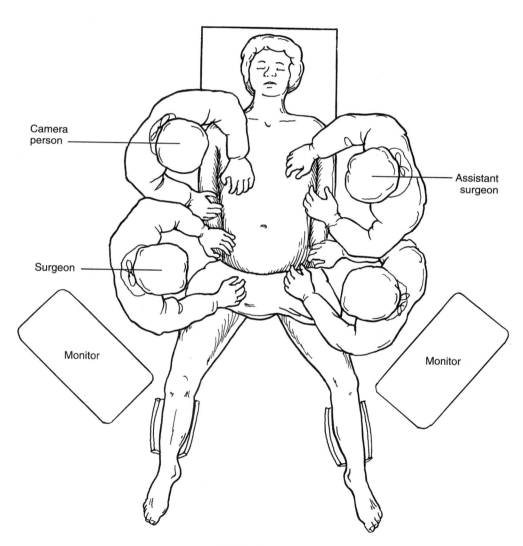

FIGURE 32-1

FIGURE 32-2. As shown in this figure, five trocars are usually used. The telescope is generally placed at the umbilicus, and the working ports are generally located on the right side of the patient beyond the rectus muscle; they are placed either above or below the umbilicus or splitting the umbilicus depending on the location of the tumor and how low a resection is to be performed. The telescope is generally a 10-mm, 0-degree telescope, but occasionally a 30-degree scope is useful, particularly for splenic resections and for delivering difficult adhesions out of the pelvis. The trocars on the right side and at the umbilicus are usually 10 mm in diameter. The trocars on the left side may be 5 or 10 mm, depending on the anticipated difficulty of the procedure and specific patient situations, as well as the size of the patient. Should a subxyphoid trocar be used, it is generally 10 mm in size to allow higher placement of the telescope and/or additional instrumentation to aid in mobilization of a difficult splenic flexure.

IX. Narrative of Surgical Technique

Access to the abdominal cavity is usually obtained with a Veress needle, which is usually placed away from the umbilicus, preferably in the right upper quadrant or the right lower quadrant depending on the presence of any

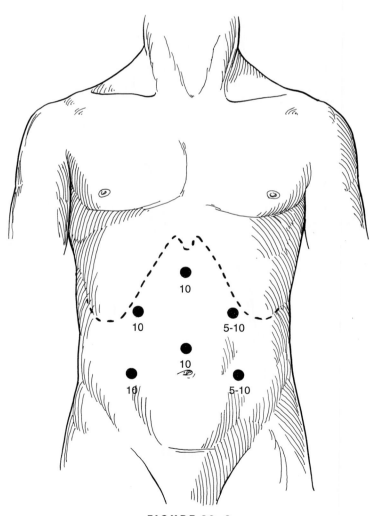

FIGURE 32-2

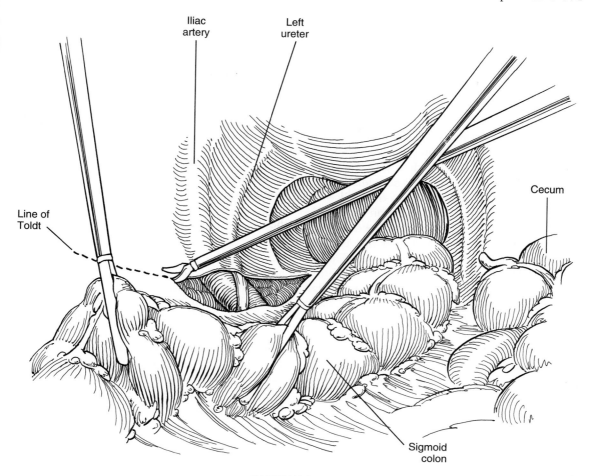

Iliac
artery

Left
ureter

Cecum

Line of
Toldt

Sigmoid
colon

FIGURE 32-3

prior surgery. As a general rule, we avoid primary umbilical placement of a trocar initially unless special circumstances are present because we have frequently encountered omentum, umbilical hernias, or similar difficult situations that have remained undiagnosed, particularly in more obese patients. The left upper quadrant and right upper quadrant, unless the patient has had prior surgery, are usually clear of adhesions. A 10-mm trocar is placed initially on the right side, and surveillance of the abdominal cavity together with, if at all possible, an ultrasound examination of the liver, is carried out.

FIGURE 32-3. After additional trocars have been inserted, the patient is placed in a relatively severe Trendelenburg position with the left side elevated a slight amount. The quality of the bowel preparation is immediately assessed, and the amount of fluid and air in the

small and large bowel is evaluated because this is one of the determining factors in the extent of severity of the Trendelenburg positioning. Additional dissection is usually carried out along the white line of Toldt at the embryonic attachments of the sigmoid colon to the pelvic brim. These are taken down in a step-wise fashion until the sigmoid colon is freed and the ureters as well as the spermatic vessels are identified. If the lesion is lower than this, this is the extent of dissection at the current time, and the sigmoid colon is mobilized well past the midline, taking particular care to avoid injury to the common iliac artery and vein, over which dissection is carried out in a very close manner. If the resection is to be very low, below the peritoneal reflection, the dissection on the left side is now carried out below the peritoneal reflection. No attempt is made to clear the anterior peritoneal reflection in this initial dissection.

FIGURE 32-4. (A) Following this, the colon is elevated, and the location of the right ureter is noted, after which a window is developed beneath the rectum. This procedure should be relatively easy to perform if adequate dissection has been carried out from the left side. After the window has been formed, a long instrument in the assistant's right hand is placed in this window to elevate the colon. This alleviates the need for external devices such as sutures or any other device from the anterior abdominal wall. Dissection is then carried out on the right side to complete the inferior dissection as far as necessary. At this point, the lower line of dissection should be fairly clear, and if this is true, dissection can be carried up to the colon, identifying, doubly clipping, and dividing the superior hemorrhoidal vessels as well as the lateral rectal vessels. After the superior hemorrhoidal vessels have been identified and divided, dissection is continued up the anterior surface of the common iliac vessels until the inferior mesenteric artery is identified. Here, care must be taken to ensure that the ureter is not included in the dissection by visualizing it through the window and positioning it below the dissection plane.

The gonadal vessels can be reflected posteriorly in a similar manner. This is also a good opportunity to continue the dissection beneath the previously dissected white line of Toldt behind the colon. The inferior mesenteric artery is identified, isolated, and ligated with an externally tied suture, using the Westin knot, which was developed in our laboratory. The vessel is doubly clipped proximally, singly clipped distally, and then divided only partially to ensure complete hemostasis. Additional hemostasis may be required should the vessel not be completely ligated. We have not used an Endo GIA stapler for this portion of the procedure because of its expense and because of the fear of incorporating too much tissue in the initial firing of the stapler.

(B) The proximal line of dissection should be established; if the lesion is low, additional mobilization of the colon may not be needed above the midportion of the colon. However, if the lesion is somewhat higher or if a very low anterior anastomosis is anticipated, the dissection should be carried up to the splenic flexure, and the splenic flexure should be mobilized liberally, allowing a lengthy amount of colon to be brought into the pelvis with a minimal amount of difficulty. If the lesion is very high, the left colic artery may have to be sacrificed to establish adequate length. High ligation of the inferior mesenteric artery can produce extra length.

After mobilization of the colon has been completed, intraoperative colonoscopy is performed. Laparoscopic bulldog Glassman clamps are applied across the proximal colon to prevent air leakage into the proximal colon. In intraoperative colonoscopy the proposed proximal and distal lines of resection are noted and the adequacy of bowel preparation is checked. Betadine irrigation is uniformly carried out in patients with cancer and in most of those with diverticulitis.

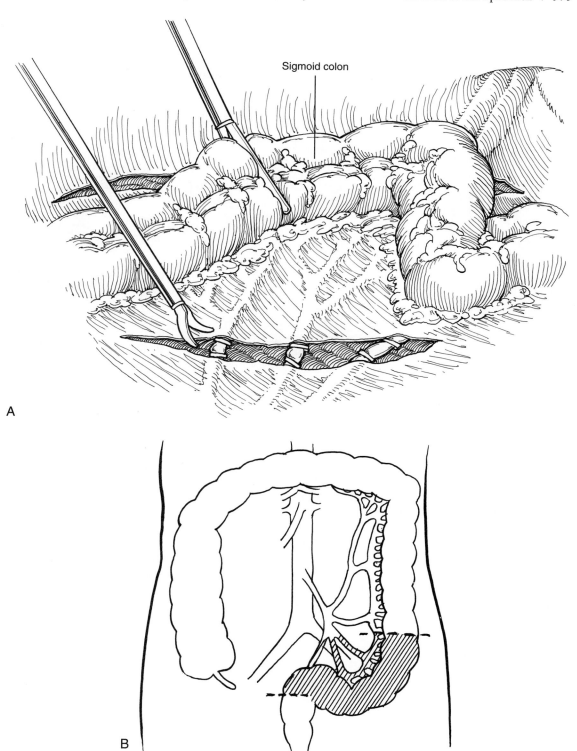

Sigmoid colon

A

B

FIGURE 32–4

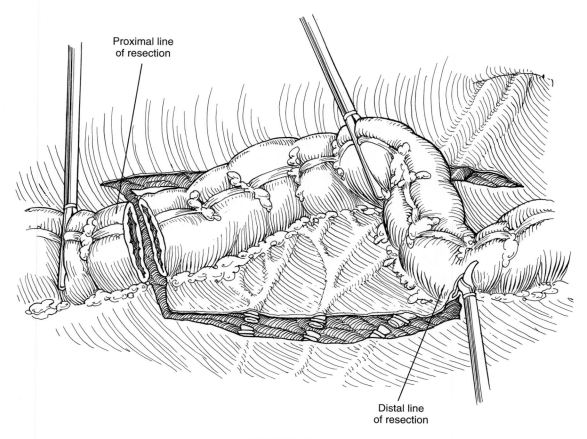

Proximal line
of resection

Distal line
of resection

FIGURE 32–5

FIGURE 32–5. After the proximal and distal lines of resection have been established, the distal bowel is divided using the scissors. The lumen is again immediately irrigated with Betadine supplied from standard irrigation sources. The distal end of the resected specimen is immediately closed with an endo-loop to protect the abdominal cavity from spillage. The proximal line of resection is then identified, and the bowel is transected at this point. It is important to emphasize that a minimal amount of bowel should be cleaned to protect against ischemia and a subsequent higher risk of stenosis at the anastomosis. As soon as the proximal bowel is divided, this end of the resected specimen is also closed with an endo-loop.

FIGURE 32-6. A specimen bag is then brought in through a 10-mm trocar site and opened, and the bowel is deposited in the bag, leaving a small nubbin sticking out of the now closed end of the sac. We use a sac that has been specifically designed for this purpose and has a purse-string suture that allows easy closure around the bag; the suture is then clipped, and an endo-loop is applied to trap the neck of the colon in the bag. We usually place the end with the diseased segment in the bag first so that the more supple portions of the bowel are removed first.

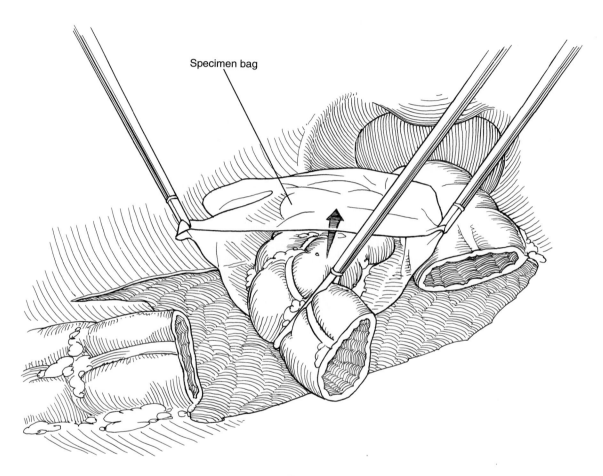

Specimen bag

FIGURE 32-6

FIGURE 32–7. The specimen and the bag are then turned around so that the endo-looped end of the bag is facing the rectum. A ring forceps is brought through the rectum, and the size of the rectum is compared with the size of the tumor. An exceptionally large tumor obviously cannot be removed transanally, but most tumors up to about 5 cm can be readily removed through this route.

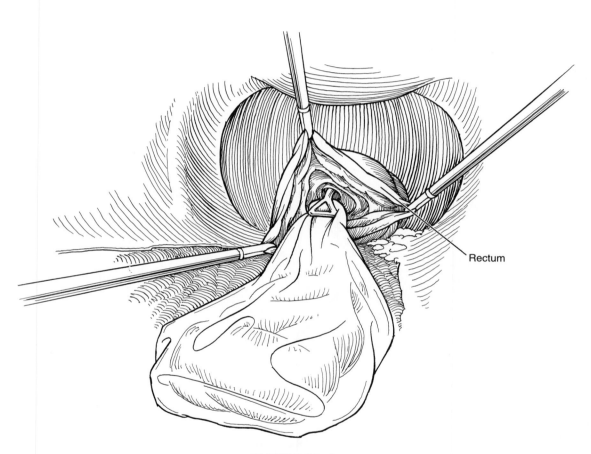

Rectum

FIGURE 32–7

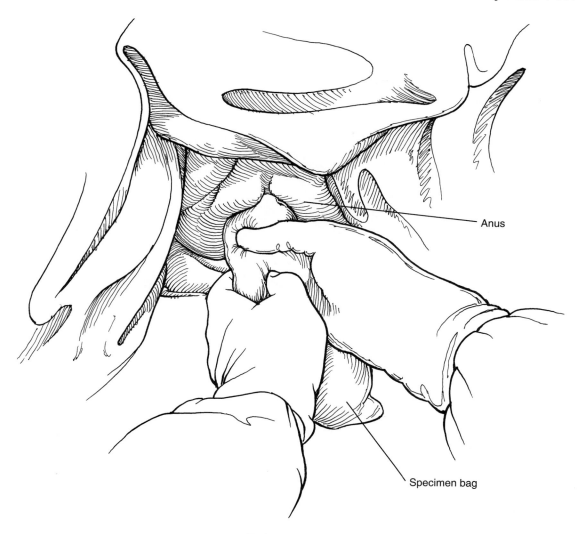

Anus

Specimen bag

FIGURE 32-8

FIGURE 32-8. In all patients the anus is carefully and slowly dilated. This should be carried out regardless of whether the specimen is to be removed transanally. Anal dilatation aids insertion of the anvil into the rectum. The bag and the colon are then grasped and slowly "snaked" out through the rectum and anus using the bag as a sheath in the rectum and not pulling directly on the bag. To have a bag that is strong enough to sustain very strong traction, the size of the bag is increased significantly, which diminishes the size of the tumor that can be removed transanally. Thus, the bag is used more as a sheath, and the colon is literally "snaked" out of the bag through the rectum. The bag is then removed, and the pelvis is inspected for bleeding. It is irrigated with Betadine solution, as is the remainder of the colon.

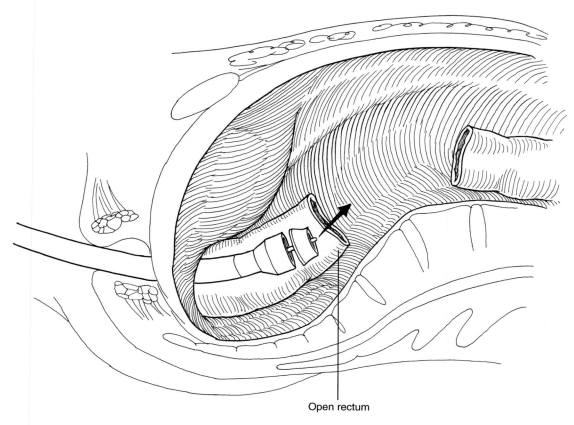

Open rectum

FIGURE 32–9

FIGURE 32–9. The circular stapler is then brought into the rectum. The size of the proximal end of the colon has been previously determined and an appropriately sized stapler chosen. We have found that a size 28-mm or 29-mm stapler usually allows passage of the anvil proximally and results in a very adequate lumen.

FIGURE 32–10. The anvil is brought into the abdominal cavity through the rectum, washed with Betadine, and then placed in the proximal colon.

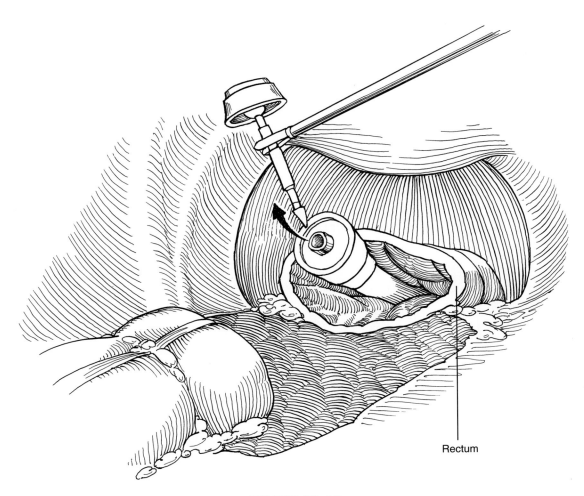

Rectum

FIGURE 32–10

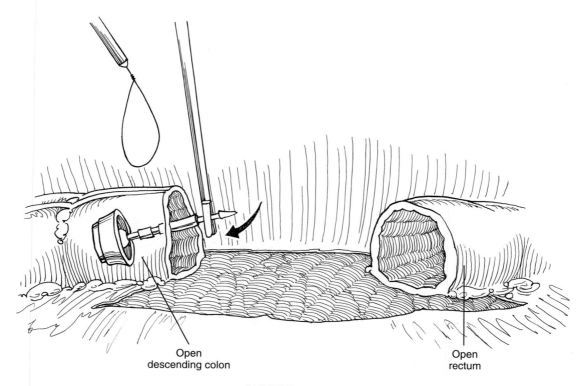

Open
descending colon

Open
rectum

FIGURE 32-11

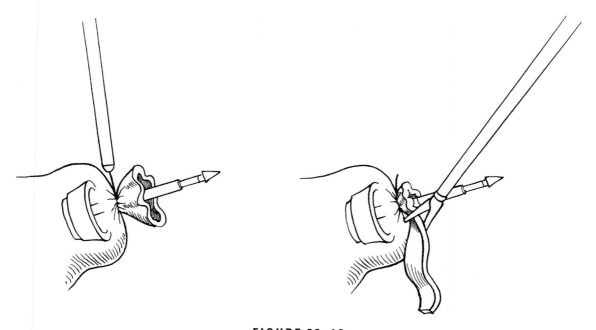

FIGURE 32-12

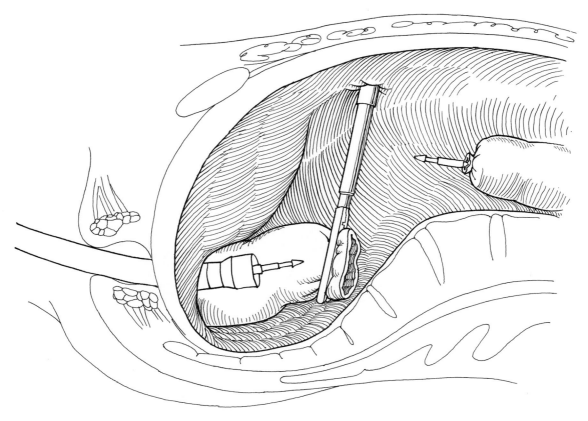

FIGURE 32-13

FIGURE 32-11. Endoloops are placed around the anvil, holding it securely in the colon.

FIGURE 32-12. Excess tissue is trimmed, and the anvil is ready for placement in the stapler.

FIGURE 32-13. The distal colon is visualized, and an Endo GIA 35 or 45 is brought into the abdominal cavity through the right lower quadrant; it is maneuvered into position over the colon and fired, and the rim of tissue thus separated is removed. The area is checked for bleeding. The end-to-end anastomosis (EEA) device is brought in through the rectum, and the spike is slowly advanced so that the staple line is near the center portion of the EEA.

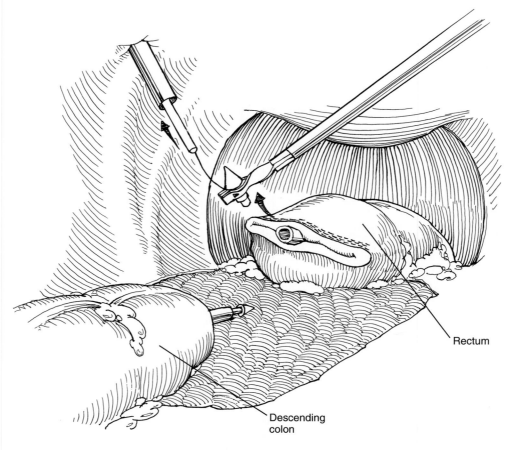

Rectum

Descending colon

FIGURE 32–14

FIGURE 32–14. The spike is removed.

FIGURE 32–15. The anvil and stapler are reconnected.

FIGURE 32–16. The stapler is closed. The stapler should be checked circumferentially to ensure that no tissue is entrapped, and the device is then fired. The amount of tension is then double checked, and a second intraoperative colonoscopy is performed to check the integrity of the anastomosis, the lack of bleeding at the anastomotic site, and the absence of leaks. Any leaks should be repaired immediately by sutures placed intracorporeally. The clamps on the colon that were left in place during this procedure are removed after colonoscopy has been completed. These clamps serve not only to prevent leakage of the colon contents upstream but also to help orient the colon because they were applied initially on the antimesenteric surface and

still should be in this position. The clamps prevent rotation of the bowel and a 180- or 360-degree misplacement of the staple line.

The entire abdominal cavity and particularly the trocars are then irrigated with a 3.5 per cent Betadine solution before fascial closure sutures are placed using a suture passer with 0 Vicryl suture. A 10-mm drain is placed in the pelvis and brought out through a left lower quadrant trocar. The entire abdominal cavity is then reinspected; all Betadine is washed free with normal saline, and the peritoneal cavity is suctioned dry. The patient is placed in a slight reverse Trendelenburg position, and the abdomen is de-insufflated. After the trocars are removed, all port sites are immediately closed. The subcutaneous tissue is irrigated thoroughly with Betadine solution and closed with 3–0 monocryl sutures, and the skin is closed with Steri-Strips.

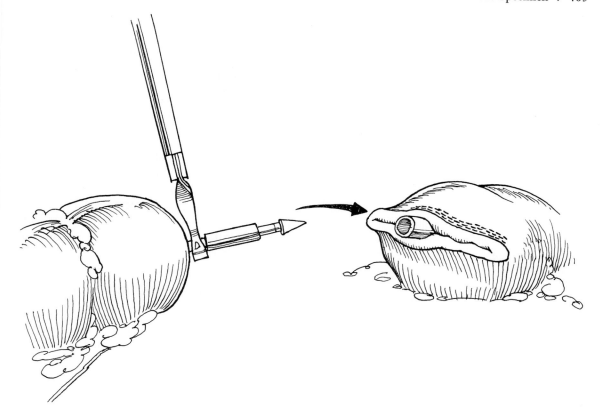

FIGURE 32–15

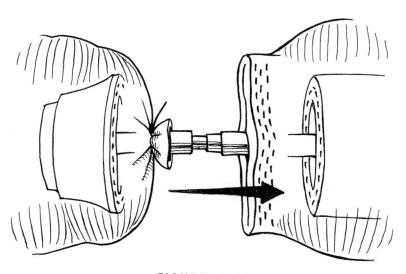

FIGURE 32–16

X. Postoperative Medications

Postoperative medications are the standard agents used in all colon resections. The patient is given fluids intravenously (IV). A nasogastric tube may or may not be left in place depending on the number of adhesions that were taken down in a given case, the length of surgery, age of the patient, and so on. This determination can only be made intraoperatively. The patient is usually given IV antibiotics for 24 hours, and then these medications are stopped. Additional medications include a minimal amount of analgesia, particularly in the realm of narcotics, as well as something for the inevitable nausea. Obviously, any previously prescribed medications should be included in the medication regimen such as antihypertensives, antiseizure medications, cardiac medications, and diabetic medications.

XI. Advancement of Diet

Although many laparoscopic surgeons empirically begin diets on the day of surgery, we have found this deleterious, particularly in an aging population. Thus, we wait at least 12 hours to start a diet and have found that most patients can tolerate clear liquids the next day. This tolerance is, of course, based primarily on the presence of bowel sounds. Liquids are not started until bowel sounds are present, and the diet is then advanced as the patient has increased bowel activity. Passage of flatus allows advancement to a full liquid diet, and passage of the first bowel movement signifies advancement to a low-fat diet with solid food.

XII. Determinants of Discharge

The patient is considered for discharge when he or she is making satisfactory progress. No attempt is made to discharge patients before they can tolerate a regular diet or have bowel movements. Other requirements are that (1) their medical problems are under control, (2) they have no fever, (3) they are ambulating satisfactorily if they are able to do so, (4) pain is under good control, and (5) the wounds are clean and healing and all drains are removed. This time period usually averages 3.5 days for patients under 50 years of age and 5.5 days for those over 50 years of age for most sigmoid and low anterior resections.

XIII. Return to Normal Activity and/or Work

Timing of return to normal activity is a gray area and is very loosely determined depending on the individual practitioner. Most patients are able to return to normal activity (depending on the type of activity) within 7 to 10 days. We do not recommend returning to work any sooner than 5 to 7 days postoperatively unless the patient has a sedentary occupation. Most patients are able to tolerate returning to full activity and/or work within 7 to 10 days. Some patients who have particular problems may not be able to return to work for 2 weeks. Patients with very heavy labor-related occupations require 10 days to 2 weeks before they can return to full, unrestricted work activities.

Chapter 33

Laparoscopic Proctopexy

RICHARD PERRY, M.D.

I. Indications

Full-thickness circumferential rectal prolapse

II. Contraindications

A. Cardiac or respiratory insufficiency
B. Large fibroid uterus or other pelvic mass
C. Too frail to tolerate general anesthesia

III. Factors Important in Patient Selection

A. Risk of infertility (women) or impotence (men)
B. Previous pelvic surgery
C. Presence of other intra-abdominal pathology including
   1. Extensive adhesions
   2. Diverticular disease
   3. Inflammatory bowel disease
   4. Uterine or ovarian pathology

IV. Preoperative Preparation

A. Full mechanical bowel preparation is mandatory
B. Most patients can be admitted the same day following routine preanesthetic work-up and bowel preparation. Frail or elderly patients may be better admitted the day before surgery for intravenous rehydration accompanying bowel preparation.
C. Prophylactic antibiotics are given intravenously within an hour of anesthesia.

V. Choice of Anesthesia

Full endotracheal general anesthesia is required. Supplementary epidural anesthesia is an advantage because it increases small intestinal tone, thereby reducing gut volume and making it easier to keep the small intestine out of the pelvis.

VI. Accessory Devices

A. An indwelling urinary catheter is used routinely.
B. TED stockings and pneumatic compression device are used for thromboprophylaxis.

VII. Instruments and Telescopes

A. 30-degree telescope (5 or 10 mm)
B. Atraumatic bowel-grasping forceps (5 mm)
C. One curved dissecting forceps (Maryland, 5 mm)
D. One pair sharp laparoscopic dissecting scissors
E. Two laparoscopic needle holders (5 mm)
F. One laparoscopic knot pusher
G. Strong monofilament thread, 0 gauge, on a robust curved needle

VIII. Position of Monitors and Placement of Trocars

FIGURE 33-1. Patient is in the supine position with the monitor at the feet. The surgeon stands on the patient's right. A 10-mm Hasson cannula is placed in the umbilicus, a 10-mm port in the right flank, and 5-mm ports in the right iliac fossa and left flank.

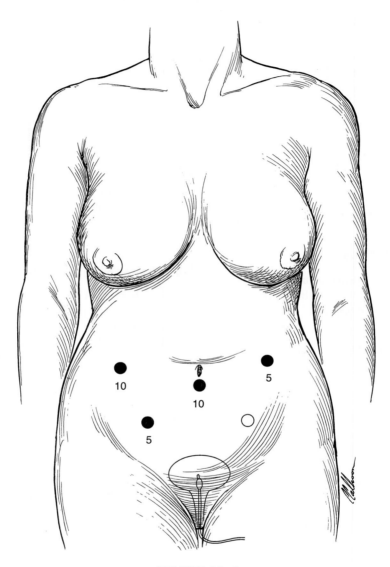

FIGURE 33-1

IX. Narrative of Surgical Technique

FIGURE 33–2. After the cannulas have been placed and pneumoperitoneum has been established, the patient is placed in the Trendelenburg position with sufficient tilt to draw the small bowel out of the pelvis so that it lies unrestrained in the upper abdomen. Any sigmoid adhesions at the pelvic brim are divided with sharp dissection. An atraumatic grasper inserted through the left port is used to draw the mesosigmoid anteriorly to the left, which stretches the peritoneum over the sacral promontory. The peritoneum is incised over the sacral promontory, just medial to the right ureter, which is identified routinely. The peritoneal incision is continued down the right side of the rectum and across the anterior peritoneal reflection. The avascular presacral space is dissected under direct vision, taking care to identify and preserve the hypogastric nerves.

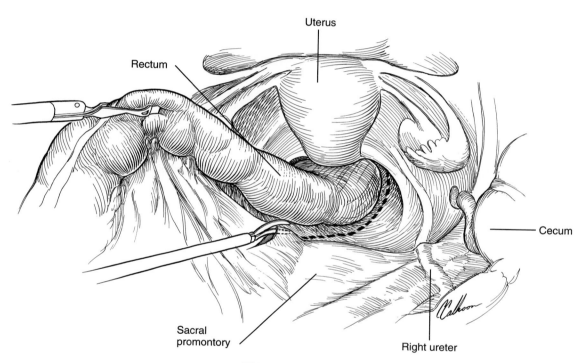

FIGURE 33–2

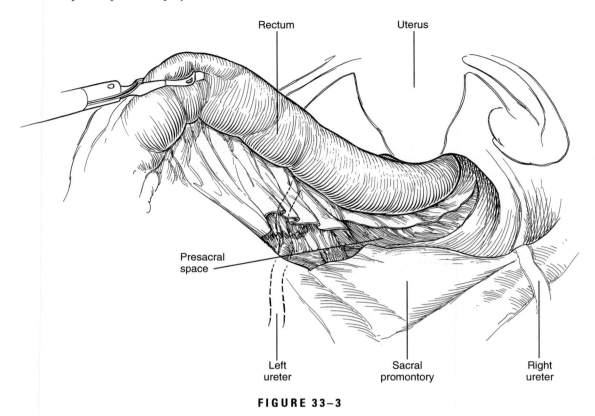

Rectum

Uterus

Presacral
space

Left
ureter

Sacral
promontory

Right
ureter

FIGURE 33-3

FIGURE 33-3. When dissecting the presacral space from the right side, care must be taken to identify and preserve the left ureter as it comes into view behind the elevated mesosigmoid.

FIGURE 33-4. Posterior dissection is continued down to the level of the fascial condensation of Waldeyer.

FIGURE 33-5A and B. The peritoneum on the left side of the rectum is incised, again carefully identifying and preserving the left ureter.

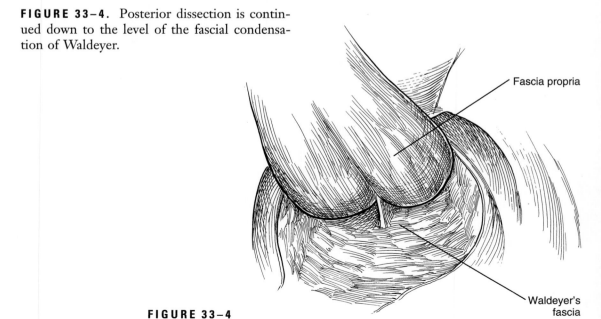

Fascia propria

Waldeyer's
fascia

FIGURE 33-4

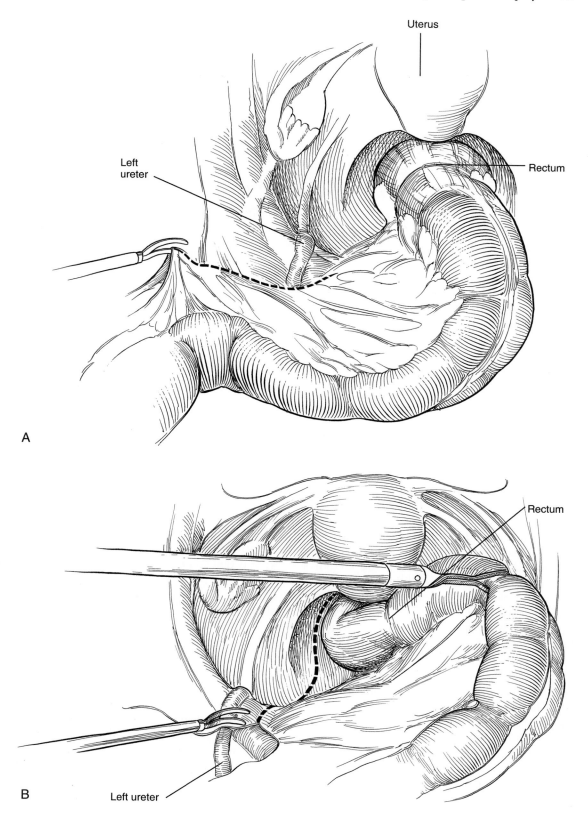

Uterus

Left
ureter

Rectum

A

Rectum

Left ureter

B

FIGURE 33–5

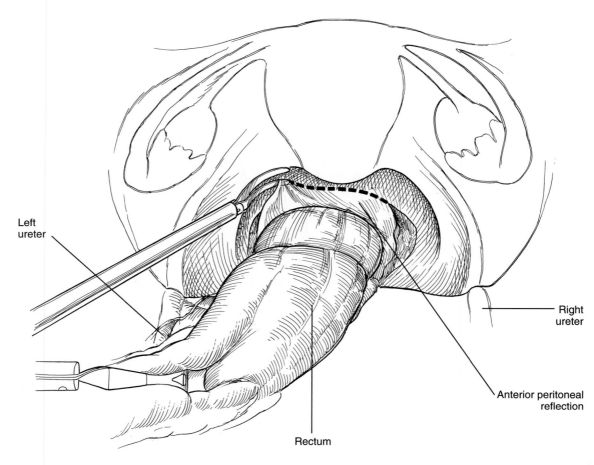

Left
ureter

Right
ureter

Anterior peritoneal
reflection

Rectum

FIGURE 33-6

FIGURE 33-6. This incision continues inferiorly to meet the incision across the anterior peritoneal reflection. Anteriorly the rectum is mobilized for a distance of approximately 5 cm below the peritoneal reflection. The lateral rectal attachments are divided a little further if necessary, until the rectum can be drawn taut without restriction by any remaining attachments.

FIGURE 33-7A. The monofilament suture (full length) is introduced through the 10-mm port. A suture is placed through the presacral fascia (or the annulus of the L5–S1 disc) at the level of the sacral promontory on the right side, with care taken to avoid the right common iliac vein and the median sacral vessels. The rectum is drawn up to the sacral promontory, and the needle is passed through the lateral rectal tissues, close to but not through the rectal wall.

The needle is then brought back out through the 10-mm trocar, and an extracorporeal Roeder knot is tied and run down with the knot pusher.

FIGURE 33-7B. The second suture is placed about a centimeter above the first. If the rectum is still not securely bowstrung across the sacral hollow, a third suture may be placed on the left side. However, in placing this suture it is important to ensure that the lumen of the rectum is not stretched out across the sacral promontory and mesorectal tissue because this can result in postoperative rectosigmoid obstruction. The pelvic cavity is then irrigated with saline and aspirated until it is dry. When possible it is desirable to close the pelvic peritoneum across the rectum using continuous 3–0 absorbable suture. The ports are withdrawn under direct vision, and the umbilical fascia and skin are sutured closed.

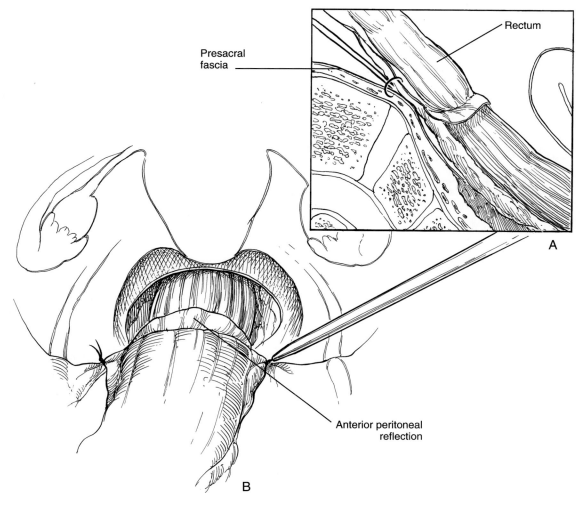

Rectum

Presacral
fascia

Anterior peritoneal
reflection

A

B

FIGURE 33–7

X. Postoperative Medications

Stool bulking agents (fiber)

XI. Advancement of Diet

Patients can take fluids ad libitum on return to the ward and may commence eating a light diet the next day. Postoperative ileus is rarely a problem.

XII. Determinants of Discharge

The patient is fit for discharge once he or she can tolerate a normal diet and has had a spontaneous bowel movement (usually 2 to 3 days).

XIII. Return to Normal Activity

Return to normal activity or work is usually possible after 3 weeks.

Chapter 34

Laparoscopic-Assisted Anterior Resection for Rectal Prolapse

DAVID BARTOLO, M.D.

I. Indications

A. Full-thickness rectal prolapse
B. Internal rectal intussusception
C. Solitary rectal ulcer syndrome

II. Contraindications

A. Unfitness for abdominal surgery (unusual)
B. Other contraindications to laparoscopic surgery (e.g., dense adhesions)
C. Mucosal prolapse, including isolated sphincter injuries
D. Failed rectopexy using prosthetic materials
E. Incontinence is not usually a contraindication
F. Severe slow transit constipation is a relative contraindication; subtotal colectomy may be more appropriate

III. Factors Important in Patient Selection

A. Barium enema examination or colonoscopy is indicated if there is any suspicion of tumor, polyps, or colitis.
B. Transit studies using ingested radiopaque markers help identify patients with slow transit constipation (see section II F above).
C. Anorectal manometry and pudendal nerve terminal motor latency measurements are performed routinely. Patients often have low resting anal canal pressures and prolonged nerve conduction times. Inconti-

nence often improves after correction of the prolapse, but this may take 12 months or more.
D. Associated anterior sphincter defects may be repaired if incontinence persists after resection rectopexy. We usually defer repair for 6 months.
E. Patients with solitary rectal ulcer syndrome are warned that symptomatic improvement is not guaranteed, particularly in the absence of significant prolapse.

IV. Preoperative Preparation

A. Admission on day before surgery. Same day admission is also possible.
B. Routine subcutaneous sodium heparin prophylaxis
C. Intravenous (IV) broad-spectrum antibiotics are given after induction of anesthesia.
D. Bowel preparation (day before surgery)
   1. *10 AM:* one envelope of sodium picosulfate magnesium citrate (Picolax, Ferring AB, Malmo, Sweden)
   2. *12 noon:* one envelope of Picolax
   3. Afternoon: one liter of Klean-Prep (iso-osmotic solution containing polyethylene glycol) (Norgine, Oxford, UK)

V. Choice of Anesthesia

A. General anesthesia with full muscle relaxation and endotracheal intubation

B. Port sites infiltrated with 0.5 per cent bupiv-acaine hydrochloride

C. Rectal nonsteroidal anti-inflammatory drug suppository inserted at end of procedure

VI. Accessory Devices

A. Urinary catheter with burrette
B. Antiembolism stockings
C. Electric stimulated calf compression
D. We do not place a nasogastric tube routinely

VII. Instruments and Telescopes

A. Three-chip camera with 30° laparoscope
B. Atraumatic Babcock clamps (two)
C. Curved diathermy scissors

D. Large polydioxanone clip applicator (Abso-lok, Ethicon, Edinburgh, UK)

E. Laparoscopic linear staple gun (3.5- and 2.5-mm cartridges)

F. Conventional purse-string clamp

G. Conventional 31/33-mm circular staple gun

VIII. Position of Monitors and Placement of Trocars

FIGURE 34–1. The patient is placed in a modified Lloyd-Davies position. The left arm is extended, and the right is tucked next to the side. The primary monitor is placed on the left side of the patient near the hip. The surgeon and camera holder stand on the right side of the patient and the assistant surgeon on the left.

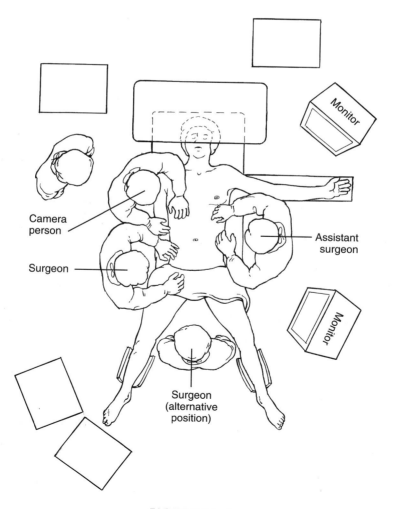

Camera person

Surgeon

Assistant surgeon

Surgeon (alternative position)

FIGURE 34–1

FIGURE 34-2

FIGURE 34-2. Four trocars are used. The trocar for the video camera is placed below the umbilicus. Two trocars are inserted on the right for use by the surgeon with one on the left for the assistant surgeon.

IX. Narrative of Surgical Technique

The patient is positioned in a modified Lloyd-Davies position with the legs kept low to allow freedom of movement of the laparoscopic instruments. The thorax is strapped to the operating table to allow steep tilting during the procedure. The skin is prepared with aqueous povidone-iodine solution. A Hasson port is inserted subumbilically, and a pneumoperitoneum is established with a pressure of 13 mm Hg.

General laparoscopy is performed, and further ports are inserted as illustrated. The rectouterine pouch is typically very deep, the lateral ligaments are scarred, and the sigmoid colon is redundant.

FIGURE 34-3. (A) Ligation of inferior mesenteric artery. A steep Trendelenburg tilt allows the small bowel to retract out of the pelvis. The sigmoid mesocolon is elevated to expose the root of the sigmoid mesentery, and the right ureter is identified. The peritoneum at the root of the mesentery is incised to expose the origin of the inferior mesenteric artery (B). The artery is skeletonized using diathermy scissors, sweeping the preaortic autonomic nerves posteriorly, and is ligated with polydioxanone artery clips before it is divided.

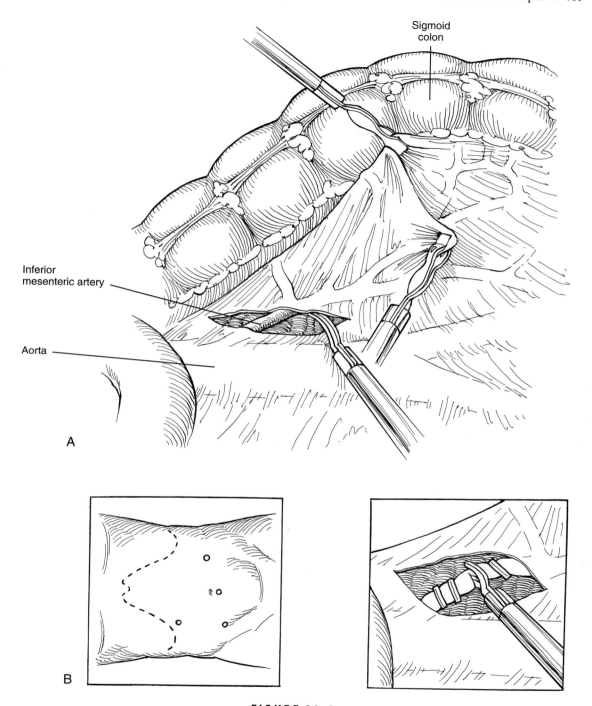

Sigmoid colon

Inferior mesenteric artery

Aorta

A

B

FIGURE 34-3

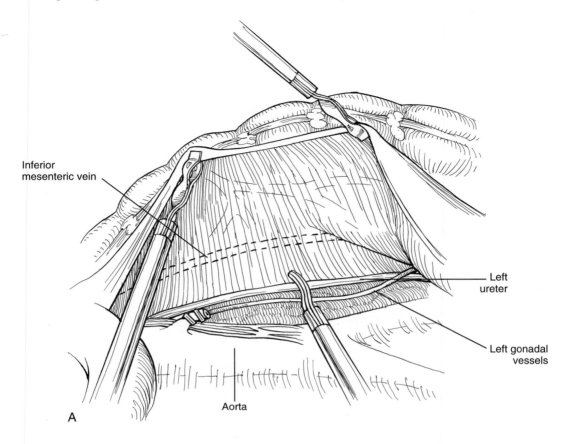

Inferior
mesenteric vein

Left
ureter

Left gonadal
vessels

Aorta

A

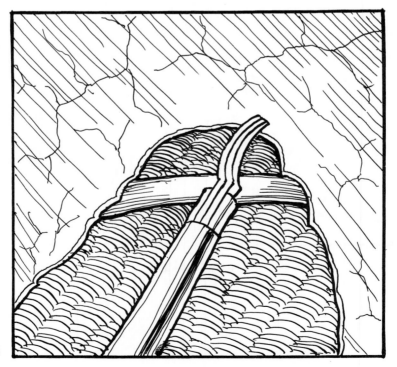

B

FIGURE 34–4

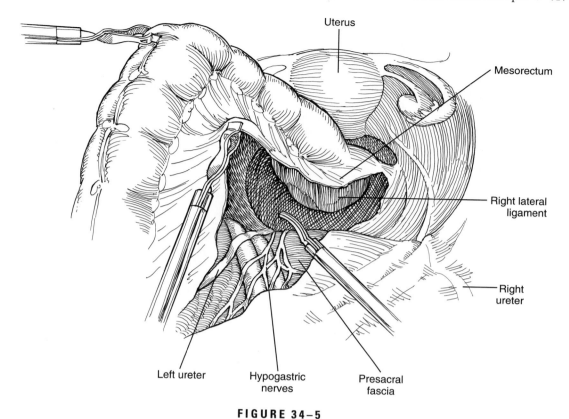

FIGURE 34-5

FIGURE 34-4. (A) Retroperitoneal dissection. The dissection is continued beyond the aorta, elevating the descending and sigmoid colon. The ureter and gonadal vessels are readily identified using this technique and are swept posteriorly, dividing loose areolar tissue until the undersurface of the left leaf of the mesocolon is reached. (B) The left ureter is preserved

FIGURE 34-5. Mesorectal and right lateral ligament dissection. The peritoneal incision at the root of the sigmoid colon is continued down into the pelvis beside the rectum. The plane between the mesorectum and the presacral fascia is entered. Using anterior retraction of the upper rectum, this dissection is carried down to the pelvic floor muscles beyond the mesorectum. The hypogastric nerves are clearly seen and are swept posterolaterally. The entire right lateral ligament is divided with diathermy scissors, alternating between posterior and lateral dissection. At this stage, much of the left lateral ligament can be conveniently divided from behind.

FIGURE 34-6. Left lateral and anterior dissection. The sigmoid colon and rectum are retracted to the right, and primitive adhesions with the pelvic side wall are divided. The previous retroperitoneal dissection is visible through the left leaf of the sigmoid mesocolon and can be divided now. Care is taken to ensure that the ureter is clear of the dissection. Division of the left lateral ligament is completed from above, and the peritoneal division is carried round the rectouterine pouch to meet the peritoneal incision on the opposite side. The vaginal wall usually separates fairly easily from the lower rectum using countertraction and sharp dissection. Attention is directed now to the left paracolic gutter, where the peritoneum is divided as far cranially as is convenient.

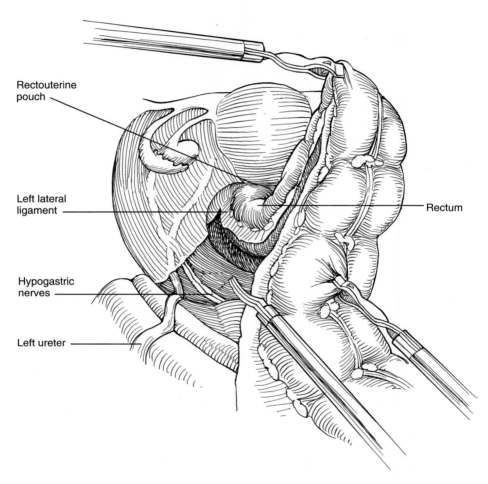

Rectouterine pouch

Left lateral ligament

Hypogastric nerves

Left ureter

Rectum

FIGURE 34-6

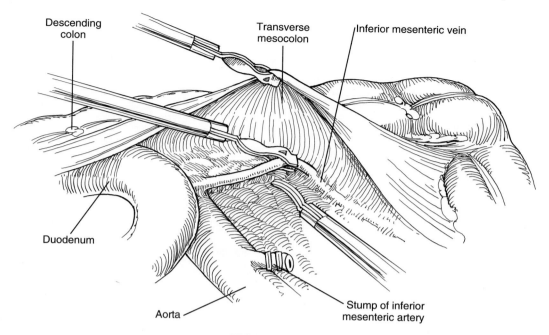

Descending colon

Transverse mesocolon

Inferior mesenteric vein

Duodenum

Aorta

Stump of inferior mesenteric artery

FIGURE 34–7

FIGURE 34–7. Division of the inferior mesenteric vein. The surgeon now sits between the patient's legs. Using the reverse Trendelenburg position and tilting the table to the right, the small bowel falls away from the left upper quadrant. The transverse mesocolon is retracted anteriorly exposing the duodenojejunal junction and inferior mesenteric vein. The duodenum is mobilized by sharp dissection, and the vein is skeletonized and ligated with polydioxanone clips above its first branch to achieve full mobilization.

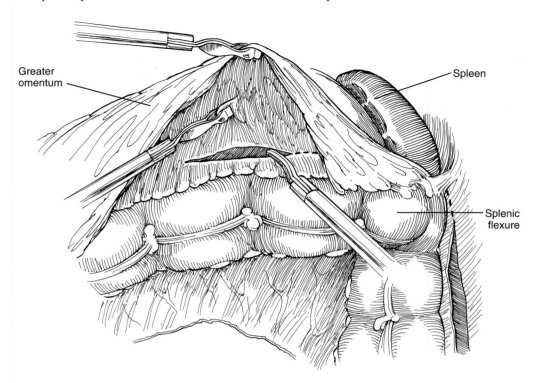

FIGURE 34-8

FIGURE 34-8. Mobilization of the splenic flexure. The greater omentum is grasped from underneath close to its attachment to the transverse colon and retracted anteriorly. The lateral half of the transverse colon is detached from the omentum, and the dissection is carried around the splenic flexure to meet up with the previous paracolic dissection. Several layers of fascia require gentle dissection to allow full mobilization almost as far proximally as the middle colic vessels. A significant vein from beneath the pancreas may require separate ligation.

FIGURE 34-9. Rectal transection. The surgeon moves back to the right side, and the patient is tipped head down again. A sigmoidoscope is inserted through the anus to 15 cm to mark the level of rectal transection. Transection is achieved using two to three sequential firings of an endoscopic linear stapler fitted with 3.5- or 2.5-mm cartridges depending on tissue thickness. Repeated trials of closure of the staple gun allow more tissue to be included with each bite. Before proceeding to the open phase of the operation, the mobility of the descending colon is checked from beneath. The divided proximal bowel is grasped with Babcock clamps inserted through the right upper port to facilitate its delivery.

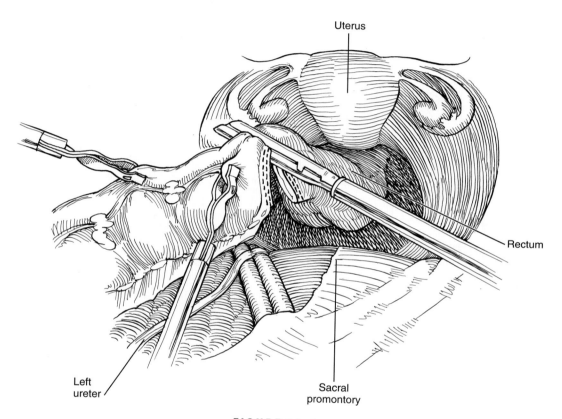

FIGURE 34-9

FIGURE 34-10. Open phase. A 4- to 5-cm transverse muscle-splitting incision is made at the left lateral port site, and the divided colon is delivered. The bowel is divided at a point where it will comfortably reach the sacral promontory. Approximately 40 cm of bowel is excised normally. The mesentery is prepared by cutting across the marginal artery beyond the intended level of ligation to ensure pulsatile bleeding. The bowel is divided using a purse-string clamp and the anvil of a 31- or 33-mm circular stapler. The bowel is then returned to the peritoneal cavity, grasping the spike of the anvil with Babcock clamps inserted through the right upper port. The transverse incision is closed in layers with absorbable suture.

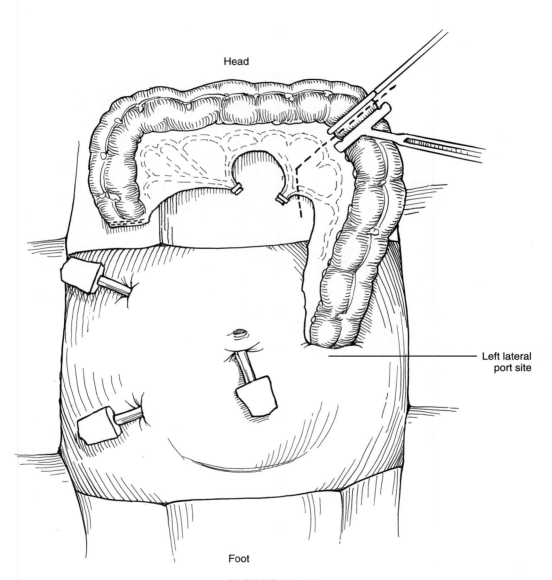

FIGURE 34-10

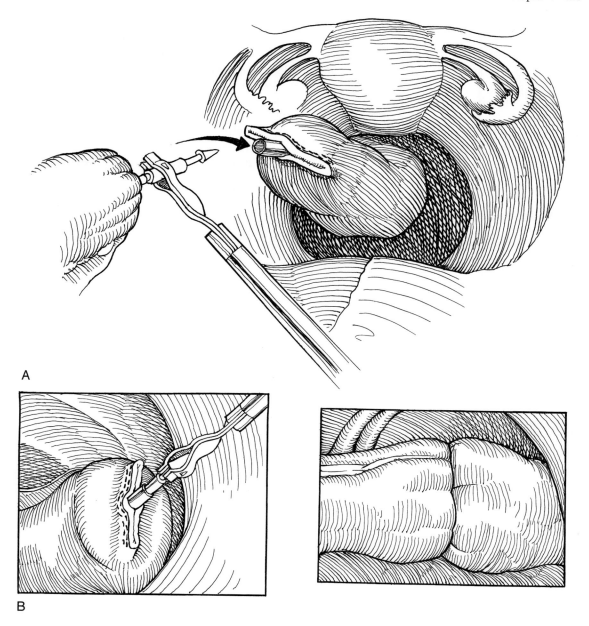

A

B

FIGURE 34-11

FIGURE 34-11A. Anastomosis. The rectal stump is cleansed with dilute aqueous povidone-iodine, and the shaft of the circular staple gun is introduced, bringing the spike through the anterior end of the linear staple line.

FIGURE 34-11B. Using Babcocks inserted through the right lower port, the spike is detached and removed from the abdomen. The anvil spike is regrasped with Babcocks inserted through the right lower port and engaged in the staple gun. Once complete, the anastomosis is air-tested, and the doughnuts are checked for completeness.

The peritoneal cavity is lavaged with antibiotic solution, a suction drain to the pelvis is left in place, and all port sites are closed with absorbable suture.

X. Postoperative Medications

A. Broad-spectrum antibiotics for 24 hours
B. Low dose sodium heparin prophylaxis until discharge from hospital
C. Bupivacaine hydrochloride 0.5 per cent to port sites
D. Suppository of a nonsteroidal anti-inflammatory drug at completion of operation
E. Opiate analgesia usually required for 24 hours

XI. Advancement of Diet

A. Free fluids are given from postoperative day 1
B. Regular diet allowed from postoperative day 1 or 2

XII. Determinants of Discharge

The urinary catheter, IV drip, and drain are usually removed by day 2, allowing early mobilization. Discharge from the hospital normally occurs on day 3 or 4, depending on patient mobility and comfort. Patients generally go home before their bowels have opened.

XIII. Return to Normal Activity/Work

No special guidance in regard to physical activity is given. Patients are usually fully mobile by 1 week and return to their normal activities by 2 weeks, depending on occupation.

Chapter 35

Laparoscopic-Assisted Total Abdominal Colectomy

JOHANN PFEIFER, M.D., and STEVEN D. WEXNER, M.D.

I. Indications

A. Inflammatory bowel disease
   1. Mucosal ulcerative colitis
   2. Crohn's colitis
   3. Indeterminate colitis
B. Neoplasia
   1. Familial adenomatous polyposis
   2. Synchronous colonic polyps
C. Functional disorders
   1. Colonic inertia
   2. Megacolon

II. Contraindications

A. Relative
   1. Acute toxic colitis
   2. Perforation
   3. Fistula
   4. Multiple previous surgeries
B. Absolute
   1. Severe concomitant cardiac or pulmonary disease
   2. Intolerance for general anesthesia
   3. Bleeding disorders
   4. Concomitant pregnancy
   5. Curable colonic malignancy

III. Factors Important in Patient Selection

A. Body habitus
B. General condition of the patient
C. Patient's preference

IV. Preoperative Preparation

A. Admission morning of scheduled surgery, unless otherwise indicated
B. Preoperative medications
   1. Fluid: morning of surgery: 1 liter of Ringer's lactate, 80 ml/hr
   2. Antibiotics (evening prior to surgery)
      a. Oral: metronidazole 1 g and neomycin 1 g at 1 PM, 2 PM, and 11 PM
      b. Intravenous: Cefotan 2 g in operating theater before surgery begins
   3. Miscellaneous
      a. Subcutaneous enoxaparin sodium (Lovenox) 20 mg in patients at high risk for deep venous thrombosis
      b. Steroids (if necessary): Solu-Cortef 100 mg prior to onset of surgery
C. Bowel preparation: sodium phosphate 45 ml at 4 PM and again at 8 PM the evening prior to surgery

V. Choice of Anesthesia

General anesthesia for all patients

VI. Accessory Devices

A. Pneumatic compression stockings are used in all patients from admission to hospital until the patient is fully ambulatory after surgery.
B. Intraoperative orogastric tube is inserted after induction of anesthesia and prior to

placement of the first port; it is removed prior to transport to the recovery room.

C. Bladder catheter is placed in the operating theater after induction of anesthesia.

D. Mushroom catheter for rectal washout is placed in operating theater after induction of anesthesia.

VII. Instruments and Telescopes

A. Laparoscopic
  1. 10-mm, 0-degree telescope
  2. Five 10/12-mm trocars
  3. One disposable 10-mm ultrasonic dissector
  4. One 10-mm extra long suction/irrigation set
  5. Two to three 10-mm Babcock clamps
  6. Two 10-mm noncrushing bowel clamps
  7. Two 10-mm Kelly clamps
  8. Two 10-mm diameter 10-mm long clip appliers
  9. One 12-mm diameter 30-mm long endoscopic linear cutter with two vascular cartridges
  10. One 18-mm diameter port
  11. One 18-mm diameter 60-mm long endoscopic linear cutter with two vascular cartridges

B. Open
  1. Laparoscopic-assisted total abdominal colectomy with end ileostomy and Hartmann pouch
    a. 3–0 chromic stoma maturation sutures
    b. Stoma supplies

  2. Laparoscopic-assisted total abdominal colectomy with ileoproctostomy
    a. One 29-mm or 33-mm diameter circular stapler
    b. One purse-string device or suture
  3. Laparoscopic-assisted total abdominal colectomy with restorative proctocolectomy with ileal J-pouch and loop ileostomy
    a. One 100-mm long linear cutter with two cartridges
    b. One 30-mm long linear stapler
    c. One 0 Prolene suture with an SH needle
    d. One 29-mm or 33-mm diameter circular stapler
    e. One modified Allis (anvil grasping) clamp
    f. 3–0 chromic stoma maturation sutures
    g. Stoma supplies

VIII. Position of Monitors and Position and Size of Trocars

FIGURE 35–1. Two video monitors are used; one is usually positioned on the right and one on the left side of the patient. Normally, the surgeon's monitor is moved toward the shoulder or the pelvis depending on the phase of the operation. The surgeon should always have a view parallel with the camera toward the operative field. We use five 10/12-mm trocars so that every instrument can be inserted into every port without the need for reducer caps.

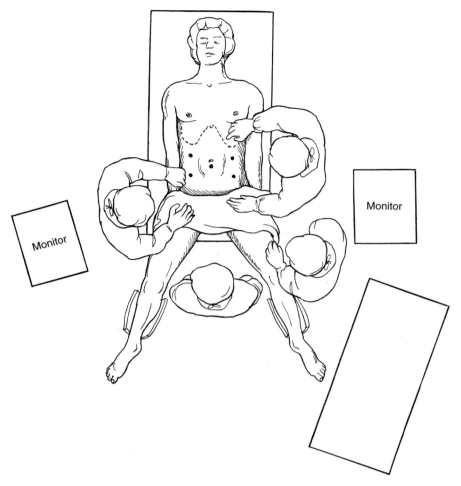

FIGURE 35-1

IX. Narrative of Surgical Technique

In principle, this operation can be modified in three ways:

1. Laparoscopic-assisted total abdominal colectomy with end ileostomy and Hartmann pouch
2. Laparoscopic-assisted total abdominal colectomy with ileoproctostomy
3. Laparoscopic-assisted total abdominal colectomy with restorative proctocolectomy with ileal J-pouch and loop ileostomy

After induction of general anesthesia, the patient is placed in the supine modified lithotomy position with the legs in Allen stirrups (Allen Medical Inc., Bedford Heights, OH). After a mushroom catheter has been inserted into the rectum a complete washout with approximately 1 liter of normal saline and subsequently povidone-iodine is performed. After the abdomen has been prepared in the usual manner, a 1-cm vertical infraumbilical incision is made, and the Veress needle is inserted into the peritoneal cavity. After carbon dioxide has been insufflated to a pressure of 15 mm Hg, a 10/12-mm trocar and the 0-degree camera are inserted. Under direct vision, four more 10/12-mm ports are placed in the left and right upper quadrants as well as in the left and right lower quadrants; all ports are lateral from the rectus muscle.

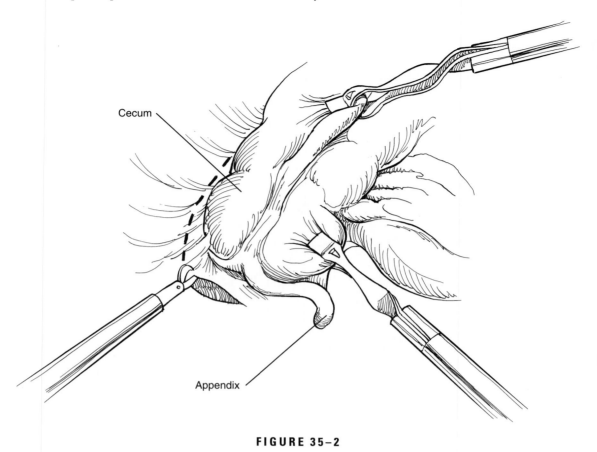

Cecum

Appendix

FIGURE 35–2

FIGURE 35–2. Using the Babcock clamp, the cecum and ascending colon are gently grasped and retracted toward the midline.

FIGURE 35–3. With the patient in the Trendelenburg position, mobilization of the colon is started at the right iliac fossa and proceeds up to and around the hepatic flexure. The dissection is performed with ultrasonic scissors, taking care to identify both the duodenum and the right ureter.

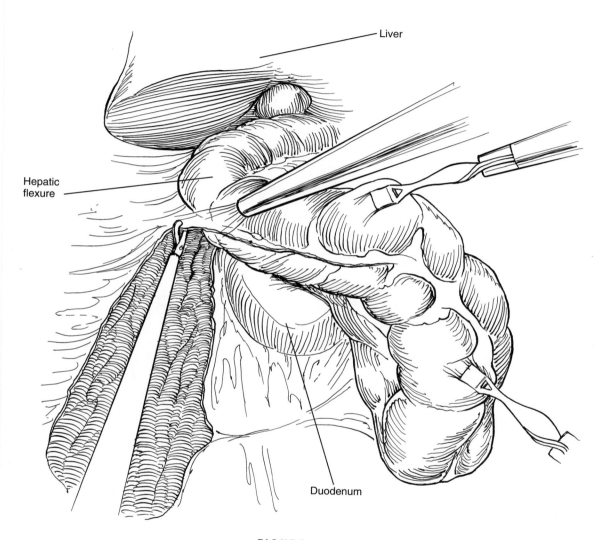

FIGURE 35-3

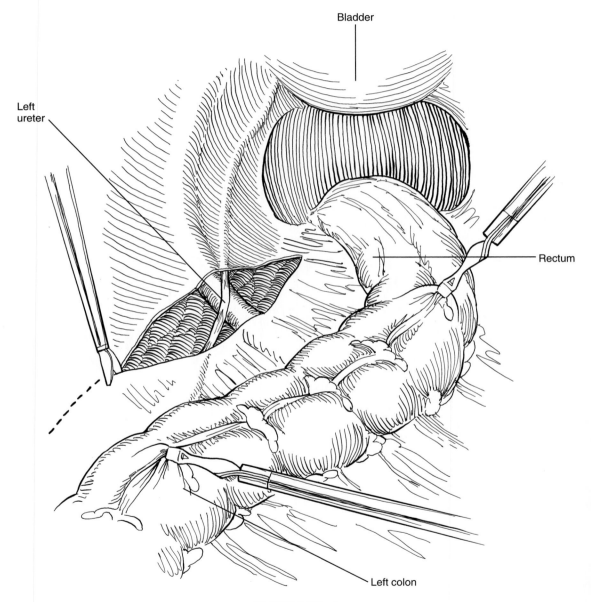

FIGURE 35-4

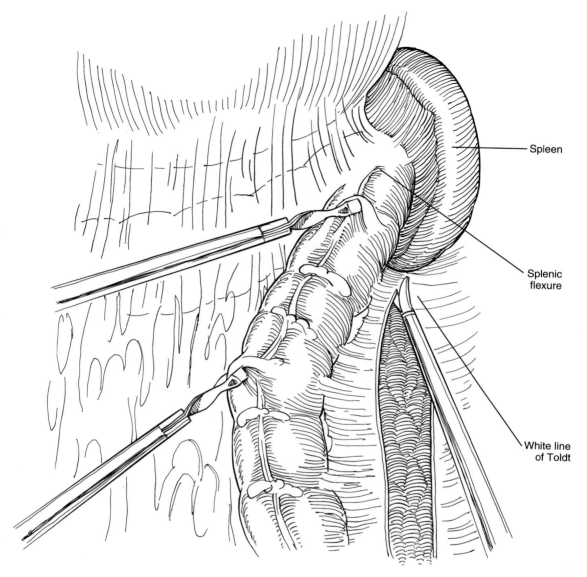

Spleen

Splenic
flexure

White line
of Toldt

FIGURE 35–5

FIGURE 35–4. The next step is mobilization of the left colon.

FIGURE 35–5. Following the white line of Toldt, the sigmoid and descending colon are freed to approximately the splenic flexure. Again, medial traction is provided with the bowel clamps.

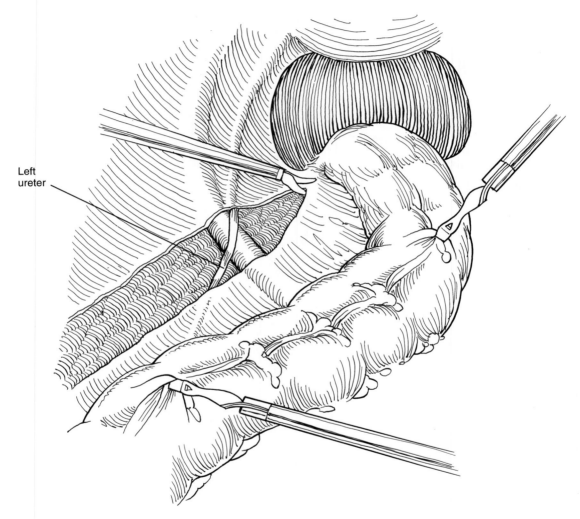

Left
ureter

FIGURE 35–6

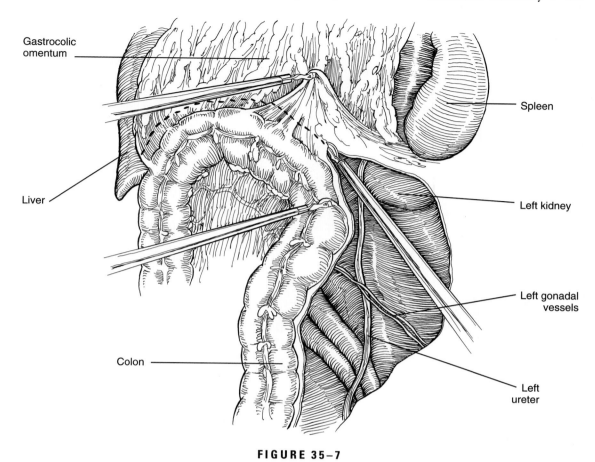

Gastrocolic
omentum

Liver

Colon

Spleen

Left kidney

Left gonadal
vessels

Left
ureter

FIGURE 35–7

FIGURE 35–6. The left ureter is always identified.

FIGURE 35–7. The entire gastrocolic omentum is then divided, visualizing the gastroepiploic vessels and dividing the vessels in the gastrocolic omentum sequentially, using two clips on the proximal side and one clip on the specimen side; endoloops can be used.

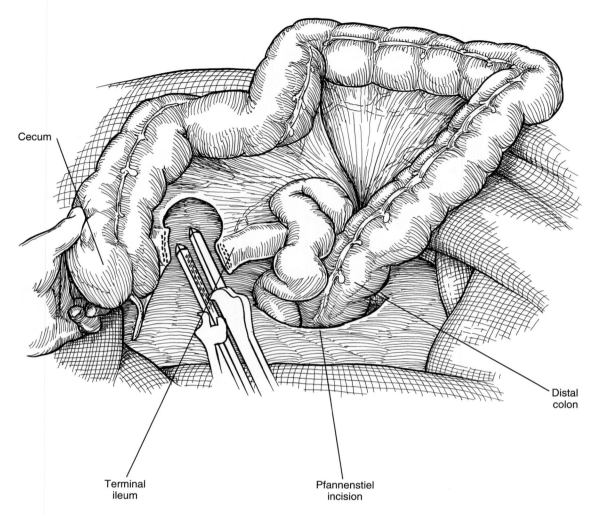

Cecum

Terminal
ileum

Pfannenstiel
incision

Distal
colon

FIGURE 35–8

FIGURE 35–8. After the entire colon has been mobilized, a Pfannenstiel incision is made. The entire colon is then delivered through the wound, and the mesentery is scored and the vessels divided and ligated in the usual manner.

FIGURE 35–9. Alternatively, intracorporeal division of the mesenteric vessels using a laparoscopic linear cutting device may be performed.

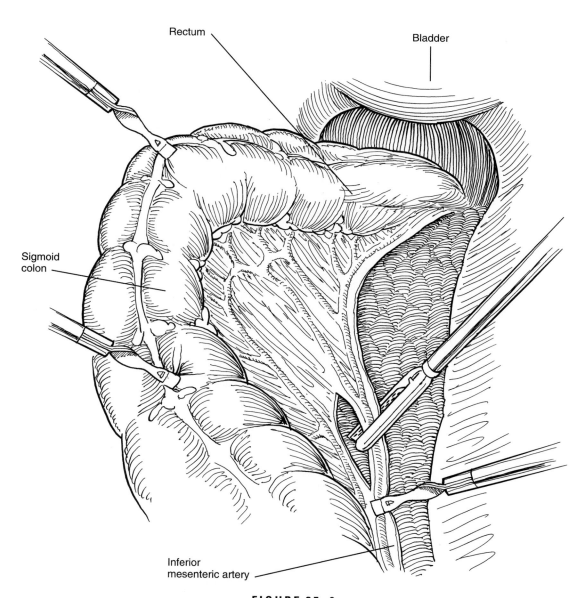

Rectum

Bladder

Sigmoid
colon

Inferior
mesenteric artery

FIGURE 35–9

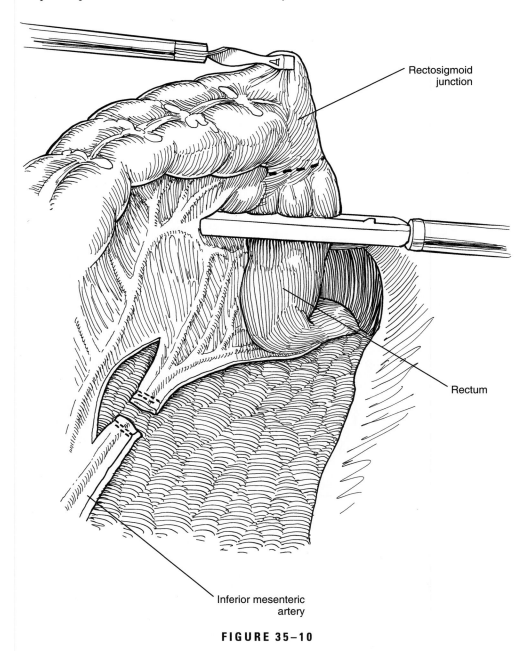

Rectosigmoid junction

Rectum

Inferior mesenteric artery

FIGURE 35–10

FIGURE 35–10. In performing an abdominal colectomy and ileorectal anastomosis, intracorporeal division of the rectum can also be accomplished using a laparoscopic linear cutting device.

FIGURE 35–11. If a J-pouch is planned (see Chapter 36), it is much more cost effective, in terms of both operative time and instrument cost, to perform extracorporeal vascular division. In addition, the rectal dissection and tran-

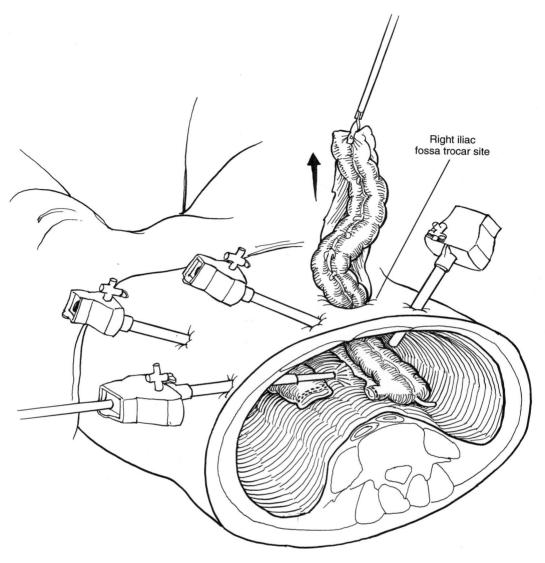

Right iliac
fossa trocar site

FIGURE 35-11

section, pouch construction, and anastomosis can all be performed through the Pfannenstiel incision. Alternatively, if an end ileostomy or an ileoproctostomy is planned, intracorporeal vascular division is more justifiable. In these situations the laparoscopic stapling device, while expensive, allows rapid vascular control. In a Brooke ileostomy, the rectosigmoid junction is transected with a 60-mm long stapling device. The right iliac fossa ileostomy site is then prepared, and the entire specimen is delivered through that site. At the end of the specimen, the terminal ileum is delivered in continuity.

Extracorporeal bowel division is then accomplished using a 75-mm linear cutter. Before the stoma matures, the abdomen is reinsufflated to verify orientation of the terminal ileum and its mesentery. Hemostasis is verified as well.

With an ileoproctostomy, the identical procedure is performed as far as transection at the rectosigmoid junction. At that point, the 10/12-mm left iliac fossa port is exchanged for a 33-mm port. The specimen is then delivered until the terminal ileum is retrieved. After the purse string has been applied, the anvil of the 29-mm or 33-mm circular stapler is placed in the lumen, and the bowel is returned to the abdominal cavity. After pneumoperitoneum is reestablished, the modified Allis (anvil grasper) clamp is used to replace the anvil over the receptable port. The anastomosis is then fashioned. The doughnuts are inspected, and anastomotic integrity is verified by performing the saline and air insufflation test during direct transanal endoscopic visualization of the anastomosis. After verification of hemostasis, the ports are removed. Regardless of approach, all fascial port sites are closed under direct vision.

IX. Postoperative Medications

A. Cefotan 2 g IV/day × 1
B. Intravenous patient-controlled anesthesia (PCA) pump: meperidine hydrochloride up to 10 to 15 mg per hour or morphine sulfate up to 6 mg per hour for 2 to 3 days
C. Corticoids (if necessary): hydrocortisone 100 mg IV every 8 hours for 24 hours, then 50 mg every 8 hours for 24 hours; if patient is eating, oral steroids are given as needed

XI. Advancement of Diet

A nasogastric tube is inserted if the patient vomits more than 100 ml more than two times in 24 hours. In all other patients, a clear liquid diet is started on postoperative day 1 with advancement to a solid diet as tolerated within 48 to 72 hours.

XII. Determinants of Discharge

The patient should have eaten a solid diet for at least 24 hours and should have had at least one normal bowel movement. The abdomen should be soft, flat, and nontender, and the wounds should be clean. The patient should be afebrile and have a normal complete blood count.

XIII. Return to Normal Activity/Work

Depending on the patient's overall general condition, normal activity or work should be resumed within 2 to 3 weeks.

Laparoscopic Total Proctocolectomy with Ileoanal Anastomosis

DAVID N. ARMSTRONG, M.D., and WAYNE L. AMBROZE, M.D.

I. Indications

A. Chronic ulcerative colitis
   1. Intractable symptoms despite maximum medical therapy.
   2. Side effects of medications (prednisone, 6-mercaptopurine, cyclosporine).
   3. Dysplasia, carcinoma in situ, or early colonic carcinoma (T2, N0, or less).
   4. Acute toxic dilatation unresponsive to medical therapy. This usually requires a three-stage procedure: total abdominal colectomy and end ileostomy, subsequent J-pouch and diverting loop ileostomy, and third-stage reversal of ileostomy).
B. Familial adenomatous polyposis
   1. Multiple symptomatic rectal polyps
   2. Dysplasia, carcinoma in situ, or early colonic carcinoma (T2, N0, or less).

II. Contraindications

A. Anorectal sphincter dysfunction. Normal sphincter function is a prerequisite for construction of an ileal J-pouch. Mechanical sphincter disruption or pudendal neuropathy is a contraindication for creating a J-pouch.
B. Senility or mental retardation. Construction and subsequent management of an ileal J-pouch is a prolonged and involved undertaking. A motivated and informed patient is an absolute prerequisite.
C. Crohn's disease. Recurrence in the ileal J-pouch and anastomotic leaks result in eventual resection and end ileostomy in about 50% of patients.
D. Rectal carcinoma. The presence of a biopsy-proven rectal carcinoma raises the possibility of subsequent chemotherapy and radiation. Radiation of the pouch results in a high incidence of pouch dysfunction. Prestaging using endorectal ultrasound may identify early (T1 and T2) carcinomas, and these patients could be candidates for an ileal J-pouch since chemotherapy and/or radiation is unnecessary. Nonetheless, preoperative lymph node involvement remains unknown.

III. Factors Important in Patient Selection

A. Age and general health. The ideal patients are young, motivated individuals in excellent health. Although advanced age is not a contraindication, senility certainly is. In addition, good general health is necessary to embark on any extensive laparoscopic surgery such as proctocolectomy and J-pouch formation. Coexisting pulmonary disease such as chronic obstructive pulmonary disease (COPD) may be a contraindication because of hypercapnia resulting from carbon dioxide insufflation. Hypercapnia may also result in acidosis, hyperkalemia, and cardiac arrhythmias. Satisfactory cardiorespiratory function is therefore a prerequisite.

B. Motivation and IQ. A highly motivated patient with a basic understanding of the postoperative management of the ileostomy and J-pouch is a prerequisite. Mental retardation is a contraindication not only because of the lack of understanding but also because of the high incidence of anorectal incontinence associated with it.

C. Occupation and hobbies. Occupations such as long distance truck driving make frequent trips to the bathroom a difficult undertaking. Patient selection should involve inquiry into the patient's occupation and hobbies that make a permanent ileostomy a more suitable choice of procedure.

IV. Preoperative Preparation

A. Patients are admitted on the morning of surgery after having performed bowel preparation at home. Dehydration is very common, and intravenous (IV) fluids are started at least 2 hours before surgery. At least 1 to 2 liters of IV isotonic fluid are given to compensate for the loss in electrolytes incurred during bowel preparation.

B. Preoperative medications include enteric antibiotics taken the day before surgery. The traditional neomycin/erythromycin combination taken three times on the day before surgery is often confusing to the patient. A simpler and equally effective regimen involves taking 2 g of metronidazole (Flagyl) in the late evening after the bowel preparation.

C. Prophylaxis for deep venous thrombosis (DVT). At least four risk factors are present in all proctocolectomy patients—laparoscopic surgery, prolonged surgery, pelvic surgery, and inflammatory bowel disease. If additional risk factors are present (e.g., previous DVT), enoxaparin sodium (Lovenox) 30 mg is given subcutaneously preoperatively.

D. Bowel preparation. One gallon of ethylene glycol (Colyte) is drunk over a period of 2 to 3 hours the evening before surgery. This

is the gold standard against which all other bowel preparations are compared. Although unpatatable to the patient, reassurance can be given that this is the last time they will have to drink the preparation. Magnesium citrate is an adequate preparation for closure of the loop ileostomy.

V. Choice of Anesthesia

General anesthesia with endotracheal intubation is the simplest and safest form of anesthesia. In rare circumstances, epidural anesthesia may be necessary, although surgical traction on the greater omentum often causes patient discomfort. Postoperative pain control by epidural anesthesia is, however, the postoperative analgesic of choice.

VI. Accessory Devices

A. After general anesthesia has been induced and endotracheal intubation has been completed, an orogastric tube is placed for the duration of the operation; it is removed after the procedure. Nasogastric tubes are uncomfortable, and the low incidence of gastroparesis or gastric emptying problems makes routine nasogastric decompression unnecessary.

B. A Foley catheter is inserted for postoperative fluid monitoring and to prevent early postoperative urinary retention resulting from traction and dissection within the pelvis. In females the urinary catheter can be discontinued after the second day, although because of the proximity of the bladder to the rectum, a longer period usually is necessary in males.

C. Thigh-high pneumatic compression stockings are applied to the legs prior to induction of anesthesia. If there are additional risk factors for thromboembolism, the stockings are supplemented by subcutaneous Lovenox.

VII. Instruments and Telescopes

A wide variety of telescopes, trocars, and laparoscopic instruments are now available. Surgeon preference is the first priority, although the relative costs of instruments have become an important selection factor. Use a nondisposable Hassan trocar through which the laparoscope is inserted. Twelve-millimeter disposable trocars (Ethicon Endosurgery, Cincinnati, OH) and anchoring screws are used for the lateral trocar sites and a 5-mm nondisposable trocar is used as the suprapubic port. The Ethicon Endoshears and Endo-Babcock provide large atraumatic grasps of tissue and are comfortable to handle.

VIII. Position of Monitors and Placement and Size of Trocars

FIGURE 36–1. If the operating surgeon is right-handed, a position on the patient's left side facilitates the pelvic dissection, since the operating hand can be pointed toward the operative field. Mobilization of the ascending and descending colon is easily accomplished from the left, although mobilization of the transverse colon may require standing between the patient's legs temporarily.

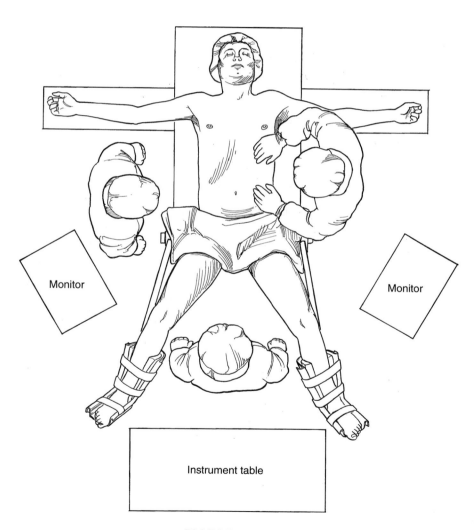

FIGURE 36–1

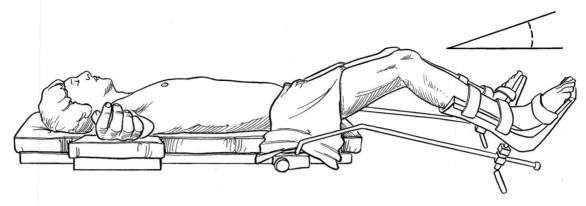

FIGURE 36-2

FIGURE 36-2. The patient is placed in a modified lithotomy position with the legs in stirrups at the same horizontal plane as the torso. Care is taken not to produce excessive internal or external rotation of the hips, and pressure on the gastrocnemius muscle from the leg supports is avoided. Both arms are tucked by the sides of the body, and both hands are wrapped to avoid inadvertent electrical contact with the table. Tucking the arms provides room for the surgeon to maneuver; otherwise he or she is restricted if the arms are placed on arm boards.

FIGURE 36-3. The Hassan trocar is inserted through an umbilical incision, which allows the greatest arc length within the peritoneal cavity. Twelve-millimeter trocars are placed in the left and right lower quadrants, and the right-sided trocar is placed at the planned loop ileostomy site. The 5-mm suprapubic trocar is used to retract the rectum during dissection of the presacral plane. The monitors are placed cephalad to the patient during dissection of the ascending, transverse, and descending colon and are subsequently moved caudad to the patient during dissection of the pelvis. Both the surgeon's and the assistant's monitors are placed in the same plane to avoid confusion and disorientation between the two operators.

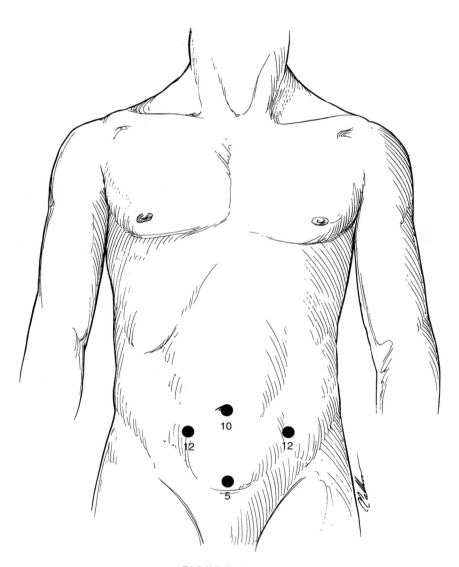

FIGURE 36–3

IX. Narrative of Surgical Technique

FIGURE 36-4. The terminal ileum or cecum is grasped by Endo-Babcock clamps placed through the right lower quadrant trocar and is placed on stretch by exerting traction toward the midline. The surgeon, standing on the left, divides the lateral peritoneal attachments of the cecum and the ascending colon toward the hepatic flexure. The terminal ileum is mobilized by dividing the base of the mesentery. Care is taken not to divide the mesentery too close to the ileum since the mesentery may be entered. The terminal ileum, cecum, and ascending colon are mobilized entirely on the ileocolic artery.

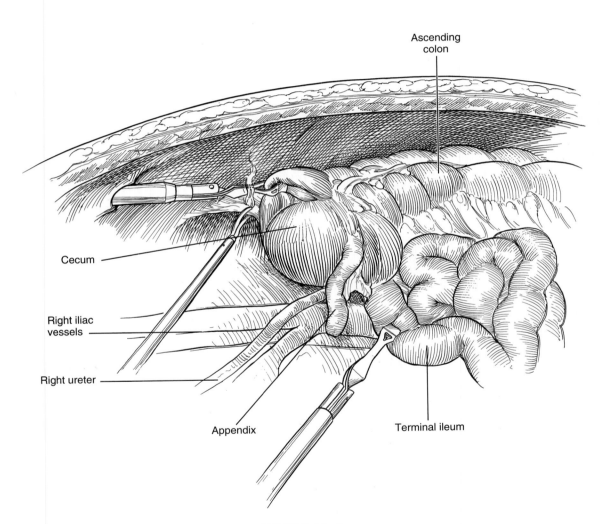

FIGURE 36-4

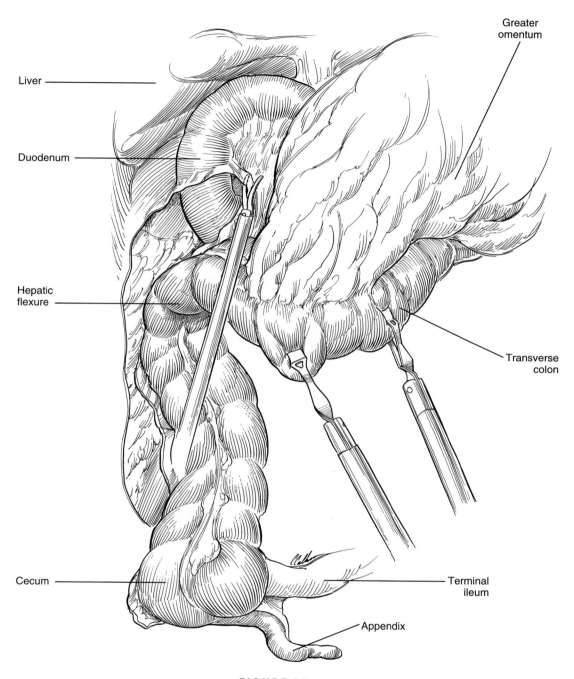

FIGURE 36–5

FIGURE 36–5. The hepatic flexure is mobilized by grasping the greater omentum, which is flipped into the upper abdomen to lie anterior to the stomach. This exposes the entire transverse colon and makes the avascular plane accessible. The greater omentum is grasped by one Endo-Babcock, the transverse colon is grasped by a second Endo-Babcock, and the avascular plane is divided to the right of the midline. Toward the hepatic flexure a number of thin-walled omental veins are encountered, and these require individual clipping before they are divided.

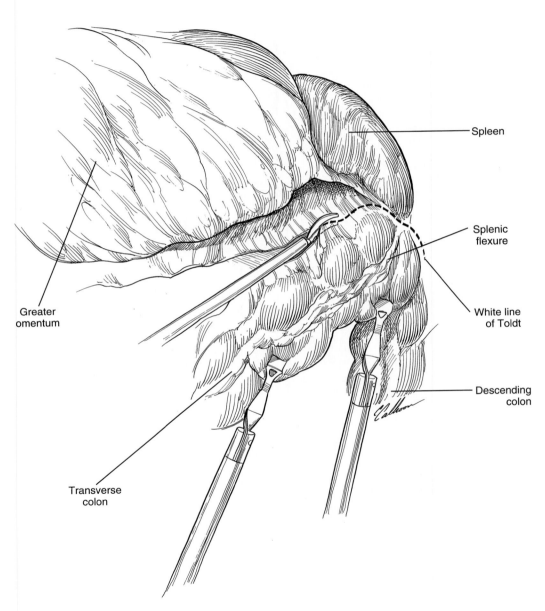

Spleen

Splenic
flexure

White line
of Toldt

Descending
colon

Greater
omentum

Transverse
colon

FIGURE 36-6

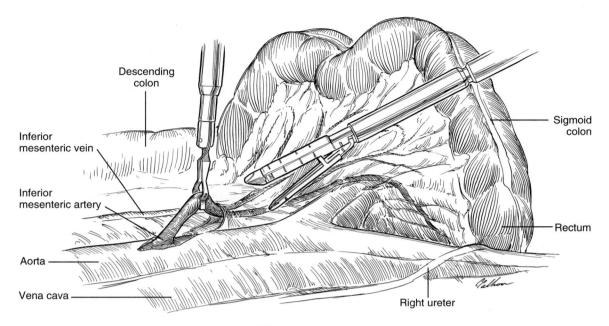

Descending colon

Inferior mesenteric vein

Inferior mesenteric artery

Aorta

Vena cava

Sigmoid colon

Rectum

Right ureter

FIGURE 36–7

FIGURE 36–6. The transverse colon is mobilized most easily by continuing in the avascular plane and entering the lesser sac to the left of the midline. Again, the greater omentum and the transverse colon are each grasped by Endo-Babcocks, and the avascular plane is developed using Endoshears. This surgical plane avoids the tedious cautery or clipping of numerous omental vessels that would be required if one entered the gastric colon plane.

Because the lesser sac has been entered to the left of the midline, the avascular plane provides a surprisingly easy route to the mobilization of the entire transverse colon including the splenic flexure. Difficulties may be encountered in extremely thin individuals because the omentum contains little fat, and the avascular plane is difficult to identify. The splenic flexure is mobilized by extending the dissection in the avascular plane to the left of the midline. This is facilitated by mobilizing the proximal descending colon by dividing the white lateral peritoneal attachment, the white line of Toldt. After remobilizing the distal transverse colon and the proximal descending colon, the splenic flexure is mobilized from the adjacent spleen and the underlying retroperitoneum.

FIGURE 36–7. The descending and sigmoid colon is mobilized by grasping the sigmoid colon with the Endo-Babcock from the right lower quadrant trocar and applying traction toward the midline. Care is taken as always to identify the left ureter. The inferior mesenteric artery can be isolated by grasping the rectosigmoid mesentery with Endo-Babcocks and placing the base of the vessels on traction. The peritoneum over the inferior mesenteric vessels can be divided, and the vessels can be dissected circumferentially. Care is taken to identify the left ureter, which lies in very close proximity. An Endo GIA stapler is fired across the base of the vessels, providing surgical access to the presacral plane through an avascular route.

FIGURE 36-8. The pelvis is dissected by grasping the proximal rectum through the suprapubic site. A second Endo-Babcock clamp can be placed in the presacral plane after the inferior mesenteric artery has been divided. Using Endoshears, the avascular plane can be entered with relative ease, and this is dissected as far as possible distally. Switching from left to right, the lateral ligaments are divided using Endoshears and cautery. The rectovaginal septum or rectovesical plane is developed in a similar manner by placing an Endo-Babcock in the posterior uterus in females or in the base of the bladder in males. Care is taken to identify the seminal vesicles during dissection in males.

After the rectal dissection has been completed as far as possible toward the levators, the laparoscopic part of the procedure is finished, and a small longitudinal incision is made in the umbilicus. The cecum is delivered through the incision, and the terminal ileum is divided as close to the cecum as possible. The terminal branches of the ileocecal artery supplying the cecum and ascending colon are serially divided and ligated.

This preserves the maximum length of the ileocolic artery to provide maximum mobility of the terminal ileum. The ascending and proximal transverse colon is then delivered through the umbilical incision, and the supplying arteries are divided and ligated. The middle colic branches are divided, and the splenic flexure and descending colon are delivered through the umbilical incision. If the inferior mesenteric artery was divided sufficiently proximal on the aorta, very few branches will remain to supply the descending colon, thereby facilitating surgical mobilization of the left colon. After the entire colon has been delivered and devascularized, the terminal ileum is transected using a GIA stapler and a Babcock clamp applied to prevent it from slipping back into the abdomen. The rectosigmoid junction is then transected, again using a GIA stapler, after the terminal branches of the inferior mesenteric artery have been divided in the proximal mesorectum. This allows the bulky colon to be removed from the surgical field and facilitates subsequent construction of the pouch.

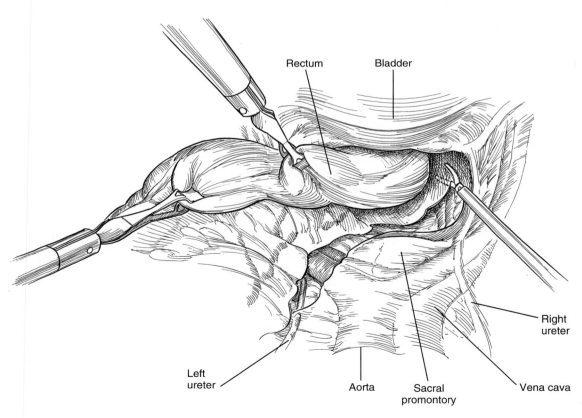

Rectum   Bladder

Right ureter

Left ureter   Aorta   Sacral promontory   Vena cava

FIGURE 36-8

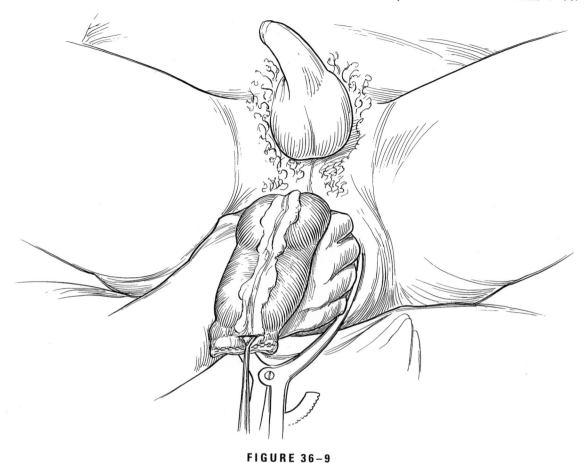

FIGURE 36-9

FIGURE 36-9. The rectal dissection is then completed by a perineal operator. A Pratt speculum is placed in the anal canal with the patient in a steep Trendelenburg position. The anoderm is infiltrated with 0.25 per cent Marcaine with epinephrine, and the presacral space is entered posteriorly, just proximal to the dentate line. The remaining lateral attachments at the level of the levators are divided using cautery, and the rectum is delivered posteriorly through the surgical defect. The anterior dissection is then completed, and the rectum is delivered. Irrigation is then performed using warm saline, and attention is turned to creating the ileal J-pouch.

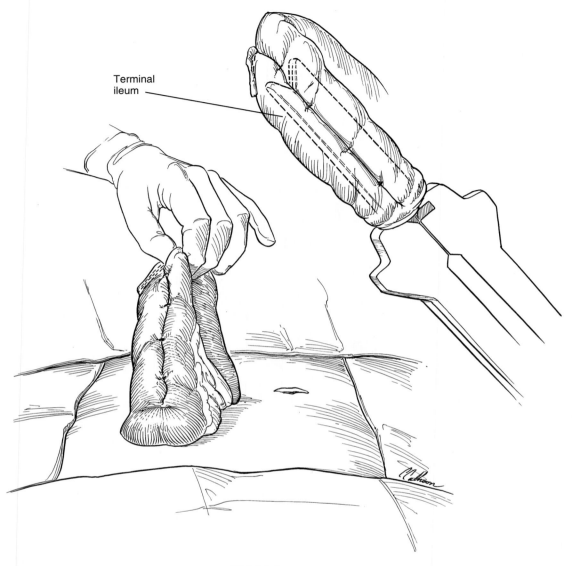

Terminal
ileum

FIGURE 36–10

FIGURE 36–10. The terminal ileum is delivered through the umbilical incision and is mobilized to the source of the ileocolic artery at the inferior border of the third part of the duodenum. A 12- to 15-cm J-pouch is created by firing two GIA staplers down each limb of the ileum. From the perineum, interrupted 2–0 Vicryl sutures are placed at the level of the dentate line at all four quadrants and at points between. The pouch is then delivered through the pelvis, and the ileal J-pouch–anal anastomosis is completed.

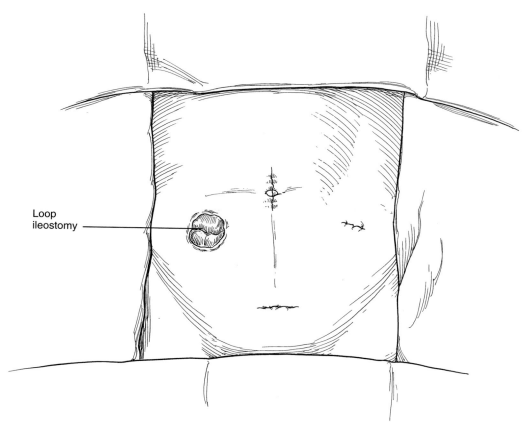

FIGURE 36–11

FIGURE 36–11. The diverting loop ileostomy is created at the right lateral trocar site as close to the ileal J-pouch as possible. A No. 10 Jackson-Pratt drain is brought out through the left trocar site, and the umbilical incision is closed.

X. Postoperative Medications

A. Postoperative analgesics are given most effectively through a previously inserted epidural catheter. Alternatively, morphine given through a patient-controlled analgesia (PCA) device produces acceptable results.

B. The patient is kept nil per os (NPO) except for ice chips until ileostomy output is noted. Tylenol (650 mg every 4 hours) is given with sips of water if a temperature of greater than 101 degrees is present. The patient is encouraged to use incentive spirometry and to ambulate on the first postoperative day. Broad-spectrum antibiotics are given for the first 24 hours and then discontinued.

XI. Advancement of Diet

Usually on the third postoperative day some output from the ileostomy is noted. At this stage, the patient is started on clear liquids and advanced to full liquids and then to a low residue diet. The patient is seen by a dietitian, who explains the need to avoid fresh fruits and vegetables to prevent blockage of the loop ileostomy. The patient is also instructed on what types of food increase or decrease ileostomy output.

XII. Determinants of Discharge

When oral analgesia is adequate and the patient is tolerating an adequate diet and is confident with stoma management, he or she is discharged home. Follow-up is arranged in 2 weeks.

XIII. Reversal of Ileostomy

Reversal of the ileostomy is usually performed 6 to 8 weeks after the original surgery. A Gastrografin pouchogram is obtained prior to closure of the ileostomy to exclude the presence of any pouch sinus or fistula. Routine examination in the office of the pouch–anal anastomosis using a pediatric sigmoidoscope is a useful precaution and serves to dilate the flimsy postoperative stenosis at the pouch–anal anastomosis. The ileostomy can be reversed using a circumstomal incision, which is then extended down to the level of the fascia, thus mobilizing the loop ileostomy in its entirety. The easiest technique of reanastomosis is to fire a GIA stapler down each limb of the stoma and then fire a second GIA stapler at right angles to it to complete the anastomosis. The anastomosis is then dropped back into the peritoneal cavity and the fascial defect is closed. The patient is warned to expect frequent and loose bowel movements in the days and weeks after ileostomy closure, although stool frequency decreases spontaneously and can be reduced further using antidiarrheal medications (Lomotil) and fiber. The patient is instructed to "juggle" the use of dietary fiber and antidiarrheal medications to produce an acceptable stool frequency. Usually antidiarrheal medication is not required after the first few weeks, when stool frequency decreases to an acceptable level. The patient continues to ingest fiber indefinitely, which serves to make the ileal content more pasty and more easily controlled. Stool frequency 6 months after surgery averages four to six stools per day.

Chapter 37

Laparoscopic Abdominoperineal Resection

JOHN E. HARTLEY, M.B., B.Sc., and JOHN R.T. MONSON, M.D., F.R.C.S.I., F.A.C.S.

I. Indications

In principle, the indications for laparoscopic abdominoperineal excision should be identical to those for the conventional procedure—that is, the treatment of low rectal cancer. During conventional open surgery the final decision about a low anterior resection versus abdominoperineal excision can be made at a late stage in the procedure after a trial pelvic dissection, and the patient is counseled accordingly preoperatively. During laparoscopic surgery much useful tactile information is lost, and if strict selection criteria are applied, the laparoscopist will not visualize those tumors that are appropriately treated by abdominoperineal resection. If inappropriate sphincter sacrifice is to be avoided, the surgeon must be certain of the intended resection preoperatively. In our practice this decision is made at a preliminary examination under anesthesia.

II. Contraindications

A. Absolute: the presence of a lesion suitable for a sphincter-saving procedure using conventional surgical techniques
B. Relative
1. Significant cardiovascular impairment
2. Cardiorespiratory problems
3. Obesity
4. Previous surgery
C. Tumor-related factors: Locally advanced disease with invasion of the contiguous pel-

vic structures need not preclude laparoscopic surgery, although it is likely to render it a difficult and perhaps hazardous venture.

III. Preoperative Preparation

A. Examination under general anesthesia. The preoperative work-up of patients undergoing abdominoperineal resection is broadly similar to that of patients subjected to conventional surgery with some important provisos. As alluded to earlier, we always undertake a preliminary examination under separate general anesthesia to confirm the diagnosis but most importantly to decide whether abdominoperineal excision or a sphincter-saving procedure is appropriate.
B. Endoanal ultrasonography. In addition, the oncologic safety of the laparoscopic approach in such circumstances is at best uncertain. We therefore undertake preoperative imaging with both magnetic resonance imaging (MRI), and endoanal ultrasonography. The results of this imaging may play a role first in the decision about the choice of surgical approach and second in considering whether preoperative chemoradiotherapy is desirable.
C. Double contrast barium enema. In addition, synchronous lesions may be overlooked at laparoscopy, particularly in the absence of serosal involvement. We therefore undertake a preoperative contrast examination of

the entire colon in all patients before laparoscopic colorectal surgery to exclude the presence of additional lesions.

D. Routine admission. The in-hospital preoperative preparation is thereafter identical to that employed prior to open surgery. The patient is admitted on the morning of the day prior to surgery.

E. Bowel preparation. We administer polyethylene glycol as bowel preparation.

F. Thromboembolic prophylaxis, in the form of subcutaneous heparin and graduated compression stockings, is also commenced on admission and continued postoperatively until the patient is mobile.

G. Antibiotic prophylaxis. Our antibiotic prophylaxis comprises intravenous metronidazole and a second-generation cephalosporin, commenced on induction of anesthesia and continued with two further doses 6 and 12 hours afterward. This regimen is identical to that which we use for open colorectal surgery.

H. Enterostomal therapist. Preoperative counseling by the stoma therapist is of course mandatory in all patients consenting to abdominoperineal resection, and the patient is marked accordingly.

I. Adequate peripheral and central venous access is requisite, and in those patients with cardiovascular impairment a pulmonary flotation catheter should be considered.

IV. Choice of Anesthesia

General endotracheal anesthesia is used

V. Accessory Devices

Graduated compression stockings

VI. Instruments and Telescopes

A. Full videolaparoscopy facilities are required with preferably two video monitors.

B. A standard 10-mm diameter, 0-degree laparoscope is used throughout the procedure.

C. A 30-degree laparoscope may be of benefit during the pelvic dissection.

D. Four standard 10-mm laparoscopy ports, with additional ports being inserted as required. The 10-mm ports are replaced by larger 12- or 15-mm ports to allow the use of stapling devices at the appropriate moment.

E. A pair of Babcock-type bowel graspers

F. Curved disposable scissors and hooked endoscopic scissors with a monopolar diathermy attachment. The latter instrument permits tissues to be held away from other structures before they are cut with diathermy.

G. One linear stapling device such as the Endo GIA 30 or 60 device (United States Surgical Corporation, Norwalk, CT) with additional cartridges

H. One multifiring endoscopic clip applicator

I. Long laparoscopy scissors for use in the pelvic dissection

J. Suction/irrigation equipment

K. A range of ultrasound transducers specifically designed for laparoscopic use are now available. These may prove to be of value in hepatic assessment during laparoscopic colorectal surgery, and this potential role is currently under investigation.

VII. Position of Monitors and Placement and Size of Trocars

FIGURE 37-1A-C. The patient is placed in a modified lithotomy position (A), which allows access to the abdomen and perineum and, by keeping the legs almost straight, prevents the legs from interfering with the movements of the long-handled laparoscopic instruments. The urinary bladder should be catheterized and a nasogastric tube inserted. These latter measures help to guard against Veress needle or trocar injury to the viscera.

As will be described later, the laparoscopic surgeon is heavily dependent on gravity as a means of exposure and retraction. In particular, there is a critical angle of Trendelenburg beyond which the small bowel falls out of the pelvis. The operating table must therefore be capable of being dropped into a steep Trendelenburg or reverse Trendelenburg position and of being rotated to the left or right. We place the patient on a bean bag, which helps to prevent the patient from sliding from the table in these extreme positions.

(B) The videomonitors are best positioned on either side of the patient's knees.

(C) The trocars are positioned as shown.

VIII. Narrative of Surgical Technique

The sequence of steps through which the surgeon proceeds during laparoscopic abdominoperineal excision is of course identical to that followed during the conventional open procedure.

First the abdomen and perineum are prepared and draped, and the anus is closed with a stout purse-string suture No. 1 silk. Carbon dioxide pneumoperitoneum to a pressure of 15 mm Hg is then achieved using either a closed or an open technique. A 10-mm trocar is then inserted, and the 10-mm telescope is introduced.

The remaining laparoscopy ports are inserted in the configuration shown above (Figure 37–1C). These ports must be inserted under direct vision if visceral injury is to be consistently avoided.

Diagnostic Laparoscopy

Preliminary laparoscopy is then performed, during which one should seek to confirm the absence of widespread intraperitoneal disease before paying particular attention to the liver. The surface of the liver must be examined carefully for the presence of metastases. The upper sur-

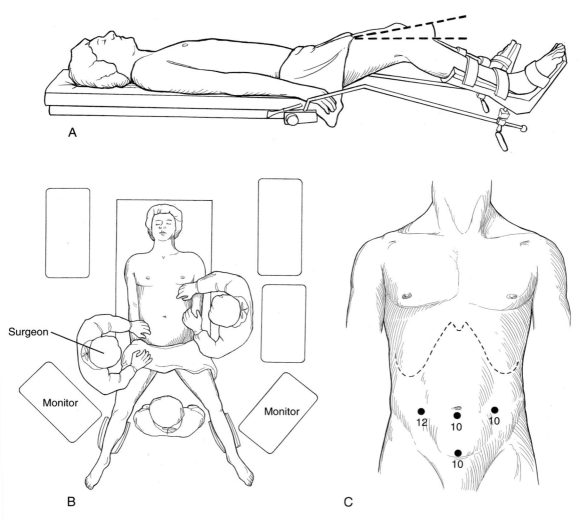

FIGURE 37–1

face of this organ is best examined with the patient in a few degrees of reverse Trendelenburg. Alternatively, a 30-degree laparoscope may be used. We perform our laparoscopic ultrasound assessment of the liver at this point before commencing the procedure itself.

Attention is next turned to the pelvic organs. These must be examined with the patient in a steep Trendelenburg position so that the small bowel falls out of the pelvis. If there are adhesions between the small bowel and pelvic structures that prevent this from occurring, these are divided. This preliminary laparoscopy should allow the surgeon first to confirm that the lesion is resectable and second to decide whether such factors as gross obesity affecting the mesenteries or extensive adhesions from previous surgery preclude a laparoscopic approach, thereby warranting early conversion to formal laparotomy.

FIGURE 37-2. Once the decision is made to proceed laparoscopically our first maneuver is to deal with the inferior mesenteric pedicle. Ligation and division of these vessels at an early stage in the procedure serves to limit blood loss during the pelvic dissection. In addition, elevation of the sigmoid and mobilization of the rectum are easier once the vascular pedicle has been divided. The left colon is held with Babcock clamps and elevated, and mesenteric windows are developed to each side of the vessels so that they can be identified and skeletonized near their origin. One of the lower quadrant ports is then replaced with a 12-mm port, and the artery and vein are separately ligated and divided using a linear cutter stapling device. We have found the Endo GIA 30 with a vascular cartridge to be eminently suited to this task. This device places six rows of staples, three on each side of the incision.

FIGURE 37-2

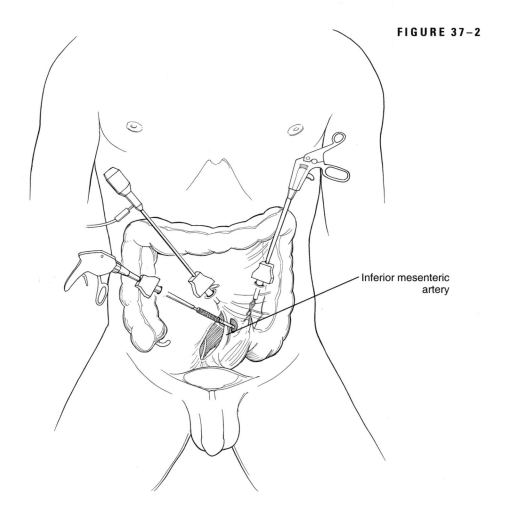

Inferior mesenteric artery

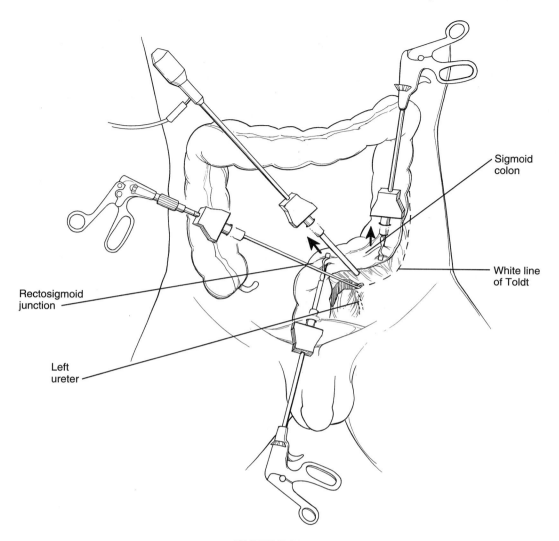

Sigmoid
colon

White line
of Toldt

Rectosigmoid
junction

Left
ureter

FIGURE 37–3

FIGURE 37–3. Next, the sigmoid colon is mobilized. The patient is placed in a steep Trendelenburg position and rolled so that the left shoulder is uppermost, maximizing exposure of the left paracolic gutter. The assistant, standing on the left side of the table, then grasps and elevates the sigmoid loop and rectosigmoid with Babcock-type instruments. The surgeon, standing on the right side of the table, while applying countertraction, again with a Babcock, incises the lateral peritoneal reflection of the sigmoid along the white line of Toldt using electrocautery scissors. As this incision is extended cepha- lad, the mesosigmoid is pushed progressively toward the midline. This lateral incision is sub- sequently continued over the pelvic brim and along the left pelvic side wall. Identification of the left ureter at all stages in this maneuver is vital if iatrogenic injury is to be avoided. In thin patients the ureter can be seen lying behind the transparent posterior parietal peritoneum. However, most often it must be deliberately sought, either at the point where it crosses the common iliac vessels or in the retroperito- neum after the left colon has been mobilized medially.

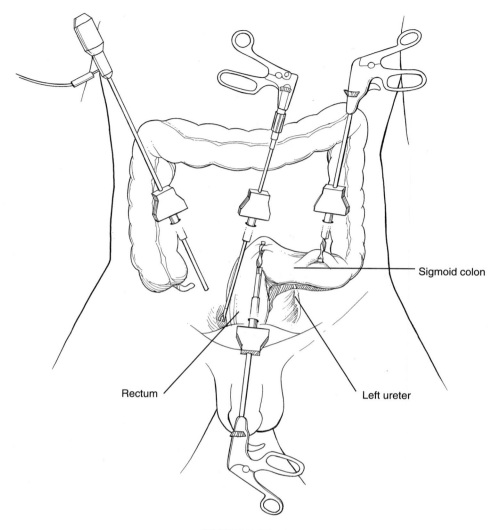

FIGURE 37–4

Sigmoid colon

Rectum

Left ureter

FIGURE 37–4. The key to laparoscopic mobilization of the rectum lies, as in open surgery, in the correct identification of the avascular areolar tissue of the presacral plane, the so-called holy plane of rectal surgery. We commence the rectal dissection at the right pelvic brim. The steep Trendelenburg position is particularly important at this stage to keep the small bowel away from the operative field. The patient's right shoulder is now rolled upward, and the surgeon stands on the right side of the table. The assistant stands opposite the surgeon and elevates the sigmoid and proximal rectum with Babcock clamps. If desired, the sigmoid

loop can be temporarily slung by its apex from the abdominal wall or, alternatively, sutured or stapled in that position. In females, stapling the uterus or fallopian tubes to the anterior abdominal wall provides an alternative means to the same end. The important factor is to provide adequate traction in an anterior direction on the proximal rectum by whatever means is chosen.

FIGURE 37–5. The surgeon then applies countertraction to the retroperitoneum and incises the parietal peritoneum just to the right of the sacral promontory, thus gaining access to the presacral areolar tissue.

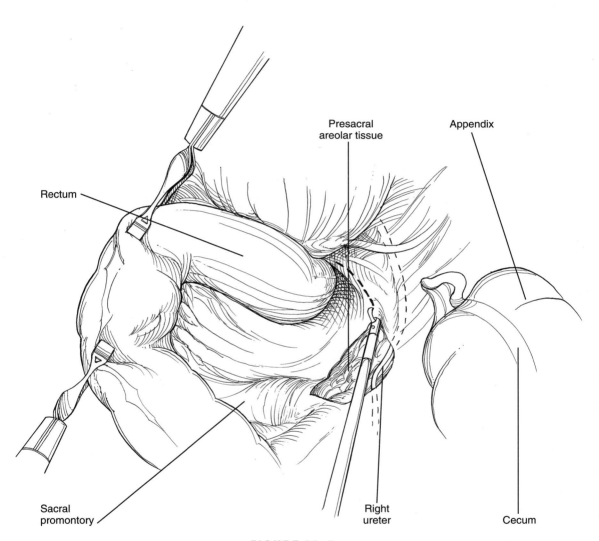

FIGURE 37–5

FIGURE 37-6. With care and meticulous attention to hemostasis, this plane can be developed by sharp dissection all the way down to the level of the pelvic floor. All this time the rectum is retracted anteriorly so that the "buttocks" of the excised mesorectum are lifted forward. In our opinion the magnified views obtained at laparoscopy deep within the pelvis are superior to those achieved during open surgery and greatly facilitate the sharp excision of the mesorectum, as advocated by Heald and coworkers. Most of the posterior mobilization of the rectum can be achieved in this way from the right side. Attention must be paid at all times to the position of the right ureter. On occasion the laparoscope may be best used through a right-sided port because the mobilized rectum lifted out of the pelvis tends to impinge on the view from the subumbilical port. Late in this stage the incision in the lateral peritoneal reflection of the sigmoid colon is continued over the pelvic brim in order to complete the posteriormobilization from right to left. The left ureter is again at risk during this stage.

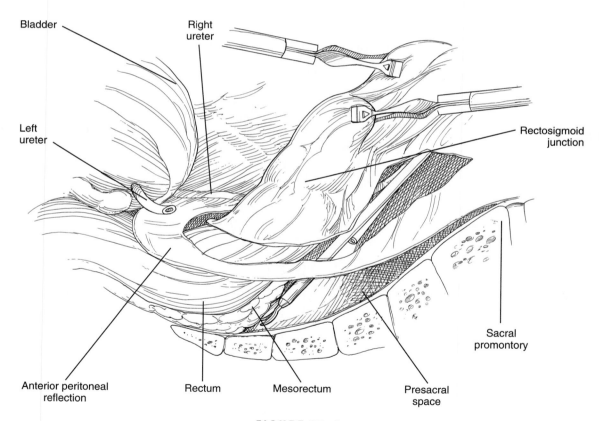

Bladder

Right ureter

Left ureter

Rectosigmoid junction

Sacral promontory

Anterior peritoneal reflection

Rectum

Mesorectum

Presacral space

FIGURE 37-6

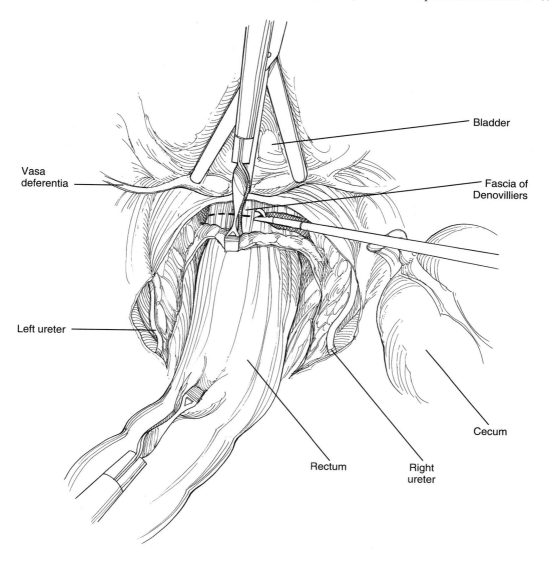

Bladder

Vasa
deferentia

Fascia of
Denovilliers

Left ureter

Cecum

Rectum

Right
ureter

FIGURE 37-7

FIGURE 37-7. When the posterior mobilization of the rectum and the mesorectal excision have been completed, attention is turned to the anterior rectal attachments. The rectum is retracted toward the sacrum by grasping the cut edge of its investing peritoneum with a Babcock. The perineal operator may place a finger or a rigid protoscope in the rectum to assist in this retraction. In men we make use of an additional suprapubic port to retract the posterior wall of the bladder and the vasa deferentia anteriorly using a fan retractor specifically designed for laparoscopic use. The fascia of Denonvilliers, thus exposed, is then incised. When this plane has been opened up, the anterior dissection is best completed by the perineal operator.

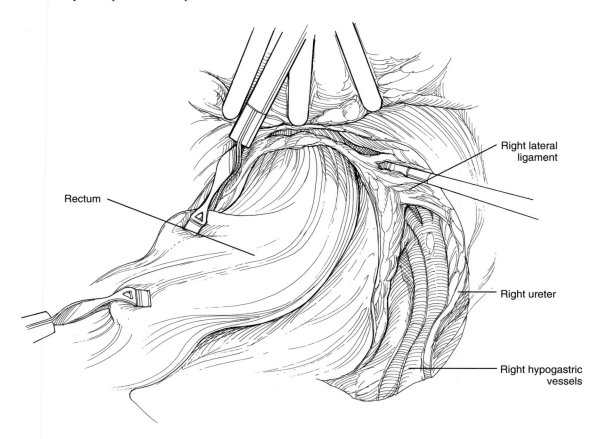

Rectum

Right lateral
ligament

Right ureter

Right hypogastric
vessels

FIGURE 37–8

FIGURE 37–8. Mobilization of the rectum down to the pelvic floor is finally completed by dividing the lateral ligaments. The assistant retracts the rectum out of the pelvis and laterally, and the lateral ligaments are divided by electrocautery under direct vision. The magnified views obtained at laparoscopy permit accurate pelvic dissection under direct vision, and with care and meticulous hemostasis the rectal mobilization can be continued down to the level of the pelvic floor. The perineal surgeon is now well positioned to complete what remains of the dissection from below.

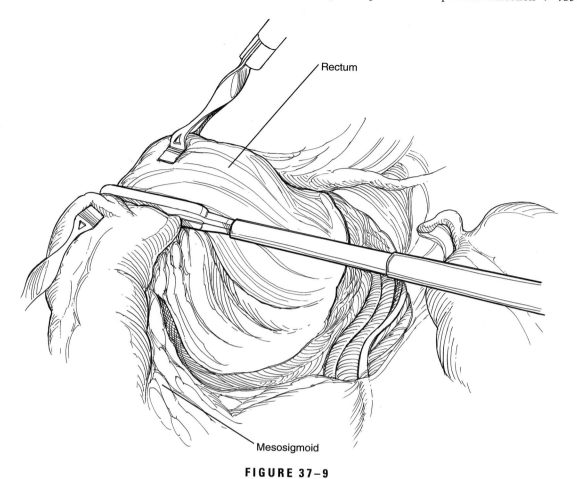

Rectum

Mesosigmoid

FIGURE 37-9

FIGURE 37-9. The proximal colon must now be transected before the perineal dissection begins, because it is impossible to perform this with any degree of safety without a pneumoperitoneum. The colon is elevated and held with Babcocks proximal and distal to the chosen point of transection. It is not necessary to fashion a mesenteric window. An endoscopic linear cutting stapler is then applied across the bowel and fired. The staple lines must be checked for hemostasis. Finally, the mesosigmoid is divided using either an endoscopic stapler or electrocautery scissors and clips.

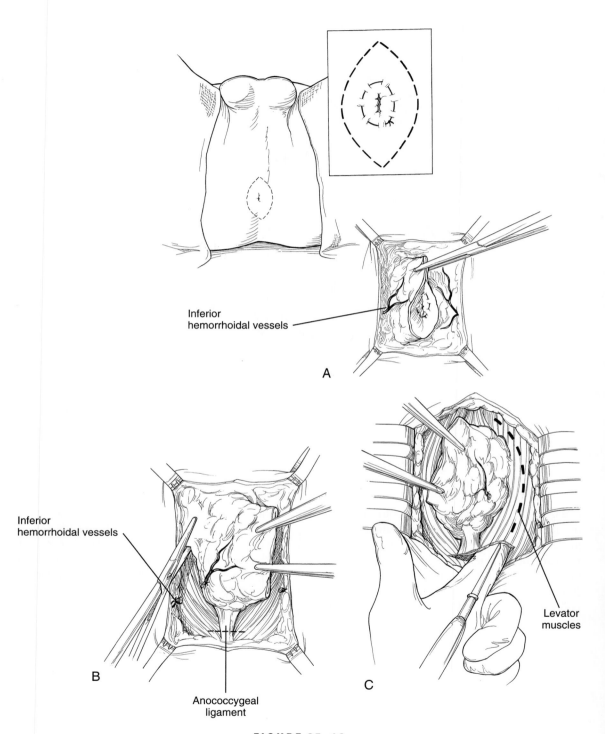

Inferior
hemorrhoidal vessels

A

Inferior
hemorrhoidal vessels

B

Anococcygeal
ligament

Levator
muscles

C

FIGURE 37–10

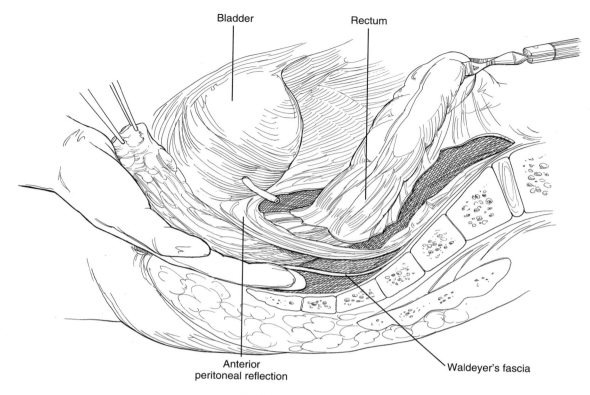

Bladder

Rectum

Anterior
peritoneal reflection

Waldeyer's fascia

FIGURE 37–11

The Perineal Stage

FIGURE 37–10A–C. The perineal phase of laparoscopic abdominoperineal resection is, in essence, identical to that which would be performed during the conventional procedure and is illustrated next. In brief, a circumferential skin incision is made around the anus and deepened through the subcutaneous fat into the ischiorectal fossa.

The inferior hemorrhoidal vessels are ligated and divided, exposing the anococcygeal ligament, which is also divided. The surgeon then passes a finger into the presacral space. This finger is swept along the superior border of the levators, freeing the mesorectum, and the levators are pulled down and divided.

FIGURE 37–11. Anteriorly, the superficial transverse perineal muscle is divided at the posterior border of the deep transverse perineal muscle, thus freeing this aspect of the rectum. The rectourethralis and puborectalis are also divided, allowing the perineal surgeon to place a hand palm upward into the presacral space behind the rectum.

FIGURE 37-12. The pneumoperitoneum is usefully maintained for a few moments by the bulk of the perineal surgeon's hand. What remains of the mobilization of the lower third of the rectum may then be completed using a combination of sharp laparoscopic dissection and blunt dissection from below. Thus, if Waldeyer's fascia was not incised during the laparoscopic phase of the operation it is now tented up by the fingers of the perineal surgeon and divided by the laparoscopist. The anterior dissection is completed by the perineal surgeon after the laparoscopist has incised the peritoneal reflection in the rectovesical or rectovaginal pouch and, ideally, the fascia of Denonvilliers. Then, with strong traction applied on the rectum and mesorectum by the perineal surgeon, any remaining component of the lateral ligaments is divided by the laparoscopic surgeon, and the middle hemorrhoidal vessels are clipped or treated with diathermy. Once the lateral ligaments have been divided, the perineal surgeon can sweep a hand around the front of the rectum, completing this blunt dissection.

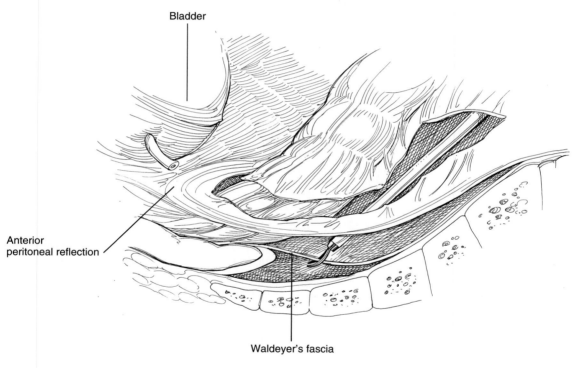

Bladder

Anterior
peritoneal reflection

Waldeyer's fascia

FIGURE 37-12

FIGURE 37-13

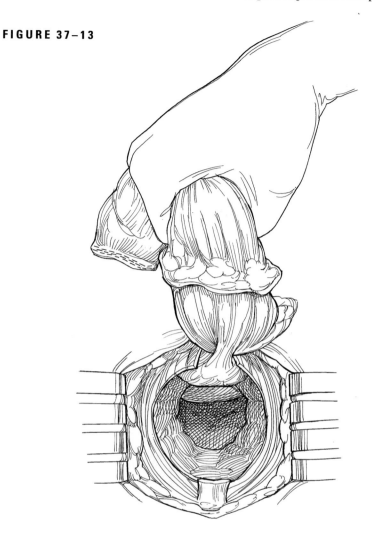

FIGURE 37-13. Finally, the staple line on the proximal end of the specimen is grasped by the laparoscopic operator and placed in the hand of the perineal surgeon, who then withdraws his hand from the pelvis along the sacrum to deliver the specimen. The remaining attachments of the specimen to the posterior vaginal wall or to the prostate in men are divided, and the specimen is delivered, at which point the pneumo-peritoneum is rapidly lost.

Closure

The pelvis is thoroughly irrigated through the perineal wound with warm saline. A careful check for the adequacy of hemostasis should be made with the patient returned to a neutral position, since venous bleeding may not be apparent in the Trendelenburg position. We place two closed nonsuction drains in the pelvis and bring these out through the abdominal wall. Alternatively, these may be passed through the levators and brought out through stab wounds in the perineal skin (anterior to a line between the ischial tuberosities to avoid damaging the sciatic nerve).

The levators and subcutaneous tissues are apposed with a stout absorbable suture, and the skin is closed with nonabsorbable interrupted sutures. The fascial sheath is closed at all trocar sites, where the skin is then closed with tissue adhesive or an absorbable subcuticular suture.

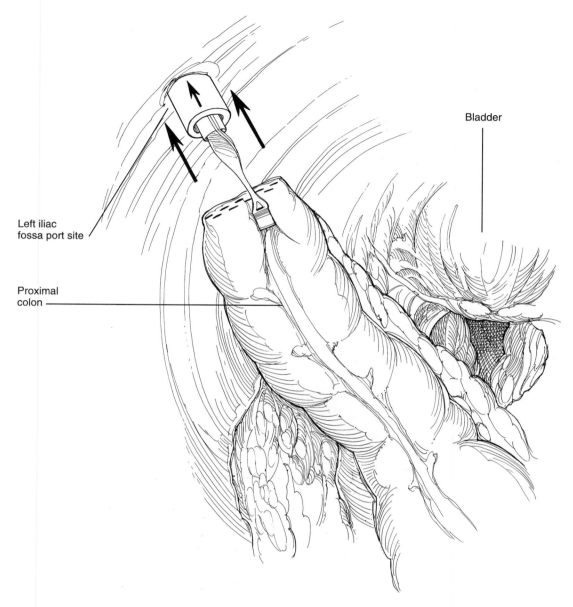

Bladder

Left iliac
fossa port site

Proximal
colon

FIGURE 37–14

Constructing the Colostomy

FIGURE 37-14. Before transecting the descending colon, it is important to ensure that the bowel will comfortably reach the anterior abdominal wall. When this is confirmed, it is a simple matter to construct a tension-free end-colostomy once the abdomen has been deflated. The bowel can then be transected. We grasp the blind stapled end of the proximal colon with a Babcock inserted through the left iliac fossa port site. The Babcock is left attached. When the abdomen is deflated, the proximal colon can be brought up to the left iliac fossa port site. The port site is then enlarged by excising a disc of skin and subcutaneous fat down to the trocar incision in the rectus sheath, which is also enlarged. Once the perineal and abdominal wounds have been closed and dressed, the colonic staple line is opened, and the end colostomy is matured in the usual manner.

IX. Postoperative Medications

The principles governing postoperative care of patients undergoing laparoscopic abdominoperineal resection are identical to those followed after conventional surgery. Antibiotic prophylaxis is therefore completed, and in our practice this comprises further doses of a second-generation cephalosporin and metronidazole, at 8 and 16 hours post induction. When fecal contamination has occurred during the operation we continue antibiotics for 5 days. The nasogastric tube is removed, and oral fluids are commenced on the first postoperative day. These are gradu-ally increased as tolerated, and a light diet is begun with signs of resolution of the ileus.

Chest physiotherapy should be routine, and the patient is mobilized as soon as practical. Thromboembolic prophylaxis should be continued until the patient is fully mobile. The patient is discharged when he or she can tolerate a normal diet and manage the colostomy; in our experience this is usually about 7 to 10 days following surgery.

X. Advancement of Diet

A. Patients take clear liquids on the first or second day after surgery.
B. They are advanced to a regular diet as tolerated.

XI. Determinants of Discharge

A. Patients are discharged when they can eat a regular diet and experience a minimal amount of pain and when the wounds, especially the perineal wound, are healing in a satisfactory manner
B. Patient have been instructed in the care of the stoma by an enterostomal nurse.

XII. Return to Normal Activity

Patients can return to their normal activities when the perineal wound and stoma have healed in a satisfactory manner.

Reference

MacFarlane J, Ryall R, Heald R: Mesorectal-excision for rectal cancer. Lancet 1993; 341:457–460.

Chapter 38

Laparoscopic-Assisted Perineoabdominal Resection

SCOTT THORNTON, M.D.

I. Indications

A. Benign disease damaging sphincter function
B. Malignant disease with sphincter invasion
C. Malignant disease that is clearly not amenable to sphincter-saving techniques
D. Other lesions or disease necessitating sphincter and rectal excision

II. Contraindications

A. Patient specific
 1. Must be able to undergo general anesthesia
 2. Extensive pelvic scarring or adhesions (relative)
B. Lesion specific: sphincter-saving approach may be possible (low anterior resection coloanal anastomosis)

III. Factors Important in Patient Selection

A. All patients are eligible
B. Desirable physical characteristics (i.e., makes operation easier)
 1. Thin
 2. Short
 3. Female
 4. Wide pelvis

IV. Preoperative Preparation

A. Evaluation for metastases
 1. CT scan of abdomen and pelvis
 2. Chest x-ray
 3. Transrectal ultrasound
B. Admission
 1. Same day admission is routine
 2. Must hydrate patients before induction of anesthesia owing to dehydration resulting from bowel preparation
 3. Elective admission before surgery
  a. Extensive cardiac disease
  b. Extensive renal disease
  c. Pulmonary toilet required
  d. Inability to prepare bowel at home
C. Preoperative medications on morning of surgery
 1. Same as for open abdominoperineal resection (APR)
 2. Broad-spectrum intravenous (IV) antibiotic (cefotetan 1 g)
 3. Antiembolic therapy (heparin 5000 units subcutaneously)
 4. Check potassium level and replace if necessary
D. Bowel preparation
 1. Mechanical: same as for open APR
  a. Begin after lunch on day prior to surgery

b. Fleet's Phospho-Soda: 45 ml orally at noon, then 45 ml orally at 7 PM

c. Potassium 20 mEq orally three times a day

d. Or, instead of *b* and *c*, use GoLYTELY 1 gallon, beginning at 4 PM and finishing by 7 PM

2. Antibiotic: same as for open APR

a. Neomycin 1 g orally at 1, 2, and 11 PM

b. Flagyl 500 mg orally at 1, 2, and 11 PM

V. Choice of Anesthesia

A. General anesthesia with endotracheal intubation

B. Must hydrate patient before induction due to dehydration resulting from bowel preparation

VI. Accessory Devices

A. Nasogastric tube

B. Urinary bladder catheter

C. Pneumatic compression antiembolic stockings

D. Ureteral catheters are strongly suggested

VII. Instruments and Telescopes

A. Laparoscopic bowel instruments
   1. Babcock clamps
   2. Shears

B. Blunt dissectors

C. Suction/irrigator
   1. 1 g cephazolin in 1000 ml normal saline
   2. 1000 units heparin in 1000 ml normal saline

D. Laparoscopic stapler/divider with vascular staples

E. Perineal dissection instruments
   1. General instrument tray
   2. Allis clamps
   3. Goulet retractors
   4. 211 and 411 malleable retractors
   5. 211 and 411 Richardson retractors
   6. Linear stapler

VIII. Position of Monitors and Patient Position

A. Modified Lloyd-Davies position

   1. Supine, with both arms tucked at the side
   2. Shoulder pads at the acromion process (to prevent sliding during table rotation)
   3. Allen stirrups, with hips minimally flexed (to allow access to the abdomen)
   4. Legs abducted as much as possible (to allow access to the perineum)
   5. Roll under the posterior superior iliac spine (to elevate the perineum)
   6. Buttocks taped apart (to ease access to the perineum, tape to be removed when closing the perineal wound)

B. TV monitors: two placed at the foot end of the patient

IX. Narrative of Surgical Technique

This procedure is designed to be performed synchronously from below and above. Thus, only lesions that have previously been deemed not to be candidates for low anterior resection or coloanal anastomosis should be considered.

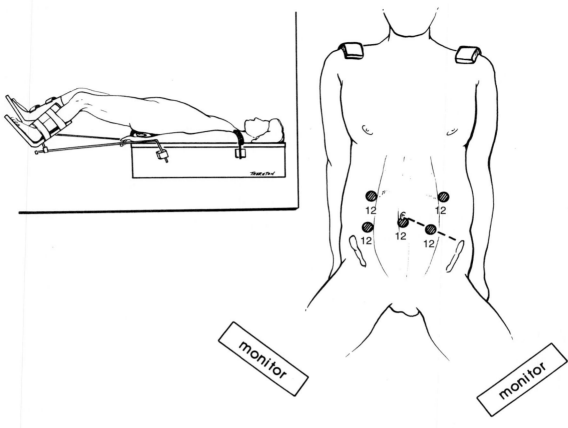

FIGURE 38-1

Laparoscopic Exploration

FIGURE 38-1. The laparoscopic part of the operation should begin first if the finding of intraoperative metastatic disease would preclude anorectal excision with permanent colostomy. If rectal excision is definitely required, the perineal dissection may begin first. The laparoscopic surgeon stands on the patient's left side and uses an infraumbilical approach to achieve pneumoperitoneum. Laparoscopic exploration is then undertaken, which with the preoperative CT scan is used to rule out metastatic disease.

Two trocars are placed in the right lateral abdomen, lateral to the rectus muscle. Ten- to twelve-millimeter trocars are used throughout; one is placed in the left upper abdomen, lateral to the rectus, and the other is placed in the previously chosen colostomy site through the rectus muscle, approximately halfway between the umbilicus and the anterior superior iliac spine. Once resectability has been established, a synchronous approach is undertaken.

Perineal Dissection

FIGURE 38–2. After resectability has been ensured, the perineal dissection is started. An elliptical incision is made, the boundaries being the ischial tuberosities laterally, the coccyx posteriorly, and the perineal body anteriorly. Posterior vaginectomy in females, especially when anterior lesions are present, will make the ante- rior dissection easier. Sharp dissection deepens the wound through the ischiorectal fat. The anococcygeal ligament is readily identified tethering the anal canal to the coccyx. Curved Mayo scissors are used to cut this, which allows access to the deep post anal space. Blunt separation in the midline separates the levator ani. The levator ani muscles are divided with cautery or division and ligation in the usual fashion.

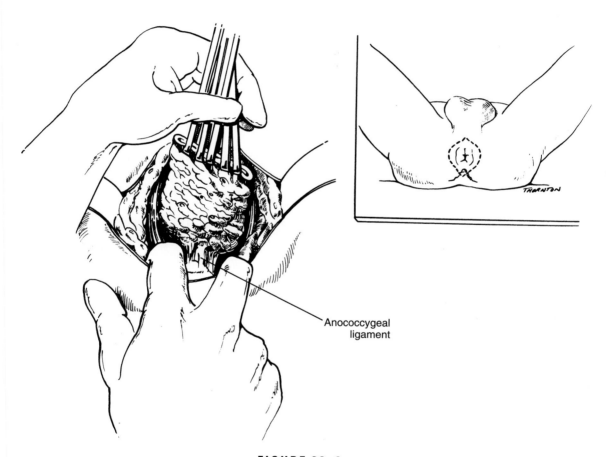

Anococcygeal
ligament

FIGURE 38–2

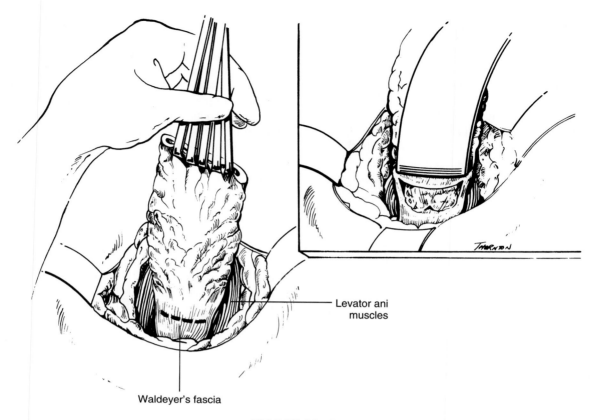

Levator ani
muscles

Waldeyer's fascia

FIGURE 38–3

FIGURE 38-3. Rigorous upward retraction of the rectum with a 2- to 3-mm malleable retractor brings the white, glistening Waldeyer's fascia into view. This is cut approximately halfway between the anorectum and its attachment to the ventral body of S2. Once cut, the bilobed mesorectal fat (covered with endopelvic fascia) bulges out. At this point, the presacral space has been safely entered.

Laparoscopic Dissection

FIGURE 38–4. Laparoscopic dissection begins with division of the left lateral (nonanatomic) adhesions between the sigmoid colon and the left lateral abdominal wall. The sigmoid colon is then grasped with two endo-Babcock clamps and retracted medially and ventrally. The surgeon divides the white line of Toldt from the mid-descending colon and continues down into the pelvis and across the anterior rectum in the cul-de-sac. Blunt and careful sharp dissection mobilizes the sigmoid colon and mesocolon from the retroperitoneum. The left ureter and gonadal vessels are left in place in the retroperitoneum. The sigmoid colon is then retracted laterally, and the peritoneum is sharply divided over the inferior mesenteric vessels on the right. This is continued down into the pelvis and over the anterior rectum to join the other incision. The sigmoid colon is now tethered only by its vascular supply, the inferior mesenteric vessels (IMA, inferior mesenteric artery; u, ureter; HP, hypogastric plexus; A, aorta).

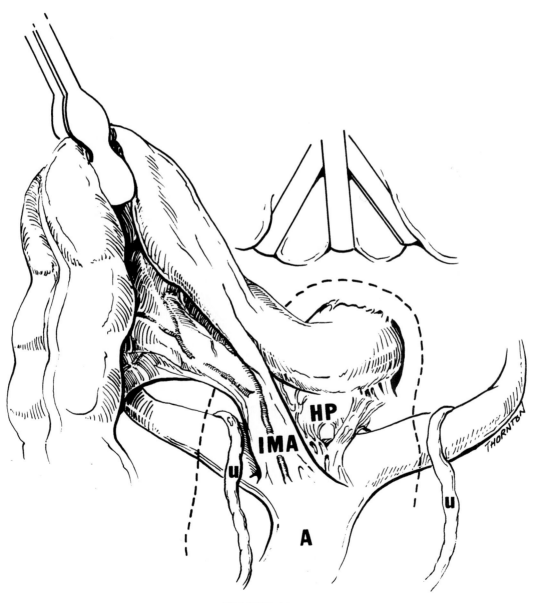

FIGURE 38–4

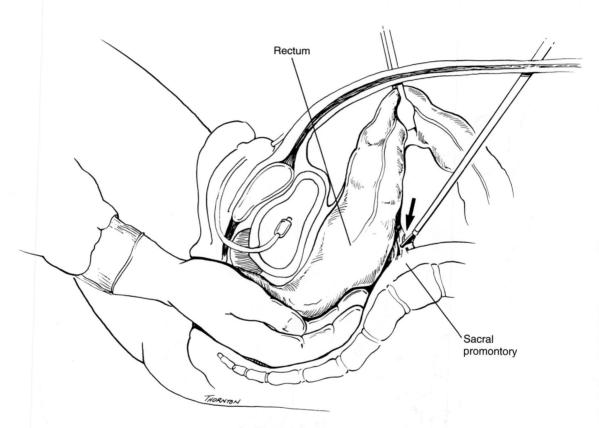

Rectum

Sacral
promontory

THORNTON

FIGURE 38–5

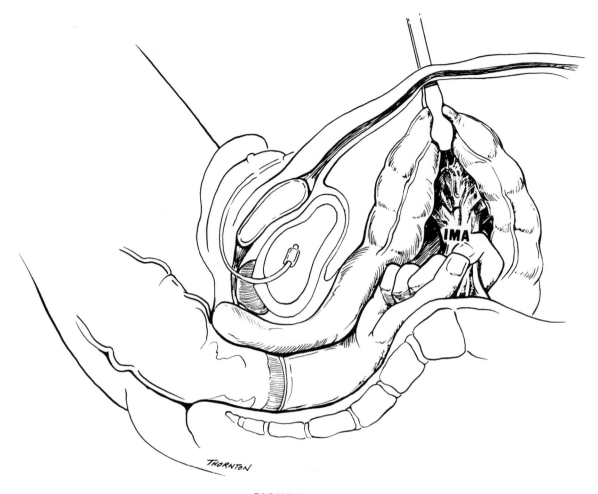

FIGURE 38-6

FIGURE 38-5. The sigmoid colon is then retracted strongly ventrally, and the presacral space is sharply entered. This space is easily seen as the flimsy connective tissue over the sacral promontory. The hypogastric plexus and nerves are kept dorsal, adherent to the presacral fascia, and thus intact. Laparoscopic sharp dissection continues distally to meet the surgeon's perineal hand. The "perineal hand" can now enter the abdominal cavity. Pneumoperitoneum is maintained by the snug fit of the surgeon's forearm and the posterior perineal wound.

Combined Dissection

FIGURE 38-6. Abdominal palpation can now be done with the perineal hand. Similarly, the perineal hand is used to identify, separate, and bluntly surround the inferior mesenteric vessels (IMA, inferior mesenteric artery).

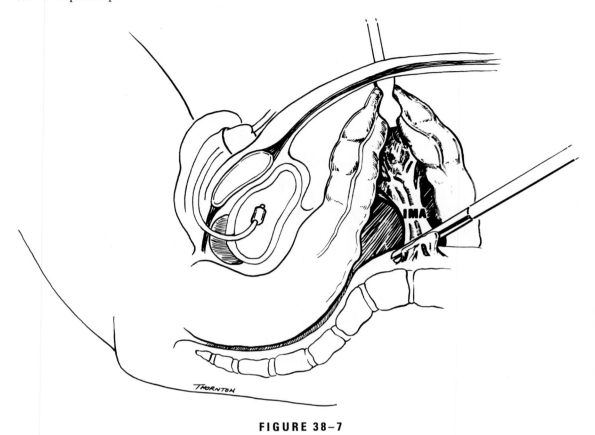

FIGURE 38-7

FIGURE 38-7. An endoscopic stapler/divider is guided by the perineal hand around the base of the vessels. Palpation of the catheters by the perineal hand ensures the safety of the ureters. The vessels are then divided just distal to the left colic artery (IMA, inferior mesenteric artery).

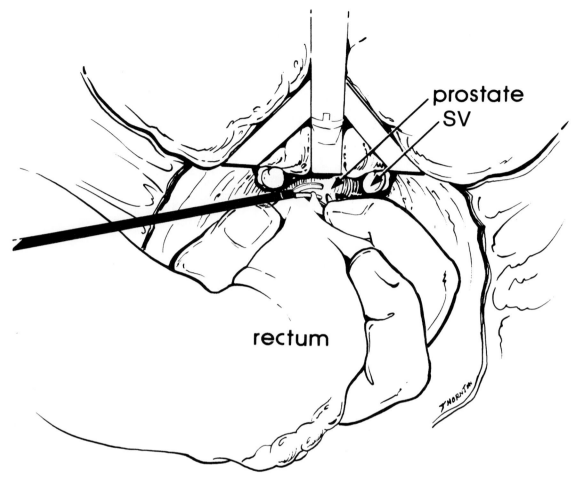

prostate
SV

rectum

FIGURE 38–8

FIGURE 38–8. Anterior dissection is then completed from below, from above, or using a combination of the two. The perineal hand greatly facilitates the laparoscopic dissection anteriorly by providing dorsal and caudal traction. The laparoscope provides an excellent view of the deep pelvis, especially with the retraction afforded by the perineal hand.

Perineal completion of the anterior dissection in males is more difficult. Blunt and occasional sharp dissection is required, and particular attention must be paid to the membranous urethra (and Foley catheter). Once the prostate is reached, Denonvilliers fascia is left in place, and dissection is continued cephalad toward the seminal vesicles (SV). The laparoscopic dissection is met here, thus completing the anterior dissection.

The anterior dissection in females is straightforward. A posterior vaginectomy allows direct entrance into the peritoneal cavity through the apex of the vagina. Otherwise, sharp dissection dorsal to the superficial and deep transverse perinei muscles allows development of the rectovaginal space. Blunt or sharp dissection in this plane will end at the peritoneal membrane, which is gray and smooth. Sharp division is used to enter the abdominal cavity.

The anterolateral dissection is completed sharply from above with retraction assistance from the perineal hand. Palpation ensures the safety of the ureters, which are surprisingly close to the perineal wound!

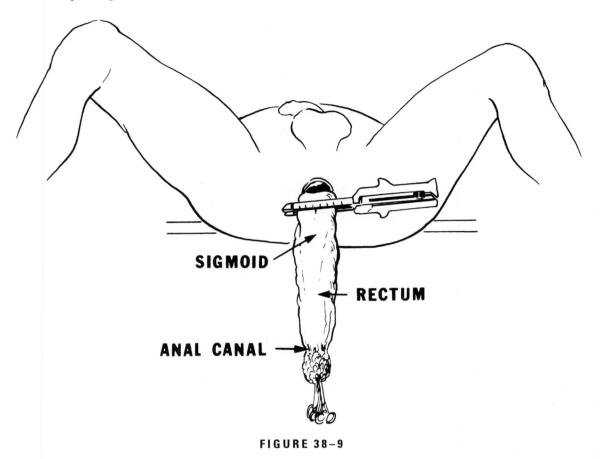

FIGURE 38-9

FIGURE 38-9. After circumferential mobilization, the entire anorectum, mesorectum, and sigmoid colon can easily be delivered out of the perineal wound. A linear stapler is used to divide the sigmoid colon, and the specimen is removed through the perineal wound.

FIGURE 38-10. The perineal hand then delivers the stapled end of the sigmoid colon to the colostomy site through the perineal wound. The fascia is incised, and the sigmoid colon is delivered through the abdominal wall. Excess sigmoid colon is removed, the colostomy is matured, and the trocar sites are closed. The perineal wound is closed in layers, with a closed suction drain inserted through a separate stab wound.

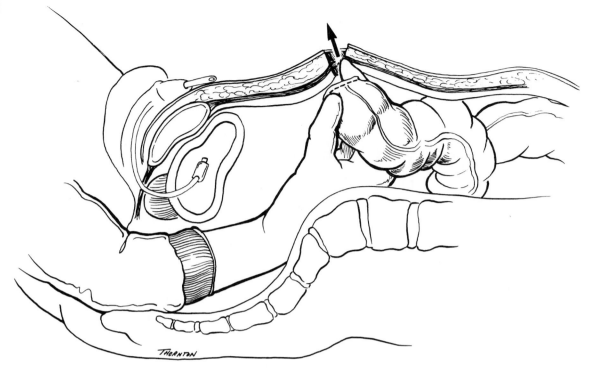

FIGURE 38–10

X. Postoperative Medications and Orders

A. Narcotics are given intramuscularly as needed
B. Propoxyphene napsylate (Darvocet N-100) is given orally (nonconstipating)
C. Broad-spectrum IV antibiotic (cefotetan) is given for 24 hours; heparin 5000 units is given subcutaneously until the patient is ambulating
D. Ducosate calcium (Surfak) is given twice a day to soften stool
E. Remove right ureteral catheter immediately after surgery
F. Remove left catheter on postoperative day 1
G. Remove drain when 50 ml of fluid or less drains in 8 hours

XI. Advancement of Diet

A. Remove nasogastric tube in recovery room
B. Clear liquid diet when awake
C. Advance to low residue diet as tolerated

XII. Determinants of Discharge

A. Tolerates low residue diet
B. Ambulates without assistance
C. Able to care for colostomy
D. Able to void or take care of urinary catheter at home

XIII. Return to Normal Activity/Work

Light activity is permitted for 4 to 6 weeks (to allow perineal wound to heal). Patient can return to work when he or she is able (1 to 3 weeks).

Acknowledgement

I would like to thank my wife, Mary Beth Thornton, A.M.I., for her expert illustrations.

Chapter 39

Laparoscopic Closure of a Hartman's Pouch

GARTH H. BALLANTYNE, M.D.

I. Indications

A. Obstructing sigmoid carcinoma
B. Acute diverticulitis
C. Sigmoid volvulus
D. Penetrating trauma of the sigmoid colon
E. Anastomotic leak

II. Contraindications

A. Severe restrictive pulmonary disease
B. Recent myocardial infarction
C. Previous lower abdominal incision that was closed with mesh

III. Factors Important in Patient Selection

A number of factors make laparoscopic closure of a Hartman's pouch more or less difficult. A surgeon early in his or her experience may wish to select patients in whom the operation may prove easier. The following factors influence the difficulty of the operation:

A. Thin patients are easier than obese patients.
B. Women are easier than men because the mesentery in women tends to have less fat.
C. Patients who did not have peritonitis may be easier than those who had feculent peritonitis following a colonic perforation.
D. Patients in whom the rectal stump extends above the peritoneal reflection are generally easier than those with a very low closure of the rectum.

IV. Preoperative Preparation

A. The colon and rectal pouch are evaluated by flexible endoscopy or contrast study prior to closure of the colostomy.
B. Patients are admitted on the day of surgery.
C. Mechanical and antibiotic bowel preparation is accomplished at home. This typically includes:
   1. Drinking a gallon of GoLYTELY over 3 hours on the day before surgery (e.g., noon to 3 PM).
   2. Taking three doses (1 g each) of erythromycin and neomycin after drinking all of the GoLYTELY (e.g., 4 PM, 7 PM, and 10 PM).
D. Patients are given Zofran 4 mg intravenously when they are first brought into the operating room.
E. Patients are given one dose of a cephalosporin intravenously prior to the operation.

V. Choice of Anesthesia

All patients receive general anesthesia. The colostomy site and the trocar sites are injected with Marcaine prior to making the incisions and again at the end of the procedure.

VI. Accessory Devices

A. Nasogastric tubes are inserted in all patients.
B. Urinary catheters are used in all patients.
C. Pneumatic compression stockings are placed on the legs of all patients.
D. An infrared lighted ureteral stent is advanced up the left ureter in patients in whom a difficult pelvic dissection is anticipated.

VII. Instruments and Telescopes

A. 10-mm, 0-degree telescope
B. Electrocautery scissors
C. Atraumatic grasper
D. Laparoscopic Babcock clamp
E. Laparoscopic fan retractor
F. End-to-end anastomosis (EEA) type circular stapling device

G. Purse-string device.
H. Luminal sizing devices (25 mm, 28 mm, and 31 mm).
I. Rigid sigmoidoscope

VIII. Position of Monitors and Placement and Size of Trocars

FIGURE 39-1. The primary monitor is placed between the legs of the patient. The surgeon stands on the patient's right side. If a robot (Aesop 3000, Computer Motion, Santa Barbara, CA) is used to hold the camera, it is attached to the left side of the operating table near the patient's left shoulder. If the operation is difficult, an assistant surgeon may prove useful to provide additional exposure. The assistant stands opposite the surgeon. The scrub nurse is best positioned opposite the surgeon near the patient's left leg.

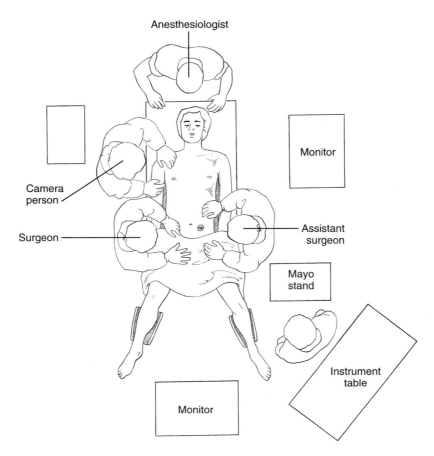

FIGURE 39-1

FIGURE 39-2. Generally, only three trocars are required. The trocar for the video telescope is placed just cephalad to the umbilicus. The surgeon uses two trocars for his or her left and right hands. These are inserted in the right lower quadrant lateral to the rectus sheath. If exposure proves troublesome, additional trocars for the assistant surgeon are inserted in the left lower quadrant lateral to the rectus sheath.

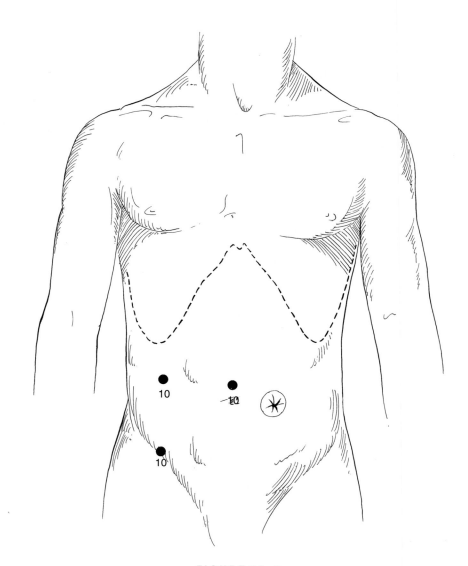

FIGURE 39-2

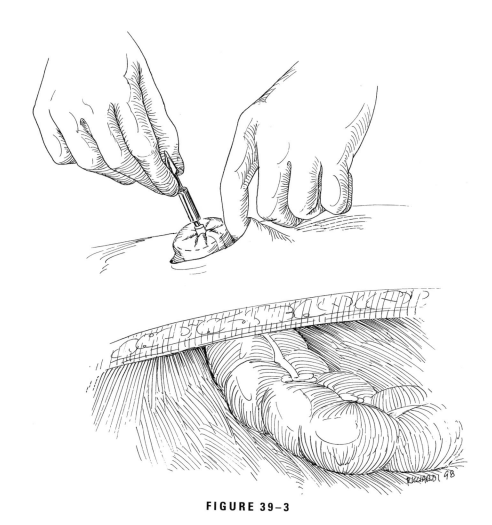

FIGURE 39–3

IX. Narrative of Surgical Technique

FIGURE 39–3. The operation commences with the mobilization of the colostomy. Since an incision is required for taking down the colostomy, this incision is used to full advantage early in the operation. The colostomy is freed from the skin, subcutaneous fat, and abdominal wall muscles. Care is taken to avoid injury to the mesentery of the colon. Any attachments of the colon to the lateral abdominal wall are freed under direct vision at this time. After the colostomy has been fully mobilized, the free edge of the colon is grasped with three Babcock clamps. The caliber of the colonic lumen is sized with the three sizers. The appropriate size of EEA stapling device is selected; the largest size is used whenever possible. An automatic purse-string device is applied to the end of the open colon and fired, stapling the purse string in place. The anvil shaft assembly of the EEA stapling device is inserted into the open end of the colon and secured in place with the purse string. The colon and anvil shaft assembly are then dropped back into the abdomen.

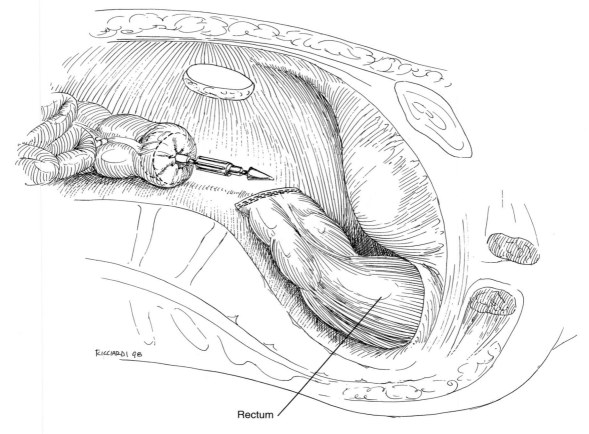

Rectum

FIGURE 39-4

FIGURE 39-4. The surgeon checks the abdominal wall under the umbilicus for adhesions both by looking directly through the open colostomy site and by inserting a finger. Any adhesions to the abdominal wall are sharply divided under direct vision. If the abdomen is obscured with dense adhesions and laparoscopy seems to be not feasible, the surgeon can elect to convert to an open operation at this time. The surgeon checks the position of the shaft of the anvil shaft assembly; this should point directly down into the pelvis.

FIGURE 39-5. A small Richardson retractor is inserted through the colostomy site and used to elevate the abdominal wall. A supraumbilical incision is made and a 10/11-mm trocar is inserted under direct vision. The colostomy site is closed with a continuous suture of No. 2 Prolene or polydioxanone (PDS). The patient is dropped into a deep Trendelenburg position. The pneumoperitoneum is insufflated with carbon dioxide to a pressure of 15 mm Hg. The abdomen is inspected with the 10-mm, 0-degree videotelescope. Two additional 10-mm trocars are inserted in the right lower quadrant lateral to the rectus sheath. The rectal pouch is identified in the pelvis. Adhesions between the small bowel and rectum are divided. Often the staple line of the rectal closure is adherent to the left lateral side wall of the pelvis; It is not necessary to free this. The anastomosis can be constructed through the anterior rectal wall. This simplifies the procedure and avoids any possible injury to the left ureter.

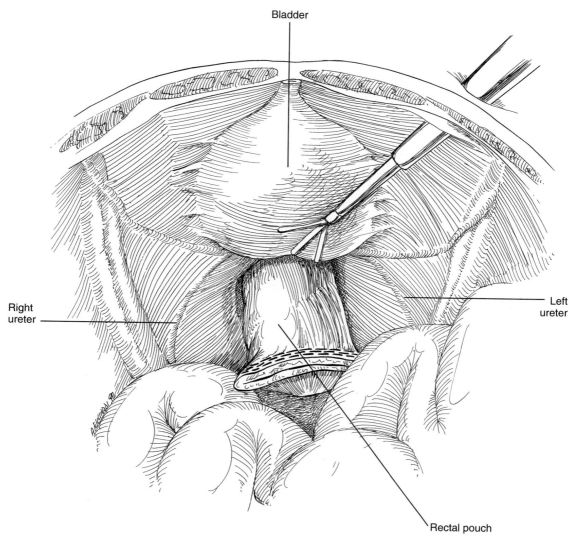

Bladder

Right ureter

Left ureter

Rectal pouch

FIGURE 39-5

FIGURE 39-6. The rectum is inspected with a rigid proctoscope. This is best accomplished after general anesthesia has been induced and prior to draping the patient. The rectal stump is irrigated with an iodine-containing solution. The rectum must be clean. Retained stool or barium is removed because it may cause misfir-ing of the EEA stapling device. The anus is slowly dilated so that it admits four fingers. The EEA stapling device is inserted into the rectum and advanced to the proximal end of the rectum. Its cartridge is pressed against the previously stapled closure of the rectum.

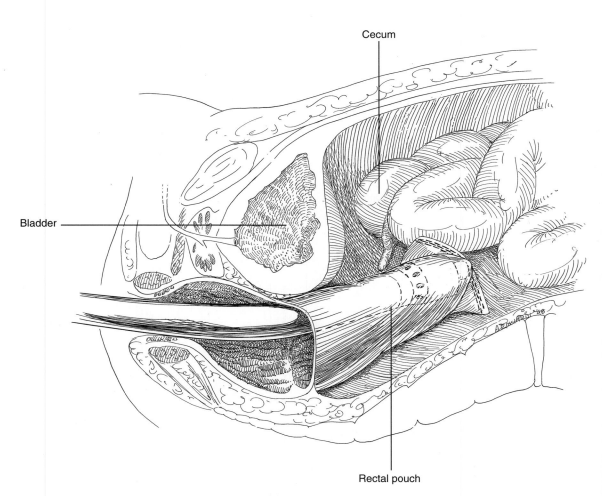

FIGURE 39-6

FIGURE 39-7. The white trocar of the EEA stapling device is screwed out through the middle of the previous staple line. If this is not feasible, it can be passed through the anterior wall of the rectum. The white trocar is removed from the center rod and retrieved through a trocar.

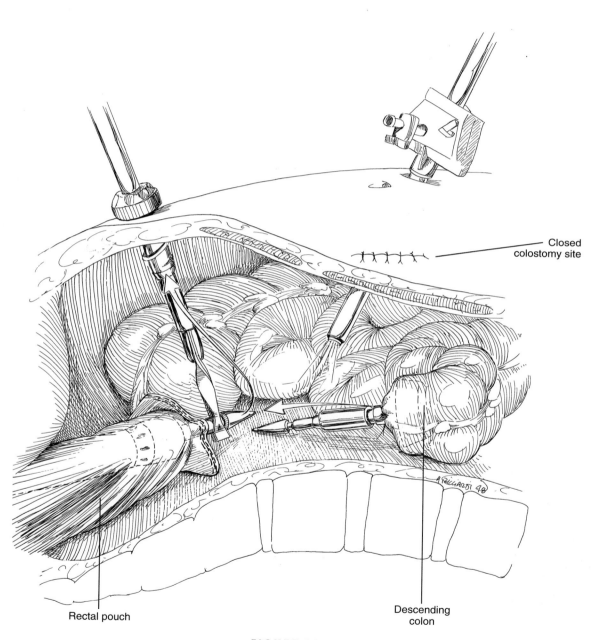

Closed colostomy site

Rectal pouch

Descending colon

FIGURE 39-7

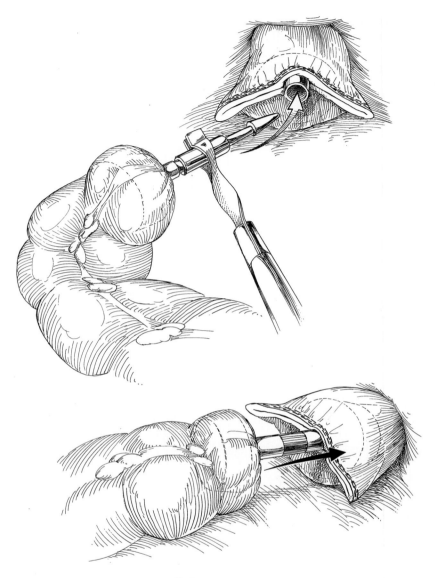

FIGURE 39-8

FIGURE 39-8. The anvil shaft assembly is grasped with a Babcock and inserted into the central rod of the EEA stapling device. The EEA is screwed closed. This process is carefully observed with the videotelescope to ensure that contiguous structures are not trapped within the stapling device. The EEA is fired, opened, and withdrawn, and the doughnuts are checked for completeness. The pelvis is then filled with irrigation fluid. The anastomosis is examined with the rigid sigmoidoscope for bleeding. The rectum is insufflated with air, checking to make sure that the anastomosis is airtight.

The abdomen is checked for hemostasis, and the pneumoperitoneum is deflated. The trocar sites are again observed for bleeding, and the trocars are removed. The fascial defects are closed with simple sutures of 0 Vicryl using a UR-6 needle. The skin edges are approximated with subcuticular absorbable sutures. The wounds are again injected with Marcaine.

X. Postoperative Medications

A. Patients are given parenteral narcotics as required.
B. Oral pain agents are started when the patient is taking liquids by mouth.

XI. Advancement of Diet

A. The nasogastric tube is left in place overnight.
B. The patient is given clear liquids the morning after surgery.
C. The patient is advanced to a regular diet on the second day after surgery.

XII. Determinants of Discharge

In theory, patients may leave the hospital when their pain is controlled with oral pain medications and they are tolerating a regular diet. Nonetheless, I generally delay discharge until they are passing flatus. This typically occurs on the third or fourth postoperative day.

XIII. Return to Normal Activity

Wounds reach 90 per cent of their ultimate strength within 10 to 14 days. Consequently, I limit patients to walking and jogging for a 2-week period. They may resume more vigorous exercise after this time period. They may return to sedentary jobs as tolerated.

Chapter 40

Laparoscopic Drainage of a Diverticular Abscess

ANTHONY V. COLETTA, M.D.

I. Indications

A. Patients who are not responding to maximal medical therapy and in whom computed tomography (CT) scans do not identify abscess formation should be considered for laparoscopy in an attempt to identify and drain occult abscesses.

B. Patients in whom the CT scan demonstrates complicated multilocular abscesses or abscesses that are not easily accessible percutaneously are candidates for laparoscopic exploration and drainage.

II. Contraindications

A. Patients with diverticulitis who are responding to bowel rest, intravenous fluids, and antibiotics

B. Patients with unilocular abscesses that are accessible to percutaneous drainage

C. Patients with a severe bleeding diathesis

D. Patients with severe cardiovascular instability due to sepsis

III. Factors Important in Patient Selection

All patients undergo a thorough history and physical examination. Careful note is taken of prior surgeries. Routine laboratory studies are performed. CT scans often not only identify peridiverticular abscess formation but also help to confirm the diagnosis of diverticulitis and identify potential involvement of surrounding organs. Barium enema and endoscopic examinations are avoided if possible in the presence of acute diverticulitis.

IV. Preoperative Preparation

A. Patients are kept nil per os (NPO).

B. Nasogastric suction is often helpful in decreasing the distention of the viscera and thus improving laparoscopic visualization.

C. Bowel preparation is not feasible in patients with acute diverticulitis associated with abscess formation and should not be instituted solely because of the contemplated laparoscopic approach.

D. Broad-spectrum antibiotic therapy is desirable, and in these patients it is instituted prior to any surgical approach and continued perioperatively.

V. Choice of Anesthesia

All patients require general anesthesia.

VII. Instruments and Telescopes

A. Laparoscopes
   1. 10-mm, 0-degree
   2. 5-mm, 30-degree

B. Trocars: one 10-mm and two 5-mm

C. Atraumatic bowel graspers

D. One irrigation-suction instrument

E. One Luken's trap on suction line

F. One high pressure irrigation system
G. Blunt-tip monopolar cautery probe
H. Monopolar scissors

VIII. Position of Monitors and Placement and Size of Trocars

FIGURE 40-1. Patients should be positioned in the dorsal lithotomy position with the legs well abducted but with hips straight (not flexed) and on a level plane with the abdomen. Easy access is necessary to the perineum for manipulation of the uterus or rectum if needed. Hips flexed in the lithotomy position often inhibit manipulation of laparoscopic instruments. The patient should be well secured on the operating table with the arms at the side if possible. It is advisable to use padded shoulder braces to avoid slipping when the patient is in a steep Trendelenburg position.

Generally only one video monitor is necessary and should be placed at the foot of the table. The video camera receiver, insufflator, and light source should be placed at the head of the table, usually at the patient's left side. Suction lines, cautery, and irrigation systems can be placed to the patient's right side. All lines should be secured to the surgical drapes to limit or minimize the crossing of lines and tubes from one side of the table to the other.

A 10-mm umbilical trocar is placed for the laparoscope. Two 5-mm trocars are placed in the right and left lower quadrants. Precise placement of these ports is based on the location of the inflammatory diverticular mass, which is determined from the initial laparoscopic examination. Small trocars are preferred to limit the size of abdominal wall incisions in the presence of the suppurative intra-abdominal process.

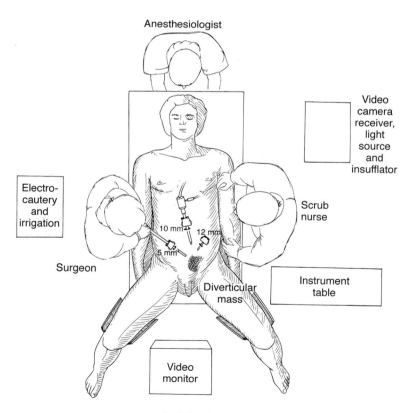

FIGURE 40-1

IX. Narrative of Surgical Technique

FIGURE 40-2. Once the patient has been properly positioned, general anesthesia has been established, and Foley catheter and nasogastric suction tubes have been placed, the entire abdomen should be carefully palpated prior to preparing and draping. The size, shape, and location of the inflammatory masses should be noted because these will have a direct impact on the techniques of blind laparoscopy. If large midline masses are palpated in the region of the umbilicus, if tympanitic loops of bowel are detected when distended, or if the patient has had prior lower abdominal surgery, then open laparoscopy using the Hasson cannula is preferred to blind puncture.

A pneumoperitoneum is established with carbon dioxide at 15 mm Hg. A 10-mm, 0-degree laparoscope coupled with a video camera is then introduced. A thorough laparoscopic examination is carried out. Free fluid is likely to be encountered and should be suctioned into a Luken's trap for culture.

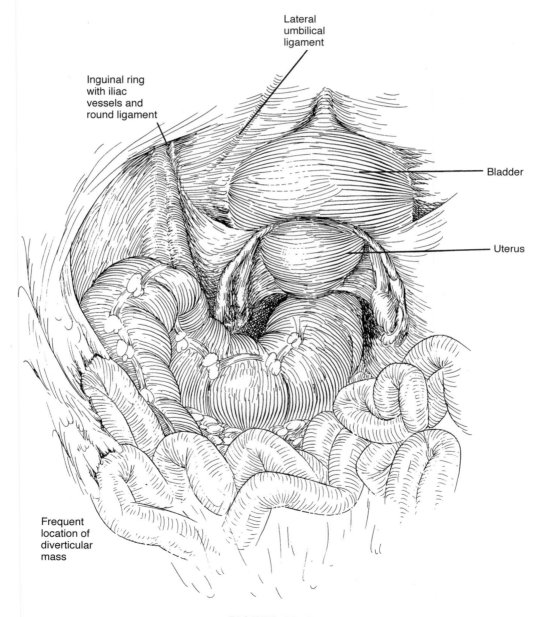

Lateral umbilical ligament

Inguinal ring with iliac vessels and round ligament

Bladder

Uterus

Frequent location of diverticular mass

FIGURE 40-2

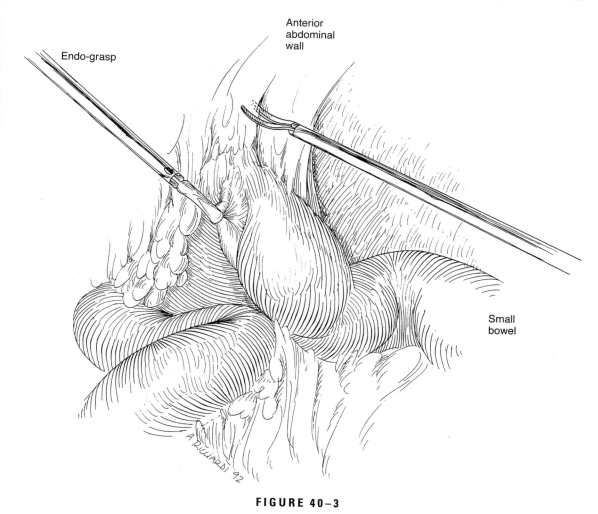

FIGURE 40-3

FIGURE 40-3. With the patient in the Trendelenburg position, note is taken of the location of inflammatory masses. There may be some bowel adherent to the anterior abdominal wall.

Right and left lower quadrant ports (usually 5 mm) can then be placed. Bowel adherent to the abdominal wall can be sharply lysed using bowel graspers and sharp scissors.

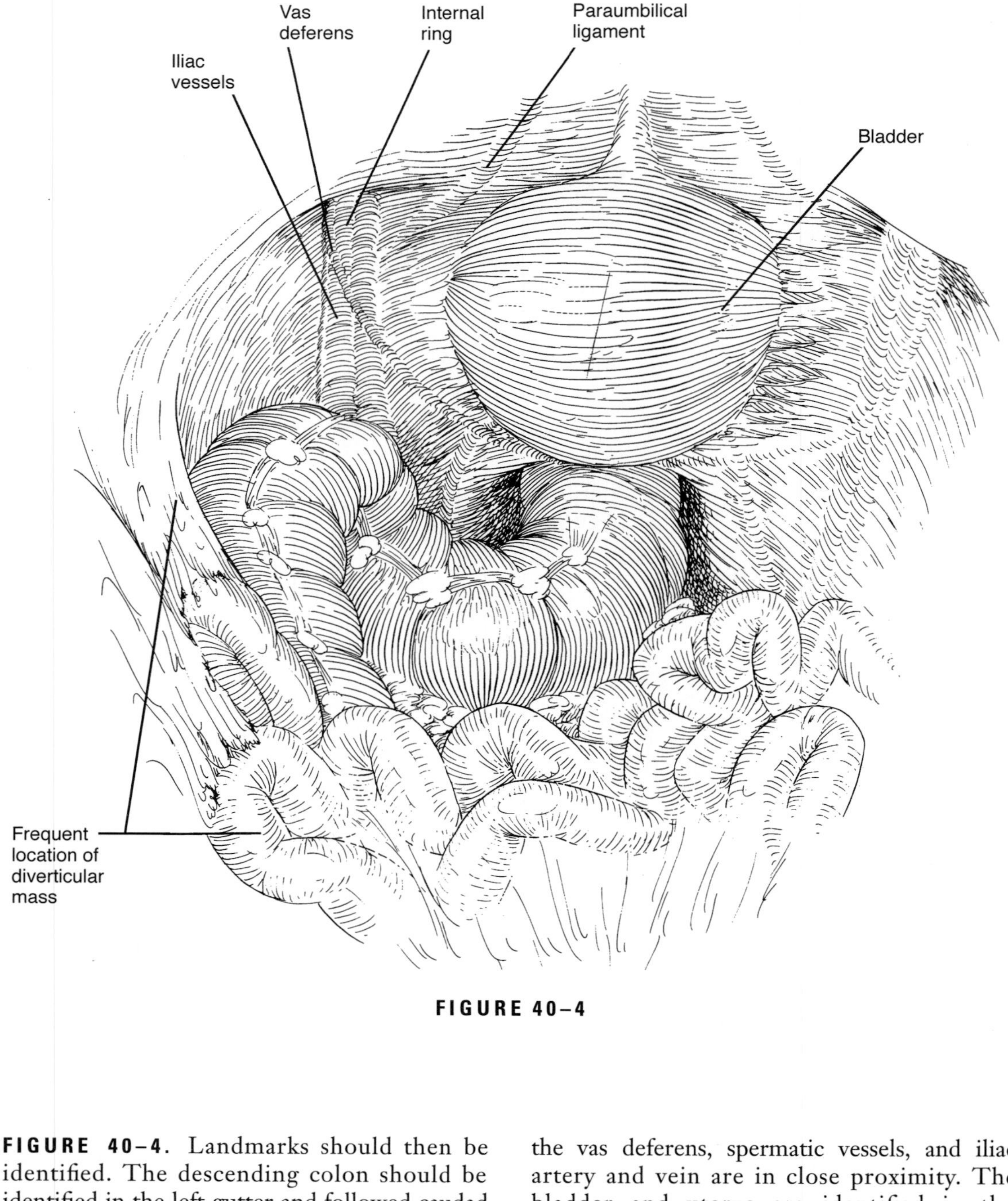

FIGURE 40-4

FIGURE 40-4. Landmarks should then be identified. The descending colon should be identified in the left gutter and followed caudad toward the sigmoid. The left paraumbilical ligament and internal ring should be noted because the vas deferens, spermatic vessels, and iliac artery and vein are in close proximity. The bladder and uterus are identified in the midline along with the adnexae in females (see Fig. 40-2).

FIGURE 40–5. As dissection of the peridiverticular tissues proceeds, it is often useful to provide countertraction of tissues using a 5-mm blunt instrument through the left lower quadrant port while bluntly dissecting with a suction irrigation probe through the right lower quadrant port. Use of the suction irrigation probe for this portion of the blunt dissection not only allows the use of aqua dissection but also provides a source of immediate suction (and therefore culture with use of an in-line Luken's trap) as soon as any abscess is encountered, thus limiting the amount of peritoneal soilage.

As in open surgery, acutely inflamed tissue planes often peel apart without force. Forceful dissection of more chronic tissues is not necessary and may be dangerous. Sharp dissection should be limited at this stage of the procedure. Once one or more abscess cavities have been identified and drained, it may be difficult to determine the end point of a dissection. In general, when these more chronic tissues are encountered, active dissection should be terminated.

An effort is then made to remove inflammatory exudate and peel that may serve as a continuing nidus of infection. High pressure (up to 200 mm Hg or more) hydrodissection is ideal for this purpose. Profuse irrigation is also carried out until the effluent is clear. An antibiotic may be added to the irrigant as in open surgery. The patient may be tilted head up and head down as well as side to side so that all dependent portions of the abdomen are well irrigated.

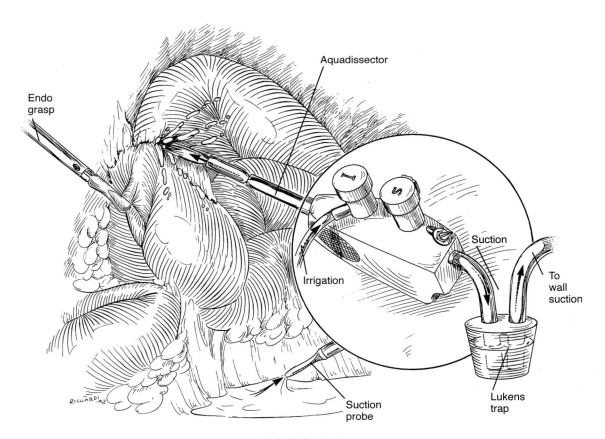

FIGURE 40–5

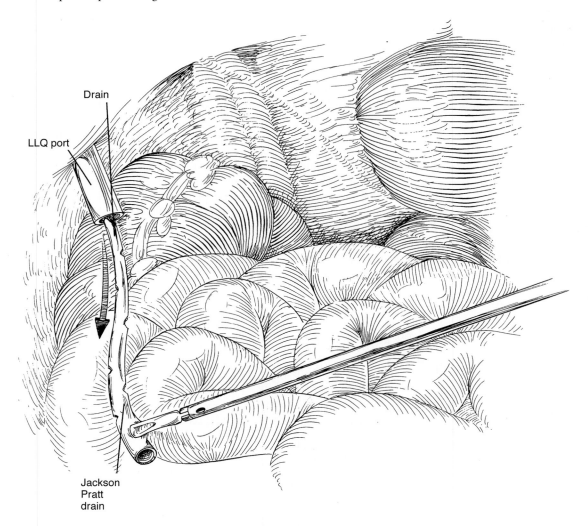

Drain

LLQ port

Jackson
Pratt
drain

FIGURE 40-6

FIGURE 40-6. Finally, a drain should be placed in the abscess cavity. A large, round Jackson-Pratt drain is ideal for this purpose and may be introduced into the abdomen through the left lower quadrant 5-mm port. Wetting the drain with saline helps it to glide through the port with ease. It can be grasped through the right lower quadrant port and placed in the abscess cavity. Prior to removing the laparoscope, the abdomen should be desufflated while the drain is visualized to ensure that it does not dislodge as the carbon dioxide is evacuated.

All port sights are then irrigated and closed with subcuticular closure. The drain is secured to the skin.

X. Postoperative Medications

A. Antibiotics should be adjusted according to the culture results obtained intraoperatively.
B. Pain medicine is given as required.

XI. Advancement of Diet

It is advisable to continue nasogastric suction, intravenous fluids, and antibiotics as clinically indicated.

A. Ileus may be encountered postoperatively in light of the inflammatory nature of the process.
B. The nasogastric tube is removed, and clear liquids are started when the patient passes flatus.
C. The Foley catheter is often maintained to assist with fluid management for several days.
D. In general, all postoperative maneuvers are similar to those expected in any patient in whom an intra-abdominal abscess has been drained.
E. A favorable response to the laparoscopic approach is heralded by an abatement of fever, pain, and leukocytosis during a period of 48 to 72 hours.
F. Persistent pain, fever, and sepsis mandate laparotomy. With improvement in the patient's status, consideration can be given to elective colectomy following proper evaluation. It may be anticipated that this could be performed as a one-stage procedure without colostomy formation.

XII. Determinants of Discharge

Patients are considered for discharge when they are eating solid foods well and have been afebrile for 24 to 48 hours after completion of IV antibiotics (usually 7 to 10 days). Oral antibiotics may be maintained after discharge if they are clinically indicated. If patients remain mildly to moderately symptomatic (abdominal pain, low grade fever, and so on), consideration may be given to further study (barium enema, flexible sigmoidoscopy), bowel preparation, and semi-elective resection of the diverticular segment prior to discharge. Otherwise, 6 to 8 weeks is a reasonable time interval prior to elective resection. If the patient becomes completely asymptomatic and barium enema and flexible sigmoidoscopy show no complicated disease (e.g., stricture, intra- or extramural tracking, fistula), elective resection may be avoided altogether after careful counseling of the patient regarding the various options.

Part VII

LAPAROSCOPIC REPAIR OF INGUINAL HERNIAS

Chapter 41

Laparoscopic Transabdominal Transperitoneal Patch Hernia Repair

JOHN CORBITT, M.D.

I. Indications

A. All primary inguinal hernias
   1. Indirect inguinal hernias
   2. Direct inguinal hernias
   3. Femoral hernias
   4. Bilateral inguinal hernias
B. Recurrent inguinal hernias

II. Contraindications

A. Inability of the patient to undergo general anesthesia
B. Inability to reduce the hernia either preoperatively or intraoperatively, in which case a trans-groin approach must be used
C. Abnormal bleeding
D. Cirrhosis of the liver
E. The need or expectation of future vascular surgery in this area, such as aortic bypass surgery, represents a relative contraindication. As a rule, grafts can be placed around the hernia repair and do not generally interfere with this repair.
F. Although extremely large hernias can be repaired laparoscopically, this does not necessarily mean that they should be done in this way, and it is up to the surgeon to decide his ability to repair the giant hernia laparoscopically.

III. Factors Important in Patient Selection

A. Ability to undergo general anesthesia. If there is a contraindication to general anesthesia, there is a contraindication to laparoscopic herniorrhaphy.
B. Patients should have a thorough understanding of the procedure and the risks involved in laparoscopy, which are added to those of the hernia repair. Patients should also be informed that at present, laparoscopic hernia repairs have been performed for approximately 5 years with excellent results; however, long term follow-up is not available at this time.

IV. Preoperative Preparation

A. The patient is admitted on the morning of surgery and discharged later that afternoon when his or her condition is stable.
B. The patient is given routine preoperative medications. Zofran (4 mg) is given to prevent postoperative nausea and vomiting.
C. Preoperatively the patient is given a prescription for a pain medication, such as Percocet, but usually very little pain medicine is required following laparoscopic herniorrhaphy.

V. Choice of Anesthesia

A. The transabdominal preperitoneal (TAPP) repair requires general anesthesia. Other types of regional anesthesia and epidural and spinal anesthesia have been attempted but are not acceptable for this repair.

B. If the extraperitoneal repair is used instead of the TAPP repair, epidural and spinal anesthesia may be used.

VI. Accessory Devices

A. TED (thromboembolic disease) hose is applied preoperatively.

B. Nasogastric tube is not necessary.

C. Urinary catheter: The beginning surgeon should use a urinary catheter to remove the bladder from the operative field. After a surgeon has become proficient in laparoscopic herniorrhaphy, the catheter may be omitted providing that the holding room nurse can assure the surgeon that the patient has voided preoperatively.

VII. Instruments and Telescopes

A. 30-degree or 45-degree, 10-mm telescope or, if a good 5-mm, 30-degree laparoscope is available, the ports may be reduced in size as indicated under that specific heading.

B. Specific to laparoscopic hernia repair is a method of fixing the mesh to the fascia and to Cooper's ligament. This is the most important part of the procedure and requires a stapler. Prior to the availability of the stapler, the mesh was sutured with interrupted sutures, and this may still be done; however, this is extremely time consuming and costly because of the necessary operating room time.

C. Polypropylene mesh is the preferred mesh for this repair because it allows extensive fibrous ingrowth. The staples simply hold the mesh in place until the fibrous ingrowth has occurred. The ingrowth of fibrous tissue is the chief component of a good hernia repair.

VIII. Position of Monitors and Placement and Size of Trocars

Generally speaking, a hernia is easier to repair if the surgeon stands on the side opposite the hernia. However, after some experience a right-handed surgeon will stand on the left side of the table, and a left-handed surgeon will always stand on the right side of the table. It is easier to view the monitor that the laparoscope is pointed toward, and therefore, initially the monitor should be placed at the foot of the table. After some experience it will not make any difference where the monitor is placed as long as it is in the convenient view of the surgeon.

There are multiple positions for trocar placement. The accepted standard is to place the primary port in the umbilicus and the secondary ports at the approximate level of the umbilicus, or slightly below, lateral to the rectus muscle. Placement of a 12-mm port in the umbilicus is preferred. This larger port is necessary because of the diameter of the stapler used in stabilizing the mesh to the floor of the pelvis. These staples cannot be passed through a smaller port. The 12-mm port is placed in the umbilicus because it is the largest port and requires closure of the fascia. The fascia in the umbilicus is easier to close than the fascia in the lateral areas. Another reason for placement of this trocar in the umbilicus is that there are fewer pain fibers in this area than in the lateral areas, and therefore the patient experiences less discomfort.

The patient will also have a better cosmetic result because the larger scar can be hidden in the umbilical area. Most important is the ability to repair a hernia on either side utilizing the hernia stapler inserted through this midline umbilical port. After the initial 12-mm port is put into place, the secondary ports are inserted under direct vision. These secondary ports should be 10-mm ports for the convenience of the operating surgeon if he is using a 10-mm laparoscope. However, if there is a desire to reduce the size of the incision, provided that a good 5-mm laparoscope is available, the two secondary ports may be 5-mm ports. My tendency at this time is to avoid larger ports whenever possible and use the 5-mm ports. If the surgeon has available the new 5-mm screw type stapler, all three ports may be 5-mm ports.

IX. Narrative of Surgical Technique

After the ports have been placed, a 10-mm, 30-degree laparoscope is inserted through the umbilical port, and the two secondary ports are used for the dissection of the pelvic floor and the placement of the mesh over the hernia defect. Only after the mesh has been put into place is the camera moved to the contralateral secondary port, and then, using the 12-mm umbilical port, the mesh is stapled in place. This port placement and procedure as described here require an assistant who may also run the laparoscope and hold the tissues being dissected. If an assistant is not available or is not desired,

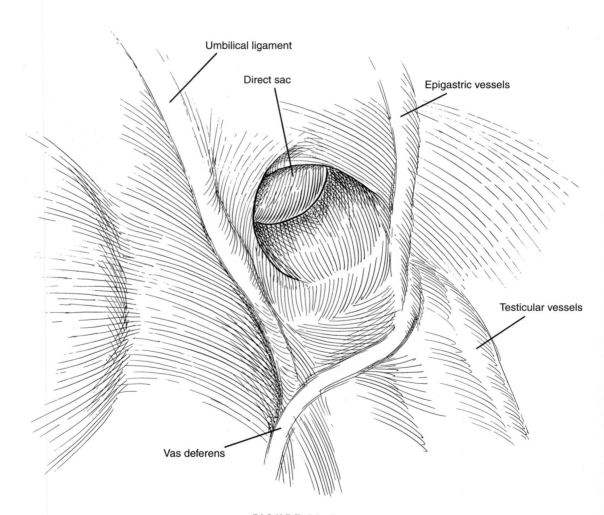

FIGURE 41–1

port placement may take a slightly different configuration with a port being placed below the laparoscope in the midline between the umbilicus and the pubis. This eliminates the secondary port at the level of the umbilicus on the side of the hernia. The surgeon always operates from the side opposite the hernia.

Using the new 5-mm stapler, the laparoscope and staplers are moved to the most optimum port for visualization and staple placement.

Direct Inguinal Hernia

FIGURE 41–1. The first description of the TAPP repair involves the dissection of a direct inguinal hernia. A right direct inguinal hernia is visualized with the camera in the umbilical port.

FIGURE 41–2. A grasper is introduced through the secondary port on the side of the hernia, and the apex of the direct sac is grasped.

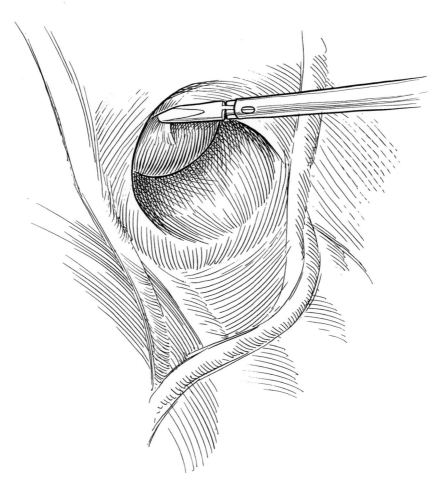

FIGURE 41–2

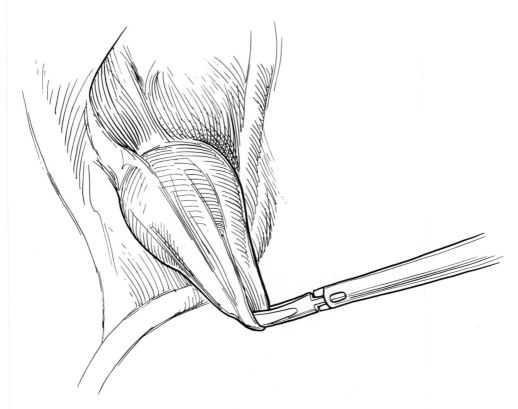

FIGURE 41–3

FIGURE 41–3. The direct sac is reduced into the abdominal cavity. The reduction of the direct sac is easy and will not jeopardize the cord structures.

FIGURE 41–4. A transverse incision extends across the top of the direct space and continues across the top of the indirect space. This transverse incision is always anterior to these spaces because there are no important structures that can be damaged in this area with the exception of the inferior epigastric vessels, which, if divided, must be ligated. Incisions are never made below the iliopubic tract because of the important anatomic structures in this area. In the case of a right-sided hernia, this incision is be- gun at the umbilical ligament with the surgeon standing on the left side of the table. It is easier to make the incision away from the surgeon. The transverse incision extends from the umbilical ligament to the anterior superior iliac spine. It is important to make a large pocket to accept a large graft in all of these hernia repairs.

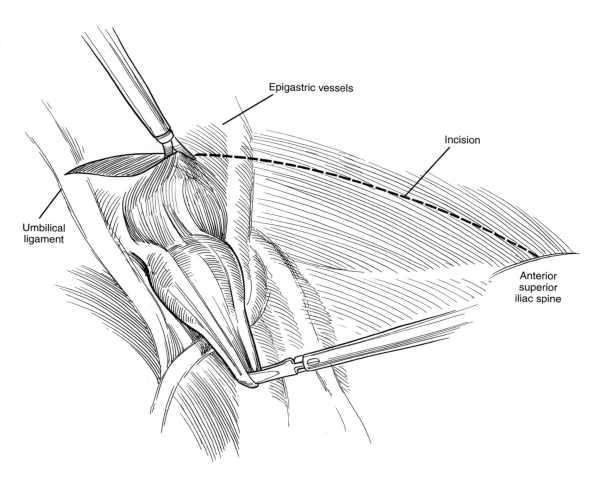

FIGURE 41–4

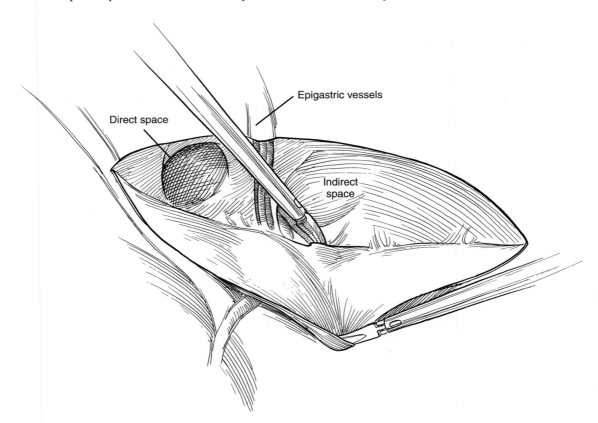

FIGURE 41–5

FIGURE 41–5. The entire pelvic floor, including the femoral space, the direct space, and the indirect space, are exposed by peeling the peritoneum posteriorly first and anteriorly second. The peritoneum is peeled off the extraperitoneal structures using a combination of traction and countertraction. It is rarely necessary to use sharp dissection or electrosurgery in this portion of the procedure.

FIGURE 41-6. An appropriate size piece of polypropylene mesh is then introduced through a 10-mm port (if the secondary ports are 10-mm), or, if the secondary ports are 5 mm, it must be introduced blindly through the 12-mm umbilical port. This mesh should not be folded but simply grasped in the middle and forced into the abdominal cavity. Folding the mesh or rolling it will require unfolding or unrolling and is additional work. The minimum dimensions of the mesh are 3 × 5 inches. This size of mesh will suffice for over 90 per cent of repairs. The mesh should be made of polypropylene to allow fibrous ingrowth. The mesh shown in this par-

ticular figure is SurgiPro mesh (United States Surgical Corporation, Norwalk, CT), which has been used with uniform success. The mesh is then placed over the entire pelvic floor. Lines have been drawn across the mesh for orientation purposes to make sure that it is placed horizontally. These lines may also be reference points for the location of the epigastric vessels and important structures when stapling the mesh in place. The mesh should lie flat on the pelvic floor and be free of wrinkles or creases. It should be noted that the corners of the mesh have been rounded. This is for easy placement under the peritoneum.

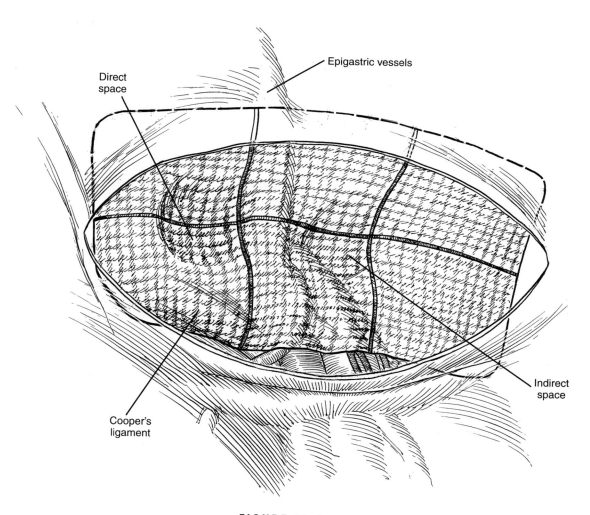

FIGURE 41-6

FIGURE 41-7. The medial corner of the mesh is placed over Cooper's ligament, which is one of the most important areas of fixation in laparoscopic herniorrhaphy to prevent recurrence of the hernia. Multiple 4.0-mm staples (United States Surgical Corporation, Norwalk, CT) are used to fix the mesh to Cooper's ligament. These staples are placed perpendicular to Cooper's ligament and should number at least three or four. The majority of recurrences in early laparoscopic hernia repair resulted from a lack of adequate fixation of the mesh to Cooper's ligament. Newer 5-mm screw type staples may be substituted and anchored more efficiently into Cooper's ligament.

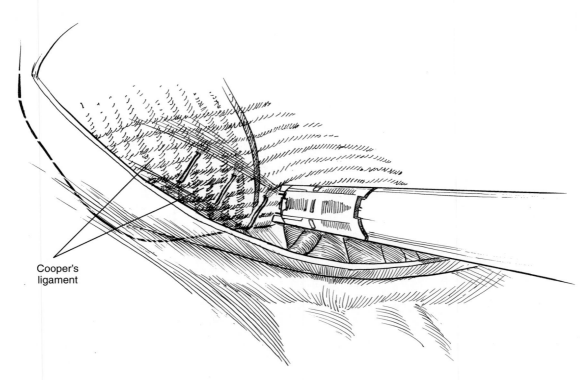

Cooper's ligament

FIGURE 41-7

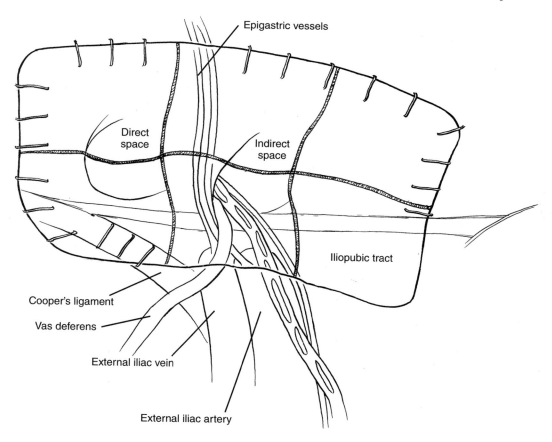

Epigastric vessels

Direct space

Indirect space

Iliopubic tract

Cooper's ligament

Vas deferens

External iliac vein

External iliac artery

FIGURE 41–8

FIGURE 41–8. Staples are placed along the edge of the mesh. If these staples are placed at a slight distance from the edge, the mesh will tend to curl. Staples are placed along the entire medial aspect of the mesh and then laterally anterior to the iliopubic tract. No staples can be placed posterior to the iliopubic tract because of the possibility of injury to the lateral femoral cutaneous nerve, the genitofemoral nerve, the femoral nerve, the cord structures, and so on. To be sure the staples are anterior to the ilio-pubic tract, the tip of the stapler is palpated by external compression of the abdomen by the surgeon's hand. If the stapler cannot be palpated, it should be considered below the iliopubic tract and should not be fired. Staples may also be placed in the body of the mesh if necessary to remove creases or wrinkles. However, these staples must be anterior to the iliopubic tract. After stapling the mesh, it should be observed to be free of wrinkles and should not curl or fold when the peritoneum is reapproximated.

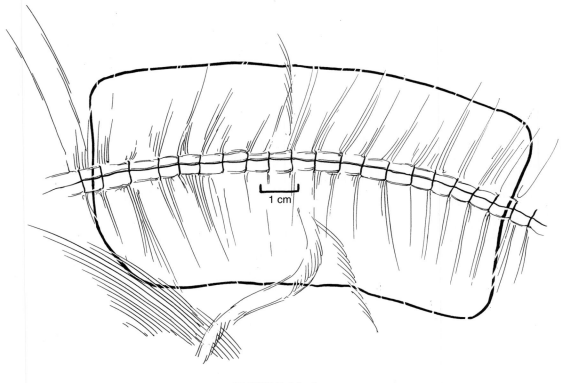

FIGURE 41–9.

FIGURE 41–9. The peritoneum is then closed tightly by placing staples and/or sutures a maximum of 1 cm apart. This is one of the more important parts of this procedure to prevent herniation of bowel between the mesh and the peritoneum postoperatively. To approximate the peritoneum, the carbon dioxide pressure is reduced to 8 mm Hg, but if there is any question about the approximation of the peritoneum, the pressure should be increased to make sure the peritoneum is tightly closed. In a bilateral herniorrhaphy, both sides are repaired with mesh before the peritoneum is stapled because if the abdomen is reinsufflated to 15 mm Hg the peritoneum may be disrupted. The peritoneum may be closed with a running suture or screw staples into the mesh anterior to the iliopubic tract and avoiding the epigastric vessels.

Indirect Inguinal Hernia

FIGURE 41–10. This figure shows a right indirect inguinal hernia, which lies lateral to the inferior epigastric vessels.

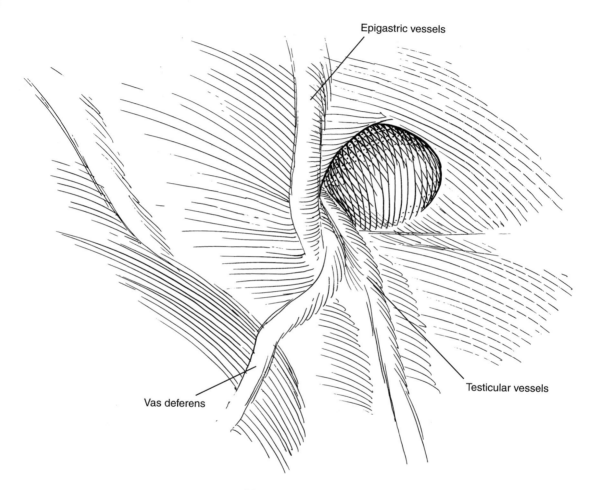

FIGURE 41–10

FIGURE 41–11. In cases of indirect hernias, the sac is amputated by making a 360-degree circumferential incision around the neck of the sac slightly inside the hernia or at the level of the peritoneal reflection. This incision should not be made away from the area of the neck of the sac or there will be difficulty in closing the peritoneum following the repair. This 360-degree circumferencial incision is made by placing one blade of the endoshears below the peritoneum just as if one were using Metzenbaum scissors, making sure that no important structures are between the blades of the scissors. The endoshears may then be used to continue the incision around the neck of the sac. These large indirect sacs are not reduced into the abdominal cavity because this is associated with injury to the genitofemoral nerve and the cord structures. These patients have been followed for a long period of time, and the formation of permanent

hydroceles has not been noted when the sac is left in place. The sac is amputated 360 degrees. The sac in this figure is seen retracted into the scrotal area. The transverse incision is then continued on to the anterior superior iliac spine, and the remainder of the hernia repair is identical to that described for the direct hernia repair.

FIGURE 41–12. It is important to place the mesh over the direct space, the indirect space, and the femoral space. With direct inguinal hernias, the mesh should be placed more medially, whereas with indirect-space hernias, the mesh is placed slightly more laterally.

At the termination of the hernia repair the carbon dioxide is evacuated from the abdominal cavity, and, under direct vision, all 12-mm trocar incisions are closed using a #1 Vicryl in the fascia.

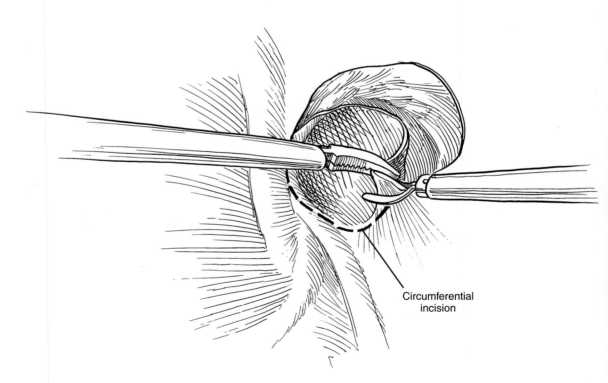

Circumferential
incision

FIGURE 41–11

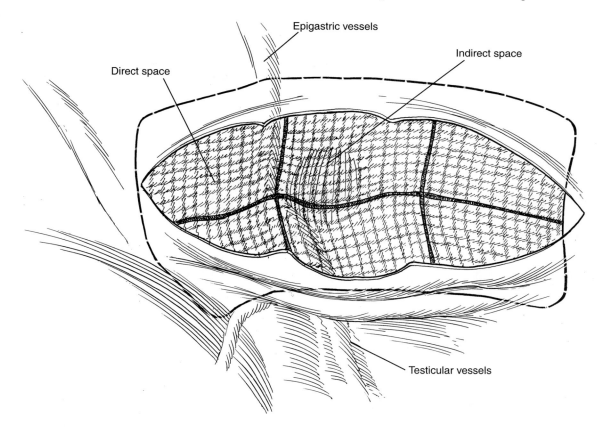

Epigastric vessels

Indirect space

Direct space

Testicular vessels

FIGURE 41–12

X. Postoperative Medications

Patients are given a prescription for Percocet postoperatively. They rarely require pain medication for 1 to 2 days, and frequently Tylenol suffices.

XI. Advancement of Diet

The patient is allowed to eat as soon as he has recovered from anesthesia and is stable. There are no restrictions.

XII. Determinants of Discharge

Patients are discharged on the day of surgery unless there are complications such as inability to void, pulmonary problems, cardiac problems, and so on. The patient is then seen in the office 1 week postoperatively and examined. If the patient does have a bulge in the inguinal area in the first postoperative week, it is probably not a recurrent hernia and should be observed. It is probably either a hematoma or a seroma and can be expected to dissipate over a 3-month period. The patient is reexamined at the 3-month interval to make sure he or she is totally asymptomatic and has returned to normal. The patient is then discharged.

XIII. Return to Normal Activity/Work

Patients are encouraged to return to normal activity within the first week. If an extremely large hernia has been repaired, heavy lifting is discouraged for 2 to 3 weeks; however, most blue collar and white collar workers with an average size hernia can return to their normal occupations after 1 week.

Chapter 42

Endoscopic Total Extraperitoneal Hernia Repair with Balloon Dissection

ROGER DE LA TORRE, M.D., and J. STEPHEN SCOTT, M.D.

I. Indications

Presence of an inguinal hernia in an adult who has not had previous retropubic surgery.

II. Contraindications

A. Patients who have undergone previous retropubic surgery (e.g., suprapubic prostatectomy)
B. Patients taking warfarin
C. Preadolescents

III. Factors Important in Patient Selection

A. Previous lower abdominal surgery may hinder balloon dissection.
B. Obesity will make initial dissection and maintenance of adequate extraperitoneal space more difficult.
C. This technique is especially useful for bilateral hernias and recurrent hernias previously repaired through an open anterior method.

IV. Preoperative Preparation

A. Same day admission for outpatient surgery
B. Preoperative medications including
 1. Prescribed oral medications taken with a sip of water on morning of surgery
 2. Continuation of medication patches.
 3. Standard preoperative antiemetics and sedatives.
C. Bowel preparation: none

V. Choice of Anesthesia

A. General
B. Spinal
C. Epidural
D. Local with intravenous sedation

VI. Accessory Devices

None

VII. Instruments and Telescopes

A. 45-degree laparoscope
B. Balloon dissector
C. 10-mm and 5-mm trocars
D. Polypropylene mesh
E. Laparoscopic hernia stapler or "tacking device"
F. Laparoscopic graspers
G. Laparoscopic scissors

VIII. Position of Monitors and Placement of Trocar

The monitor is placed at the foot of the bed.

516

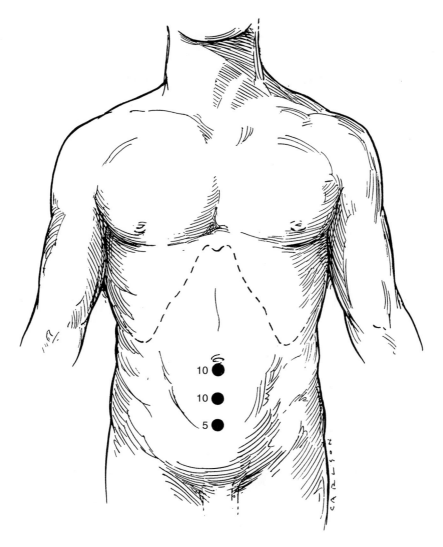

FIGURE 42-1A

FIGURE 42-1A. Midline placement. When patients are undergoing bilateral inguinal hernia repair, all three trocars are placed in the midline. This set-up is also used when the surgeon is working alone. The surgeon stands on the side contralateral to the hernia being repaired.

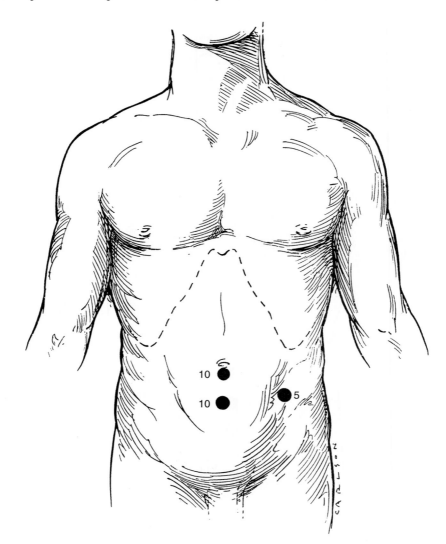

FIGURE 42–1B

FIGURE 42–1B. Lateral placement. One of the trocars can be placed laterally when the surgeon is repairing a unilateral hernia with an assistant. The surgeon stands on the side contralateral to the hernia.

IX. Narrative of Surgical Technique

The operating room is set for a laparoscopic procedure with the monitor at the foot of the operating table. Following the administration of anesthesia, the patient is placed in a slight Trendelenburg position, and the surgeon stands on the side contralateral to the hernia. Suction irrigation and electrocautery are not needed in the majority of cases.

FIGURE 42–2. A 1- to 1.5-cm infraumbilical incision is made and advanced through the subcutaneous tissues. S retractors or Army-Navy retractors are used to expose the anterior sheath of the rectus muscle on the side of the hernia (or the side of the largest hernia if bilateral). A 1-cm incision is made in the anterior sheath, and the underlying rectus muscle is then retracted laterally, exposing the posterior rectus sheath.

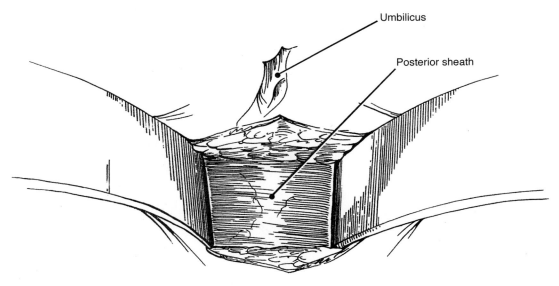

FIGURE 42–2

FIGURE 42-3. The balloon dissector is inserted through the incised tissue onto the posterior sheath and advanced toward the symphysis pubis. The balloon is then inflated with saline or air until adequate lateral dissection to the anterior superior iliac spine (ASIS) is appreciated or the balloon capacity is reached. The balloon dissector is then removed, and the created space is then maintained with gas insufflation of 8 to 10 mm Hg pressure.

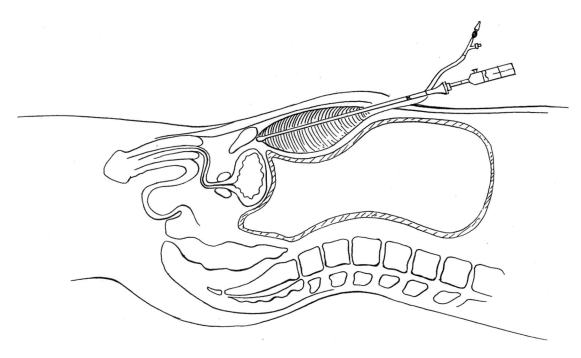

FIGURE 42–3

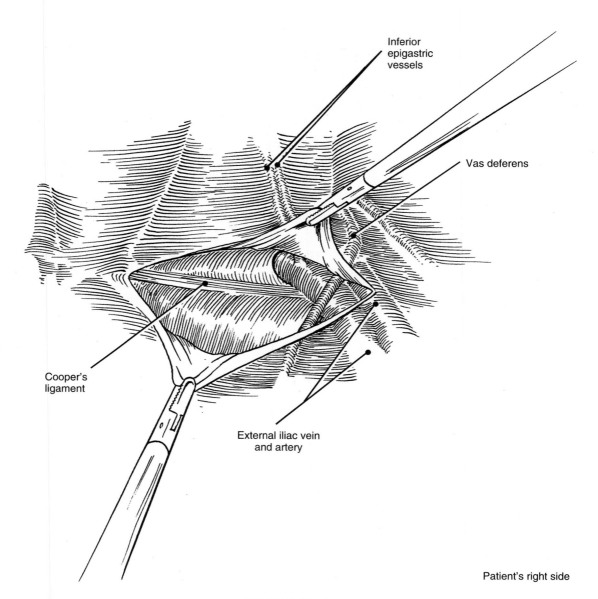

Inferior epigastric vessels

Vas deferens

Cooper's ligament

External iliac vein and artery

Patient's right side

FIGURE 42-4

Transversalis

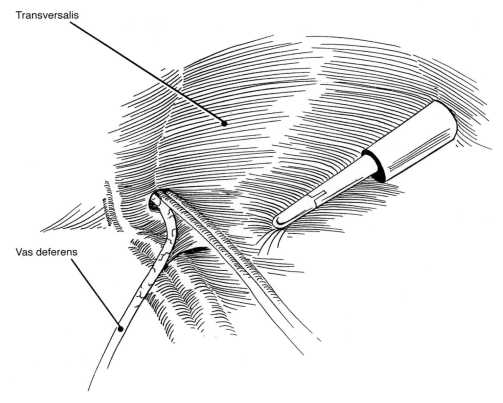

Vas deferens

FIGURE 42–5

FIGURE 42–4. Under direct vision with the angled laparoscope, a 10-mm trocar is introduced into the extraperitoneal space at the level of the ASIS, along the midline. A 5-mm trocar is introduced either in the midline approximately 3-cm caudad to the 10-mm trocar or on the side of the hernia at the level of the ASIS, along the anterior axillary line. Through these trocars, laparoscopic graspers are used to dissect and clearly delineate Cooper's ligament. Inspec-

tion is made of the direct and femoral spaces. If a hernia is noted here, it is reduced by retracting any existing preperitoneal fat within the defect and separating it from the overlying attenuated fascia.

FIGURE 42–5. The lateral aspect of the abdominal wall is bluntly dissected to the level of the ASIS. A lateral port may then be placed in the extraperitoneal space.

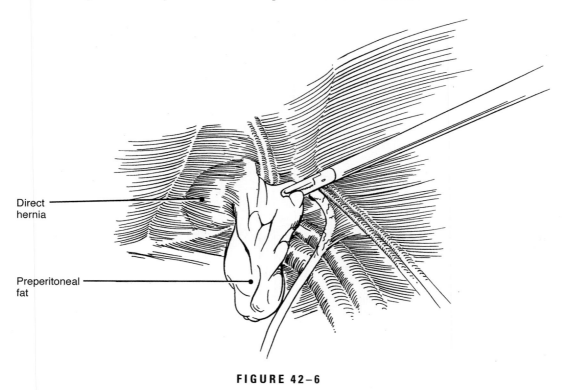

Direct
hernia

Preperitoneal
fat

FIGURE 42–6

FIGURE 42–6. If a direct hernia is present, the preperitoneal fat is retracted and separated from the attenuated fascia of the direct space.

FIGURE 42–7. Attention is then turned to the internal ring, lateral to the epigastric vessels. If indirect hernia is present, the hernia sac must be retracted from the inguinal canal and separated off the spermatic cord. The hernia sac is then pulled cephalad until the posterior peritoneal edge is brought to the level of the ASIS.

FIGURE 42–8. The indirect hernia sac can be dissected off the cord structures. Note that if an inguinal-scrotal hernia exists, the proximal sac can be ligated proximally where it has been separated from the cord and then severed distal to the ligature. The proximal end is then retracted cephalad, bringing the posterior peritoneum to the ASIS level.

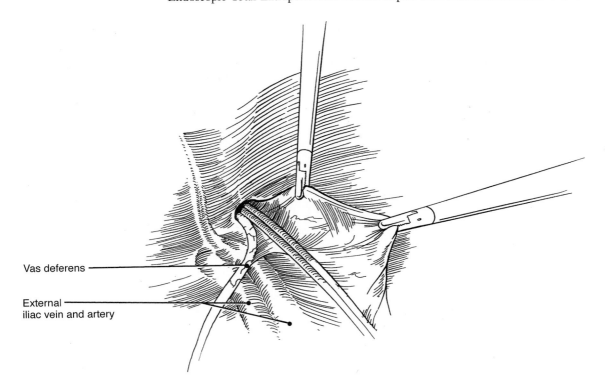

Vas deferens

External
iliac vein and artery

FIGURE 42–7

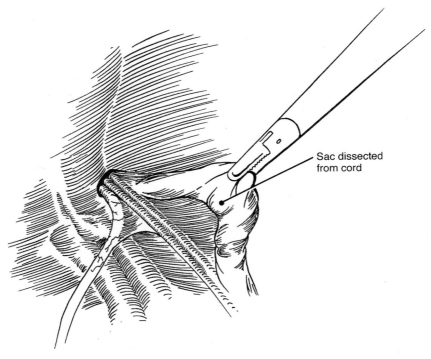

Sac dissected
from cord

FIGURE 42–8

FIGURE 42-9. The peritoneum is retracted cephalad off the spermatic cord structures to the level of the ASIS. This is termed posteriorizing the cord.

FIGURE 42-10. Next, a 12 × 15 cm sheet of polypropylene mesh is folded so that it can be introduced into the created space through the 10-mm trocar. Once in the space, the mesh is unfolded and positioned in such a manner that it covers the indirect, direct, and femoral spaces. The lower edge of the mesh is caudad to the peritoneum, and the mesh should lie directly on the cord posteriorly.

FIGURE 42-11. Alternatively, the mesh may be slit so that it can be placed around the cord. The edges of the slit must then be joined and secured together.

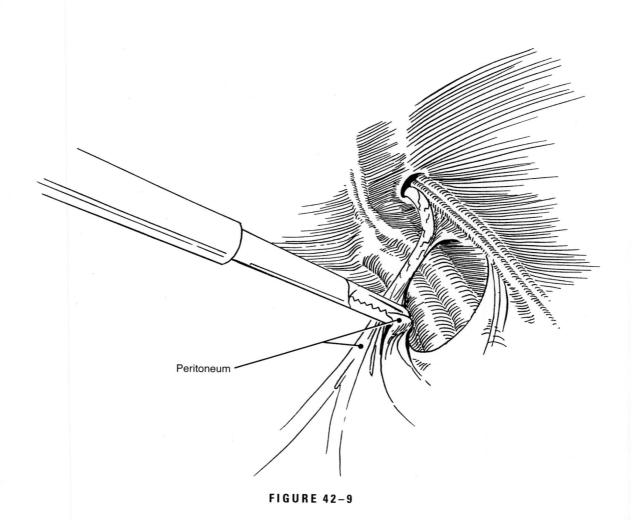

Peritoneum

FIGURE 42-9

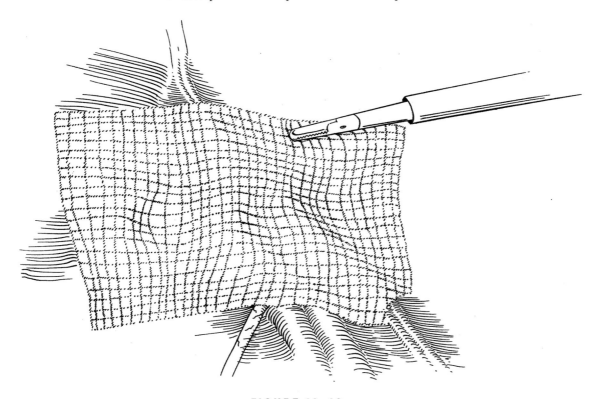

FIGURE 42–10

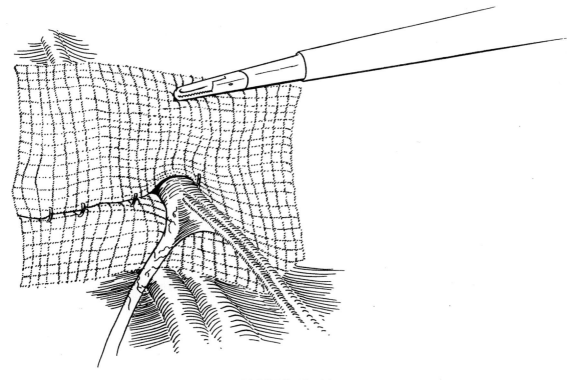

FIGURE 42–11

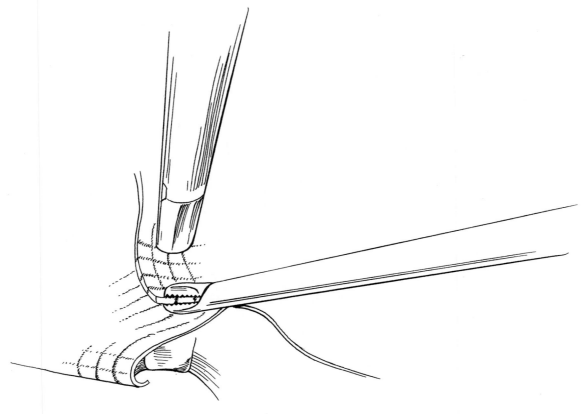

FIGURE 42-12

FIGURE 42-12. A hernia stapler or tacking device is then inserted into the space, and the mesh is secured to Cooper's ligament and the lateral abdominal wall.

For bilateral hernias, the procedure described is repeated on the contralateral side. Once the mesh is secured, the gas is allowed to escape as the patient is taken out of the Trendelenburg position, causing the peritoneum and its contents to "roll" into the mesh. The trocars are removed next, and the fascial defects from the large trocars are approximated with 2–0 Vicryl suture. The skin incisions are then reapproximated.

X. Postoperative Medication

Oxycodone 5 mg/acetaminophen 325 mg: one to two tablets every 4 hours as needed (10 tablets are prescribed)

XI. Advancement of Diet

May resume regular diet postoperatively

XII. Determinants of Discharge

A. Stable vital signs
B. Dressings dry with no evidence of bleeding
C. Tolerating oral fluids
D. Pain controlled with oral medication
E. Voiding spontaneously

XIII. Return to Normal Activity/Work

A. May return to normal activity on the evening of surgery or as soon as postoperative pain allows
B. May return to work within the first postoperative week

Index

Note: Page numbers in *italics* refer to illustrations.

ISBN 0-7216-6326-5

90038

9 780721 663265